socio

The Nature of Suffering

The Nature of Suffering

AND THE GOALS OF MEDICINE

ERIC J. CASSELL

OXFORD UNIVERSITY PRESS
New York Oxford

Oxford University Press

Oxford New York Toronto
Delhi Bombay Calcutta Madras Karachi
Kuala Lumpur Singapore Hong Kong Tokyo
Nairobi Dar es Salaam Cape Town
Melbourne Auckland Madrid

and associated companies in
Berlin Ibadan

First published in 1991 by Oxford University Press, Inc.,
200 Madison Avenue, New York, New York 10016

First issued as an Oxford University Press paperback, 1994

Oxford is a registered trademark of Oxford University Press

Library of Congress Cataloging-in-Publication Data
Cassell, Eric J., 1928–
The nature of suffering and the goals of medicine
Eric J. Cassell.
p. cm. Includes index.
ISBN 0-19-505222-6
ISBN 0-19-508912-X (pbk.)
1. Medicine—Philosophy. 2. Suffering. 3. Physician and patient.
I. Title. [DNLM: 1. Chronic Disease—therapy. 2. Philosophy, Medical.
3. Physician-Patient Relations. W 61 C344n]
R723.C42828 1991 610'.1—dc20
DNLM/DLC for Library of Congress 90-7657

Chapter 1 is adapted from "Ideas in Conflict: The Rise and Fall (and Rise and Fall) of New Views of Disease," by Eric Cassell. Chapter 2 is adapted from, and pages 73–78 of Chapter 5 are reprinted from, "The Changing Concept of the Ideal Physician," by Eric Cassell. Both articles are adapted and reprinted by permission of *Daedalus*, Journal of the American Academy of Arts and Sciences, from the issue entitled "America's Doctors, Medical Sciences, Medical Care," Spring, 1986. Vol. 115/2.

Chapter 3 is adapted and reprinted from the article "The Nature of Suffering and the Goals of Medicine," by Eric Cassell, which appeared in *The New England Journal of Medicine*, 306: 639–645, 1982, by permission of the publisher.

Pages 102–103 in Chapter 7 are reprinted from "The Relationship Between Pain and Suffering" by Eric Cassell in *Advances in Pain Research*, edited by C.S. Hill Jr. and W.S. Fields (New York: Raven Press, Ltd., 1989), pages 67–68, by permission of the publisher.

The excerpts on pages 186 and 187 in Chapter 11 and pages 100 and 101 in Chapter 7 are reprinted from *Talking with Patients: Vol. I. The Theory of Doctor Patient Communication, Vol. 2, Clinical Technique*, by Eric Cassell (Cambridge: MIT Press, 1985), pages 84 and 124–125, respectively, by permission of the publisher.

2 4 6 8 10 9 7 5 3 1

Printed in the United States of America

This book is dedicated to my mother and father

in loving memory and with profound and enduring gratitude

Preface

THE TEST OF a system of medicine should be its adequacy in the face of suffering; this book starts from the premise that modern medicine fails that test. In fact, the central assumptions on which twentieth-century medicine is founded provide no basis for an understanding of suffering. For pain, difficulty in breathing, or other afflictions of the body, superbly yes; for suffering, no. Suffering must inevitably involve the person—bodies do not suffer, persons suffer. You may read this as merely another way of saying that modern medicine is too devoted to its science and technology and has lost touch with the personal side of sickness. The argument of this book is that such criticism, as correct as it may seem, does not get at the root of the difficulty and is consequently inadequate.

The difficulty is not with medical science or technology *per se.* No solutions to important problems can be based on a return to innocence, even if that were possible. Neither do the troubles arise because the wrong students are chosen—for decades medicine has had the best and the brightest the country has to offer. Nor is it money, power, or status. The problems were present when there was plenty of all three and they are there now when all are diminished. Finally, I believe the high cost of medical care and the malpractice crisis are more likely derivative than causative.

For more than two generations remedies for medicine's dehumanization and impersonality have been a failure. Great teachers have tried, wonderful books have been written, innovative medical school courses and curricula have been established, and even new medical schools have been founded on ideas believed to offer solutions. For the most part, all these attempts, large and small, have been disappointments. Over these decades there have been many great teachers, more wonderful physicians, and nothing less than superb medical care to be found. But these islands of excellence remain just that, islands separated from the mainland.

The problem does not lie with the general diagnosis of medicine's ill. The widespread perception, growing since the 1920s, is correct that what is lacking in twentieth-century medicine is an adequate consideration of the place of the person of the patient. The common belief that medicine is mired in this fault, however, is in error. In fact, as I will discuss in detail throughout there *is* change taking place. The sick person has been coming to the fore as the focus of medical care and the disease is gradually taking second place. Why is this not better known, and why is it taking so long to become medicine's dominant idea? As with the beginnings of all elemental social change, dissatisfaction with the existing order is more evident than willingness to accept new ideas and give up old ways of doing things. The solid intellectual foundation has not yet been constructed, the ideas on which the change is based have only been articulated by a minority, and the lessons that must be learned before the transformation is routinized have not yet been taught.

How is medicine to deal with suffering that arises in the person of the sick when even the word person is problematic. Despite all these decades of concern, there is little agreement about exactly what defines a person (except that each of us knows we are persons). Further, doctors do things. If they are to act specifically on the sick *person,* then they must know what that means, what they are to do, and how and what measures there are of the consequences of their actions. And they must acquire this knowledge in a systematic way, which means that it must be taught. Without system and training, being responsive in the face of suffering remains the attribute of individual physicians who have come to this mastery alone or gained it from a few inspirational teachers—which is where we are today.

To say that the focus of medical care is the sick person (rather than the disease) is a statement of a theory of medicine—a *different* theory from when the disease is the primary concern of doctors. New theories do not arise from the genie's lamp; they have an historical genesis. In addition, theories, new and old, have not only antecedents, but consequences. For example, if the focus is on the *sick* person, what made the person sick? If the disease made the person sick, are we not back where we started? Because of these questions the journey through this book starts not with a discussion of the nature of suffering, but with the history of theories of medicine. The task of Chapter 1 is to demonstrate how important theory is to medicine (indeed, to all endeavors) and to show how the weaknesses of the theory that is being superseded—disease theory (when people are sick, it is because they have diseases)—have contributed to its obsolescence. Medicine is so bound up with society that it probably will not be a surprise to see that current concerns about the environment arising as part of the ecology movement are intellectual trends related to the changes in the focus of medicine. Similarly, the increasing importance of ethics in medicine reflects changing cultural conceptions of the nature of persons.

The hallmark of modern medicine is its dependence on science and technology, and understanding the relationship of the two is fundamental to understanding medicine's problem with suffering. Whenever I use the word science

I am referring to its more restricted, modern usage as a branch of study that relates to the phenomena of the material universe and their laws. In this usage medical science is concerned with the phenomena and laws of normal and abnormal human biology. I do *not* use it in its older, more colloquial meaning of a particular branch of study, a trained skill, or reliable knowledge. I must make it clear at this point, as I noted above and will restate throughout, that nothing I say should be seen as anti-science or against technology. They are not, in themselves, the basic problem and there is no going back, thank heavens. It is inevitable, however, that difficulties raised by science and technology will become predicaments for medicine. One of the reasons for this is that medicine is practiced by doctors and what creates dilemmas for doctors as they attempt to care for the sick creates quandaries for medicine. Theories of medicine are exemplified in the actions of doctors. (In this book the words doctor and physician are employed interchangeably.) In fact, as Chapter 2 discusses, what any era considers the ideal physician reflects an amalgam of the demands made by the reigning theory of medicine, the social forces acting specifically on doctors and sick persons, and the general social attitudes toward persons and their relations with each other. Since all of these have been changing during this century, and more rapidly since World War II, it is not surprising that the concept of the ideal physician has also been transformed. The failure of medicine to meet the test put by suffering, which is really the failure of physicians to deal adequately with the suffering of their patients, only comes to be considered a failure because of personal and social expectations that are only recently emerging.

The nature of suffering is the topic of Chapters 3 and 4 and you might wish to start the book with them.

Doctors do not deal with suffering in the abstract—they treat persons who are afflicted by something that leads to the suffering. The separation of the disease that underlies the suffering from both the person and the suffering itself, as though the scientific entity of disease is more real and more important than the person and the suffering, is one of the strange intellectual paradoxes of our times. In Chapters 3 and 4 we begin to illuminate not only what suffering is, but, because the two are inseparable, what a person is. And what it is about being a person alone and among others in a culture that leads to suffering. These chapters should also make clear that the reduction of sick persons to their physical, psychological, or social dimensions is both artificial and leads away from the relief of their suffering. We are of a piece; virtually nothing happens to one part that does not affect the others.

In addition to the intellectual and social bases of medicine and their exemplification in physicians, there is a third dimension without which any understanding of medicine and its approach to suffering will be incomplete—the relationship between patient and doctor. This mysterious relationship through which *all* medical care flows of *any* type and in *any* setting (even when there seems to be none) is the subject of Chapter 5. The relationship is mysterious if only because it is the foundation of the phenomenon of healing, itself obscure. It seems mysterious also because it points to aspects of the connections between individuals which in a rational, essentially non-spiritual culture like ours are little known and less understood. An appreciation of these connections and their disruption is required for a comprehension of suffering itself. Our expectations of physicians, sadness when they fail us, and their moral demands on themselves also arise from the nature of the doctor–patient relationship.

Because consideration of medicine, sickness, or suffering is impossible without manifest or latent notions of disease, Chapter 6 examines what it means to say that someone has a disease. Using cancer of the breast, pneumonia, and coronary heart disease as examples, it becomes apparent that while many think of diseases in their classic form, recent decades have seen profound changes in this concept.

Throughout the remainder of the book, the idea of person is heightened. Ensuing chapters discuss the work of doctors in their four fundamental tasks: finding out what is the matter (diagnosis), finding how it happened (cause), deciding what to do (treatment) and its interdependent partner, predicting the outcome (prognosis). As strange as it may seem, throughout much of the history of medicine, and certainly in the modern era, the idea has taken hold that the disease can be discovered, its cause uncovered, treatment accomplished, and predictions about its outcome made apart from the particular sick *person*. Put another way, many doctors—perhaps most people—still believe that different persons with the same disease will have the same sickness. By the end of Chapter 9 (and probably sooner) the illusion—for it is no less than an illusion—will be permanently dispelled. Once we understand the nature of suffering, we can discuss the changes in medicine necessary for its relief; this is the topic of the last three chapters and the epilogue.

To be successful in treating the sick and alleviating suffering, doctors must know more about the sick person and the illness than just the name of the disease and the science that explains it. What can be known about the sick *person* seems to make up the deficiency. To meet this requirement we want the doctor to know as much about the sick person as about the disease. On the face of it, this seems impossible—the individual is unknowable, an ancient saying goes. While this is true, Chapter 10 shows that the extent that we *do* know each other through shared ideas, beliefs, culture, and language is remarkable. With skill and training even more of the person can be known, particularly when the knowledge is focused on the task of caring for the sick. Prior to the nineteenth century, the body was largely a mystery. In the last century and in ours the wonders of the body have been revealed to the gaze of medicine with results that have reached far beyond medicial science. Just as privacy about the body held back knowledge in the past, reticence about revealing ourselves presently retards learning about persons. Nonetheless our era has seen the beginnings. The job of the twenty-first century is the discovery of the person—finding the sources of illness and suffering within the person, and with that knowledge developing methods for their relief, while at the same time revealing the power within the person as the nineteenth and twentieth centuries have revealed the power of the body.

The dominance and success of science in our time has led to the widely held and crippling prejudice that no knowledge is *real* unless it is scientific—objective and measurable. From this perspective suffering and its dominion in the sick person are themselves unreal. This is simply an unacceptable conclusion. Chapter 11 examines the kinds of information necessary to know about persons. Our perceptions of other persons are not based on elemental facts alone but also on values and aesthetic criteria. The way we think in terms of values is explored to show that along with brute facts, values are not mere prejudices but a kind of information that can be consistently and reliably employed in our knowledge of persons. Were it not so there would be no stability in our personal or social lives. Aesthetic criteria, which at first might seem foreign to medicine, are also essential for knowing whole persons within space and across time. Values and aesthetics raise the specter of subjectivity, so worrisome to medicine and medical science. In response to that problem we see further how the person of the doctor, first discussed in the relationship with the patient and interspersed in succeeding chapters, enters into the equation of medical care.

Since antiquity there has been a prejudice in favor of reason and against experiential knowledge. The long-standing dichotomy of medicine into its science and art is a medical expression of this bias. Knowledge, however, whether of medical science or the art of medicine, does not take care of sick persons or relieve their suffering; clinicians do in whom these kinds of knowledge are integrated. Chapter 12 deals with the nature of experience in general and the clinician's experience specifically. At first it appears that the problem to be solved is the relationship of knowledge to experience. In practice the more central issue turns out to be the relationship of the subject to experience. The patient and the illness are not merely experienced, they are experienced by this particular physician. The problem is that experiential knowledge is tinged with emotion and passion—it cannot be otherwise. Centuries of trying to disengage the person from knowledge born of experience through science or other means have not been successful. The solution to the problem lies in remembering that only another person can empathetically experience the experience of a person. In medicine the triad is inseparable—patient, experience, physician. It must finally be accepted that there can be no substitute for the physician as a person. The moral compulsion of their responsibilities exposes physicians to the peril of unavoidable uncertainty and overwhelming subjectivity created by serious illness and suffering. It can only be through education and method that these dangers are converted into therapeutic power. It follows that medicine needs a systematic and disciplined approach to the knowledge that arises from the clinician's experience rather than artificial divisions of medical knowledge into science and art.

The timeless goal of the relief of suffering remains the challenge to change and the enduring test of medicine's success.

New York E.J.C.
October 1990

Acknowledgments

THIS BOOK had its genesis in the project on suffering started in 1979 at the Hastings Center, an organization dedicated to research and teaching about ethical issues raised by biomedical advance. From its origins, the Hastings Center (then The Institute of Society, Ethics and the Life Sciences) had done research on ethical issues related to death and dying. As the years passed, the problems of the dying became the increasing concern of many individuals and groups in the United States and Europe. Dr. Elisabeth Kubler-Ross taught, and it had become received wisdom, that many of the problems of the dying arose from the denial of death that was widespread in the culture. If that was the case, one had to wonder, why had the subject "death and dying" become so popular throughout the United States. Courses on death and dying sprang up in schools of all levels, from grammar school to college. Newspapers and magazines ran articles, popular books were written, and even a death and dying jargon developed. It seemed a strange kind of denial. The changed attitude toward death that all this publicity suggested appeared not to have changed the dimensions of personal loss and pain that my colleagues and I observed among our dying patients and their families.

We wondered, at the Hastings Center, whether the popularity of the subject of death and dying was in itself a denial of something more painful than death itself—suffering. The project on Death, Suffering and Well-being was born of those conjectures. More than two years of excellent presentations and superb discussions during the project could not help enlarging my understanding of suffering. Particularly memorable were Darrel Amundsen on suffering in the early Christian literature, William Arrowsmith's discussion of suffering in the Greek tragedies, David Bakan on pain management, Robert Belknap on suffering in Russian Literature, Rabbi Jack Bemporad on the Jewish view of suffering, Daniel Callahan on suffering and public policy, Mary Douglas on cross-cultural perspectives on suffering, Robert Fulton's discussion of the sociological viewpoint, William May on suffering in contemporary American theatre, Thomas Murray on the special problem of the neonatal intensive care unit, Elaine Scarry on the language of suffering, Mark Siegler on the problem of suffering in the aged, David Smith on suffering in Christian theologies, Mary Vachon on suffering among caregivers and others by Arthur Caplan, James Childress, H. Tristram Englehardt, Hans Jonas, Harold Merskey, Robert Morison, Edmund Pellegrino, Martin Pernick, Issy Pilowski, Mary Rawlinson, Margaret Steinfels, David Tracy, Robert Veatch, and Patricia White. My paper, "The Nature of Suffering and the Goals of Medicine," which was subsequently published in the *New England Journal of Medicine,* was presented to the group on April 24, 1981.

Walsh McDermott died in 1981. To my personal sense of loss was added the loss of a teacher and mentor who had a remarkable prescience about medicine's future. David Rogers, then President of the Robert Wood Johnson Foundation, arranged for support for and helped edit a Festschrift in Dr. McDermott's honor that was published in *Daedalus.* While preparing the two essays for that volume, I became aware of the importance of understanding the historical trends that had led to the current era in medicine and that were foreshadowing the developments that this book is about.

Early on it was apparent to me that medicine's continued advancement would require rethinking the fundamental philosophical principles on which it was based. Twentieth-century scientific thinking as it had been incorporated into medical science, and the philosophical positivism that supported it, was the world view underlying my training and current scientific medicine. This way of looking at the world, however, seemed inadequate to the problem of suffering and the care of the sick—medicine's basic tasks. Searching for other philosophical foundations, on the other hand, looked as forbidding as it was necessary. I wanted to avoid a problem among physicians that Robert Veatch has called attention to, the generalization of expertise—because we can do one thing well, we think we can do anything. I searched for teachers to introduce me to and then help me through the philosophical literature. The teacher on whom I have leaned the most is Rabbi Jack Bemporad. In 1981 I gave a lecture on suffering to his (then) congregation in Dallas and, in our conversations afterwards, he urged me to start reading the work of Alfred North Whitehead. Rabbi Bemporad lent me some books and by the time I stepped off the plane in New York I was convinced that I ought to return to full-time study. That was not too practical, so in the ensuing years I slowly worked my way to an understanding of Whitehead's later work. Despite the difficulty for physicians like myself, unused to the language of philosophical discourse, I believe I am correct that a new understanding of medicine will not be possible without a return to basic philosophical issues.

It will be noted that this book also relies heavily on the work of the great late nineteenth-century logicians, Bradley, Bosanquet, and Lotze and on early twentieth-century philosophers such as Alexander, Collingwood, and Dewey, whose work addresses issues pushed aside by the mainstream of American analytic philosophy of this century. I turned to their work because I believe it was leading to an enlarged view of knowledge and the human condition that was diverted by the mushrooming of the scientific perspective. There is considerable evidence of a return to these ideas not only in medicine but in philosophy (as well as in literature, art, music, and other disciplines). Once again, tolerant colleagues have been of immense help in the process of my wanderings afield. This is particularly true of Daniel Callahan, Peter Dineen, Straughn Donnelly, Will Gaylin, Hans Jonas, Leon Kass, Balfour Mount, Edmund Pellegrino, Mark Siegler, Richard Zaner, and Robert Zimmerman. It was Stephen Toulmin (to the rescue once again) who steered me to R. G. Collingwood. I believe it is true to say that if there were no Hastings Center I would have done none of the writing of these last two decades. It has been a place to present ideas, engage in lively discussion, and hear excellent and helpful criticism in an atmosphere of warm and friendly intellectuality.

Kay Toombs made important contributions to my understanding of suffering which are reflected in Chapters 3 and (especially) 4. James P. Smith was extremely helpful in the discussions of cardiopulmonary pathophysiology in Chapter 8. Chapters 11 and 12 are the beginnings of my answer to issues raised by Samuel Gorovitz and Alisdair MacIntyre in their well-known essay, "Towards a Theory of Medical Fallibility," which I have been thinking about since it was presented to the Hastings Center group on the Foundations of Ethics and its Relationship to Science in 1974. Chapter 12 is in its present form primarily because of the wonderful discussions at the meeting on Experience as a Basis for Ethics organized by Warren T. Reich and as a result of the advice of Drew Leder in a long conversation in the Cleveland airport (during which we missed our plane).

The research leading to portions of this book has been aided by grants from the Robert Wood Johnson Foundation, The National Fund for Medical Education, the Commonwealth Fund, and the Mayer Foundation. I am once again grateful to Margaret Mahoney, who has been supportive of my work from the beginning.

Authors, as everyone knows, can be relentless, so one must have sympathy for those who consent to read an entire manuscript. Thus my feelings of gratitude are especially great toward Elaine Scarry, Kay Toombs, and Richard Zaner. I feel more than fortunate to have had the help and collegiality of Richard Zaner who not only read the manuscript and provided searching commentary, but with whom I have been able to share a vision of the entire intellectual project—rare good luck. Joan Cassell helped shape Chapters 1 and 2 as they originally appeared in *Daedalus*. Nancy Schlick was the primary editor for the entire manuscript. Over many years I have come to depend on her intelligent and insightful criticism, excellent editorial skills, and friendship.

The continuing laboratory in which all the ideas in this book has been tested and refined has been my medical practice. I am grateful to my patients for their patience, for teaching me so much, as well as for providing my life and livelihood. I had been a solo private practitioner for twenty-five years when Dr. Kenneth Scileppi joined me in 1986. Not only has he been a pleasure to work with, but he has been extremely generous in lifting burdens from my shoulders so that I can continue to study and write.

The last three years of this book's creation have been shared with Patricia Owens. With rare intelligence and perspicacity she has read every word of every version of every chapter—cheerfully! Her willingness to share in clarifying the ideas and her tolerance of the burdens has, with much else, made these years happy when such a vision had dimmed.

Contents

The Nature of Suffering

1

Ideas in Conflict: The Rise and Fall of New Views of Disease

AS I SAT at the battered desk in the Bellevue Clinic, the young woman opposite me implored me to believe that her back *really* hurt. Her chart contained brief scribbles recording several previous visits; each time the doctor had prescribed heat and aspirin. After her first visit X rays had been taken of her lower back, but the X rays were normal. I had seen her once before and was inclined, like the other residents who had seen her, to dismiss her complaints as unimportant—garden-variety low back pain with no evidence of disease. Because of her tone of voice, I looked at her face, perhaps seeing her for the first time. "It really, really hurts," she said. I asked her where it hurt and she twisted to point to a spot on the upper spine at about the level of her breasts. That was strange because every entry in the chart talked about low back pain and the X rays pictured her lower spine. I asked if that was where it had always hurt. She said that it had hurt in the same place since February when she fell while ice-skating. "And it's May already, and it still hurts just as much."

I was chagrined and embarrassed. In all those visits to at least three medical residents, not one of us had overcome our misconceptions about young women with back pain to find out what had happened or had examined her adequately to discover her trouble. The new set of X rays—of her upper spine—showed a healing fracture of a part of her vertebra. At her next visit I explained what the source of her pain was, that there was nothing that could be done for it, but that it was not at all serious. "I don't mind that," she said, "I'm so glad to know that there really is something wrong, that I wasn't just going crazy."

As inexcusable as the error may have been, it is important to understand that its origin was not carelessness or bias alone. As a physician in training, I was not fundamentally interested in *her.* That may sound strange since, of course, I wanted to help her, but what I was basically interested in was finding a disease in her. If there was no disease, then politeness (to the extent that Bellevue residents of that era were polite) demanded reassurance and a prescription for aspirin. But that was being polite, being a person—not being a doctor.

It was 1956; she did not act angry, threaten to sue, or announce (publicly, at least) how unfeeling doctors were. In the more than thirty years that have passed since that incident, patients have changed, doctors have changed, and medicine has changed. But the emerging concept that the *sick person* should be the focus of medicine rather than the person's disease is related to ideas about the nature of sickness that have evolved through the centuries. This chapter describes some of the theories on which medicine has been based, why theory is important, and how these ideas have been changing during our times.

The Importance of Disease Concepts to Medicine

Throughout the history of medicine a dispute has existed between those who see disease as a generalized phenomenon and those who hold that diseases are localized entities (1). The first idea, often called the physiological (most closely approximating, but less far reaching than what is now called the ecological) conception of disease, was embraced by the Hippocratic school which saw the origins of disease in an imbalance between the forces of nature within and outside the sick person. The second viewpoint, the ontological conception of disease, understands diseases to be *entities,* things that invade and are localized in parts of the body (2). One or another of these conceptions of disease has always held sway in medical thought, sometimes for centuries.

Francis Bacon envisaged science as making perhaps its most important contribution to human progress in medicine; nonetheless, science came late to medicine. Independent discoveries, such as those of the great anatomists or the early physiologists, were of unquestionable importance in understanding the human body. However, they could not be brought to bear on medicine until the manifestations of sickness were systematized in a way that allowed physicians to know when they were dealing with the same problem—does this patient with rash and fever have the same disease as that patient with rash and fever? And this could not come to pass until a theory of medicine developed that emphasized and unified the actual phenomena exhibited by sick persons. Previous theories were so concerned with ultimate causes as to be of little relevance to what was going on at the sick bed and of practically no use to clinicians—doctors who actually take care of the sick. The disputes between theorist and practitioner, between rationalist and empiricist, have pervaded Western medicine from its Greek beginnings, independent of which theory of disease—ontological or physiological—prevailed (3).

I believe that how well a theory that is fundamental to medicine *works* has a profound impact on how effective doctors are, on how they behave, on relations within the profession, on relationships with patients, and even on the power of the profession in general. This is a difficult topic, because, in defiance of reality, physicians generally view themselves as realists who disdain all theorists and philosophers. Clinicians tend to focus on other things—the practical, or what "works." They do not seem to believe that there is a theory for clinical practice. Unfortunately, when doctors dismiss theory, they often do things with unhappy result because they do not really know *why* they are doing them. For example, when a patient has a widespread cancer whose primary (place of origin) is unknown, physicians will often go to considerable lengths to find the place of origin even though it may cause the patient great discomfort without offering *any* benefit. They do this because disease theory (the concept that when people are sick a disease can always be discovered whose constant characteristics provide a rational basis for the illness and for the action of doctors) dictates the importance of making a diagnosis—knowing the disease. Widespread cancer (metastatic adenocarcinoma) is not a diagnosis in doctor's terms; metastatic adenocarcinoma from the stomach, now that's a *doctor's* diagnosis. Unfortunately, when physicians do things like this they may bring into conflict two or more of their own values. In this instance the need to know the disease conflicts with the more fundamental dictum, "Above all, do no harm." (4).

Whether doctors like the idea or not, human action is inevitably theory driven. We act as we do (we even see what we see) because we have a concept—a theory—about what will be the consequences of our actions (5). Medical actions also are dependent on theory because they are undertaken with a belief about possible causes and consequences. Thus, while clinicians tend to disregard theory, they are, nevertheless, guided by some sort of theory—the push to find a diagnosis, for example. But when individual physicians have theories that are at wide variance from one another, or theories, which, while similar, are far removed from direct clinical experience, then little basis exists for common understanding among doctors *or* patients. We are able to speak together only because of a common language for objects and events. A common language for something implies a common interpretation of the events signified by the words; the more exact our use of language, the more exact our common interpretation. Hence, the disease called catarrhal jaundice became viral hepatitis, which then split into hepatitis B and hepatitis A. Then non-A non-B hepatitis was added, and most recently delta hepatitis joined the group of diseases that had all been included originally in the category catarrhal jaundice. Each change in terminology is accompanied by a change in the internal content of the notion signified by the descriptive category (6). When several doctors talk to each other about a patient with hepatitis B they have in their minds ideas about source of infection, incubation period, course of the illness, progression to chronic liver disease, and even the possibility of ending with cancer of the liver. In fact, however, at any one moment they do not *know* whether most, or even any, of the ideas that they share about hepatitis B apply to this *particular* patient. They do not share concrete matters of fact about *this* patient, but rather abstractions and theories about hepatitis B in general. I would like to extend this notion further by suggesting that the more solidly doctors and laypersons all share the same theories about disease and its causes and treatment, and the sturdier and more resistant to attack the theory is, the more solidly united and impregnable the whole profession is. I believe Coulter is correct when he says that "professional coherence is engendered by doctrinal coherence" (7).

The opposite is implied. When the primary theories that bind the profession together begin to come apart or their weaknesses are exposed, then the profession as a whole begins to lose coherence for physicians as well as the public at large. Such is the case at the present time when the theory of medicine is in transition. One has only to see how expansive and vaunting chiropractic clinics have become to recognize how much weaker the current hold of medicine's theory is on the general population. This observation in the face of modern medicine's obvious therapeutic effectiveness should also help drive home the fact that humans act on their interpretations of events—their theories—not on events themselves.

The relation of theory to clinical practice in medicine has always been highly problematic. Scientific theory dictates diagnosis and disease understandings but says nothing about sick persons, their behavior, patient–doctor communication, and so on. If the whole point of the clinical encounter is to decide what is the right and the good thing to do for a specific patient, then traditional medical theory is sorely lacking. Which is precisely what this book seeks to remedy.

The Rise of Disease Theory

The genius of the disease theory of medicine, which came into being in France in the first decades of the 1800s, is that it provided both a common basis of understanding for doctors and one for bringing science to bear on the problems of medicine. The classication of disease has occupied such a central place in the history of medicine until the middle of this century that it is useful to quote Faber to understand why.

> The attempt to "describe the diseases" borrowed from descriptive natural history has been found to be inseparably bound up with the quest for the causes of the morbid phenomena. Clinical medicine is, therefore, at work, like the other natural sciences . . . at the great task of attempting to understand natural phenomena in an attempt to control them. . . . It does not stop short at this, however, but goes on to construct by synthesis clinical pictures of individual diseases subject to fixed laws in their course and development. . . . these clinical pictures of disease . . . denote a delimited group of natural phenomena produced by some definite cause. . . . To the physiologist and worker in the laboratory, morbid categories are subordinate concepts, but to the physician, to the clinician, the reverse is the case; he cannot live, cannot speak, cannot act without them (8).

It follows from disease theory that the purpose of the clinician is to discover in the sick patient that unique phenomenon with its unique cause that is the disease (and thus the source of the sickness), and to base diagnostic and therapeutic actions accordingly. The great clinicians of the 1930s exemplified these practices. In those years, medicine was captivated by the promise that through science it would discover the nature of diseases, their causes, and their cures. American medicine was not long out of an era of poor medical schools and inadequately trained physicians (9). Many physicians augmented their education by study in Europe, and German medical ideals were extremely influential. World War I provided the push for the development of a testing ground for new techniques and understandings. Enough specific treatments had become available to enable physicians to see medicine of the 1930s as tremendously advanced in relation to just a few decades earlier. X rays, blood tests, and other laboratory studies—generally carried out by physicians themselves—provided a precision previously lacking. A medical school graduate of 1934 recounted that he specialized in urology in part because, with the advent of the intravenous pyelogram, "when I told my patient what was wrong, I *knew* that was what was wrong" (10). This hunt for precision in diagnosis has characterized medicine ever since.

Trouble in the Temple: Weaknesses in Classic Disease Theory

But even in those early years, when the prospect of the first era of cure in the history of medicine seemed to be dawning, trouble was apparent. The trouble took the form of two weaknesses of the disease theory shared by medical science of the era. The first is the fundamental place held by the idea that each disease had one and only one cause. The second was the belief that all function (as in heart function) in the body, or elsewhere in nature, is founded on structure (as in the anatomy of the heart) and that changes in function therefore imply changes in structure. So that, for example, any change in the way the heart works must follow from a change in the heart's anatomy, microscopic or otherwise. Both ideas, on which the theory of disease is based, have been undermined by the advance of medical science.

First, let us look at the concept that every disease has a specific cause:

> The principle of etiological specificity of disease implies that every disease entity is produced by a quite particular cause, that different diseases cannot arise from the same cause, nor can different causes produce the same disease. We now conceive of each of the pathological processes as a single, gradually developing phenomenon resulting from the action of a specific etiological agent, though with variations depending on individual circumstances or external conditions. Symptom-complexes cannot pass for diseases (11).

Infectious diseases provided the perfect model for such understanding. Indeed, by the end of the nineteeth century and the beginning of this one, the discoveries of bacteriology encouraged the belief that disease would be controlled by merely preventing the transmission of microbes (12). While this idea of cause is essentially artificial (7), it has the advantage of restricting the viewpoint of physicians to the disease itself and to immediate causes. It also allowed the emphasis in therapeutics to be shifted away from the previous crude empirical therapies toward a search for treatments that got at "the cause." The degree to which this idea took hold can be seen in the extent to which modern patients prefer such treatments over those that merely get at "symptoms."

Perhaps the biggest blow to the cardinal place of "unique causes" has been the therapeutic revolution itself. With the exception of antimicrobials, *none* of the fantastic array of effective therapeutic agents is directed against the "cause" of the disease. The drug allopurinol interferes with the production of uric acid, but elevated uric acid is surely not *the* cause of gout. Tricyclic antidepressants have been a major advance in the treatment of depression. Their effectiveness *may* be related to their effects on brain neurotransmitters, but nobody believes that abnormalities in those chemicals are the *cause* of depression. Both beta blockers and calcium channel blockers have dramatically improved the treatment of angina and coronary heart disease, but neither is aimed at the cause of the disease. The list could go on and on. In fact, doctors know very well that they only rarely treat causes, whatever they may tell themselves.

The other conceptually important but basically weak aspect of classical disease theory is its dependence on the idea that all changes in the function of an organism or its parts are referable to changes in its structure. In the everyday medical world this has made the search for a diagnosis essentially the search for altered structure. If a patient had symptoms referable to the large intestine, perhaps a tumor was present. X rays were taken. If they showed the tumor, the patient had a disease. If they did not, it was possible to dismiss the patient's complaints as "nerves," or spasm—in other words, no disease. As another example, a patient lies racked with back pain on an X-ray table, but the X rays do not demonstrate an abnormality of structure—herniated disc or some similar entity. The patient can be told that there is "nothing wrong." It is obvious that *something* is the matter or the person would not be in such pain. But no disease is present, at least according to traditional theories of disease, because there is no structural change.

Disease theory has been enormously successful because much, if not most, of the time it *works*. When something is wrong, a disease is usually there to find. Yet the difficulties with this approach were already commented on by Dr. Francis Peabody in 1927 in his classic paper, *The Care of the Patient* (13). In some circumstances the approach does not work at all—despite psychiatry's enormous efforts, mental disorders almost never fit the classical criteria for disease. In other situations it works too well—the aged have many diseases that can be identified, but acting on them can lead not to benefit, but to illness from overtreatment.

As knowledge has advanced, the firmness of the distinction between structure and function has given way. For example, if people take the drug phenobarbital, enzymes in their livers are activated that effect the way their livers work toward other drugs or substances. Are these alterations in liver function based on enzyme induction caused by altered structure? Certainly not in the classical sense.

Another example of the failure of classical structural disease concepts (or their enfolding into function) is chronic obstructive pulmonary disease—the term that has come to replace the structural diagnoses of emphysema and chronic bronchitis. Epidemiologists in the United States and Great Britain could not find structural changes in the lungs that were consistently associated with functional impairment in breathing common to patients in England and America. They ended up agreeing on the *definition* of the condition to be called chronic obstructive pulmonary disease: the disease present in a patient who coughed and brought up phlegm for as much as three months a year for at least two years! No such definition previously existed in modern medicine. Chronic obstructive pulmonary disease is a reduction in the ability to breathe (characterized by certain sharply defined abnormalities in the physiologic measurement of the breathing function) that occurs in the presence of various structural changes—there is *no* unique alteration in structure.

Patients generally expect structural disease names as a diagnosis for their illnesses. And they are encouraged in this expectation by their doctors. When runners develop pain in some part of their leg and go to a physician or orthopedist, they expect to be told that they have chondromalacia of the patella, or tendonitis, or a heel spur—all names for abnormal structure. They then expect treatment to be directed at the abnormality of the body part. Their orthopedists rarely disappoint them. It is more difficult to explain that the pain in the knee does not primarily involve the knee, but muscles in the thigh and the calf that are shortened and exert too constant a force on their attachments around the knee. And that they got that way because the runner has not stretched his or her muscles properly and is running tight. Functional explanations take longer (to the uninitiated) than (say) "tendonitis." Of course, it would not be so difficult for patients if more doctors understood it.

The basic problem is that the idea of structure, while it may have some everyday utility, is an artificial one. Structure is what you see under a microscope. Structure is what pathologists tell us about. (Which is why disease theory made the pathologist the referee of medicine.) But what you see under the microscope is not what is happening in sick people. Nothing in nature holds still like that—everything is changing all the time. What we call "function" merely changes fast enough for us to measure it in a clinical setting. Even the structure of the body changes constantly.

Scientific advance, not theoretical deficiencies, ultimately undermined the fundamental place of the structure-function relationship in disease theory. The enormous and exciting advances in medical science during the last generation have not been primarily about diseases, but about how the body functions in health and disease. Knowing diseases, in the old-fashioned sense, is not nearly as important as knowing pathophysiology.* The modern physician's ability to so effectively treat heart disease depends on current knowledge about how the heart functions. The heart can be seen, and intervened in, as a muscle pump, as a hydraulic system, or as an electrical system in a manner that is vastly better than when it was considered the seat of rheumatic heart disease, syphilitic heart disease, arteriosclerotic heart disease, and so on. Because the language of structure remains common among doctors and is simpler than the language of function or process, physicians still talk structure—but they increasingly act on functional abnormalities without concern for structure. The autopsy room used to be the central theatre where disputes about the diagnoses of difficult cases were resolved—(sadly) doctors do not even bother going to see autopsies anymore. The reason that current therapies are not directed at the "cause" is that knowledge of pathophysiology—the concatenation of biological events that distinguishes abnormal function from normal physiology—provides the opportunity of designing therapies that will interrupt the abnormal chain of occurrences and meliorate the disease.

The Rise of the Ecological Perspective

The Second World War widened the horizons of medicine. For the first time in such a definitive manner, Western technological medicine reached across national and cultural boundaries. The 1930s had shown the promise of modern medicine, and during and immediately after World War II, that promise began to be truly fulfilled. Effective antimicrobial agents existed for many infectious diseases, including tuberculosis, that would previously have decimated undernourished and war-torn populations. The postwar success of medicine and its technology transmitted an image of hope and of the potential goodness of humankind. It seemed that medicine and medical science were the herald of a new world.

But with the successes came failures. By the 1950s overwhelming evidence existed that technological medicine did not easily cross cultural boundaries, if doing so required the active acceptance of the *beliefs* behind the technology (14). A frequently cited example is the difficulty in getting indigenous populations to accept the concept of microbes—to boil water or use sanitary facilities (15).

By the late 1940s and the 1950s it was commonly known that cultural and social factors were important elements in the development of disease. But this knowledge largely failed to penetrate conventional medical education. My own experience is illustrative. I had been trained in internal medicine in the

*The term pathophysiology will be used throughout to mean the biological basis of disease. It is also employed to denote the biological chain of events making up the disease process. In medicine it has come to stand for a kind of thinking about disease in which understanding basic biological mechanisms down to the molecular level is pre-eminent. Thus, it is a term used to describe not only the biological basis of a specific disease but the general scientific approach of modern medicine to all diseases.

Third Medical Division of Bellevue Hospital (in our eyes, Mecca) when I joined the Department of Public Health at Cornell University Medical College as a fellow. In 1959, in preparation for teaching a Public Health Seminar to third-year medical students entitled "Medicine Across Cultural Boundaries," my chairman, Professor Walsh McDermott, gave me a number of books, World Health Organization pamphlets, and papers about the problems of cross-cultural medicine. I read them with care. It is not an overstatement to say that they completely changed my understanding of medicine. As a result of my training, and in common with most physicians at the time, I tended to see the problems of sickness as diseases that could be discovered within patients (remember the embarrassing case with which I began this chapter). Diseases were acted on directly, to the extent that such treatments were possible. In therapeutic acts, the patient might be a help or a hindrance in achieving access to the disease, but in any event, the disease, not the patient, was the primary focus. When patients were found to have tuberculosis, I had no difficulty with the simple facts that tuberculosis was the cause of their illness and the tubercle bacillus was the cause of their tuberculosis. The material that Dr. McDermott gave me cast irrevocable doubt on such a simple formulation of the problem of sickness and the chain of causation.

I became aware of the power of social and cultural forces and their impact on health. In common with most, however, I continued to see cultural factors as encouraging the presence of certain diseases, or preventing an unquestionably effective technology from being brought to bear on the disease problems of non-Western groups. Such an understanding led to the belief that if Western scientific medicine and technology could be introduced with the aid of social scientists to ensure acceptance by the host culture, the cause of the repeated failures after World War II could be overcome. The Many Farms experiment, started by Walsh McDermott in 1955, was based on this premise. There, high technology–medicine was introduced to the Navajo in such a manner that native healing systems and Western medicine coexisted with apparent comfort. Individual and community expectations were met or exceeded. The presence of Western-trained physicians fighting the individual illnesses of individual patients was embraced by the Navajo.

When all the data was in, however, Professor McDermott saw it quite differently. In 1972 he published an important paper, *Health Care Experiment at Many Farms,* in which he makes it clear that the fundamental problem in transcultural medicine is not developing the sensitivity to requirements of the host culture that will permit access by personnel and technology, although this is unquestionably vital. Instead, the afflictions of the Navajo (with the important exception of tuberculosis and perhaps otitis media) did not fall within the ken of technological medicine. Although 1950s medicine had solutions to their major diseases, the primary causes of morbidity and mortality of the Navajo do not fall within the system of entities that count as "diseases" in our medicine. In Dr. McDermott's term, they did not have "name" diseases. For example, in common with children in many poverty-stricken areas, the Navajo children developed a combination of diarrhea and respiratory infections (in which no specific microbe could be found) that occur in the setting of malnutrition and inadequate hygiene and which are often fatal. Dr. McDermott was struck by the seeming paradox of the acceptance of the personal physician system of Western medicine by the Navajo and the ineffectiveness of the technology.

> Popular expectations and misunderstandings of what an individual physician can do operate as a formidable constraint on the rational use of biomedical technology. Indeed, because of the nature of medicine, as a practical matter its technology has to be deployed irrationally. This is largely the consequence of our tradition of having both essentials of medical care—the technology and the human support—administered by the same person, the physician (16).

What was not clear at the time is that the ideas contained in the term *rational* use of the biomedical technology might be in need of redefinition. The quotation's implication is that because of the expectations of patients, personal physicians are forced (by their patients) to use technology where it is of no value.

We are now full circle. The phenomenal development of Western scientific medicine was dependent on the "discovery" of diseases as we know them—entities with a specific cause and a specific location, whether anatomical or biochemical. Where health problems cannot be defined in those terms—such as the problems related to malnutrition and poor hygiene in much of the developing world after the Second World War—scientific medicine is a misfit.

It is apparent, however, that Western medical science has had many successes in Third-World cultures. In part these advances occurred because some of the health problems fit the technology, in part because of the westernization of these peoples. These are insufficient, however, as explanation. Medical science *without formal acknowledgment of the conceptual shift* has itself become increasingly less dependent on disease concepts, pursuing instead an understanding of biological processes apart from specific diseases. Here we have come again to a more "physiologic" concept of disease, ideas that in our time are most closely allied with the "ecological perspective," which Rene Dubos was closely identified with.

Following the war, Dr. Dubos began to write increasingly about the interdependence of organisms and their environment. in perhaps his best-known book, *The Mirage of Health,* he demonstrated that humankind's adaptation or maladaptation to its environment contained the roots of its bodily afflictions (17). In this view, to see *the* cause of tuberculosis as the tubercle bacillus is a naive interpretation that is not rescued by words sent to do the job, such as "necessary but not sufficient cause," "contributory cause," and so on. In *Man Adapting* and then in *So Human an Animal,* Dubos continued to illustrate the constantly evolving process that is the life of an individual, a culture, a nation, and even an epoch; and how that process cannot be separated from human biology and the social and cultural evolution that occurs concurrently (18)(19).

Dubos' work was widely acclaimed and taken up by the environmental movement that swept the country in the late 1960s, culminating with Earth

Day, April 22, 1970 (20). The goals of the environmental movement entered our society, as air pollution control and the reclamation of natural resources achieved a large political constituency. Public support for environmental reform was based, in part, on a perception by the population that the environment was far dirtier and more threatening than the evidence might support (21). Americans have continued to perceive many of their bodily ills to be the result of environmental toxins. They have changed their diets, significantly reducing the amount of meat and saturated fat consumed, and they have even cut down their intake of hard liquor and alcohol in general. Achieving and maintaining fitness have become widespread values. And the belief has grown that individuals are responsible for maintaining their own health. These changes in behavior and concepts are consistent with an ecological (or physiological) perspective on disease and its causation. It would not be equally true to say that the fundamental ecological concepts—the idea of chains of causation and the interrelationship of humans and their environment—have become part of everyday *acknowledged* ways of thought in medicine.

The Social Responsibility of Medicine

Not only has the theory of disease changed during this century, but the responsibility attributed to medicine by its public and by physicians has broadened during the same period. It would be an error, however, to attribute the origins of the social medicine movement solely to the decades after World War I, because already in 1848, while studying the prevalence of typhus in Silesia, Rudolf Virchow had become an outspoken believer in the idea that the origins of many diseases lay in the social conditions of the populace. Nonetheless, in the United States, despite the earlier contributions of the Public Health movement, social consciousness in medicine did not begin to flourish until the decades after World War I. The disease burdens of the poor, immigrants, and workers were seen by many to be directly the result of social conditions that medicine should be active in remedying. These beliefs were stimulated by what then appeared to be the great success of the Russian social experiment. On a more mundane level, the social medicine movement of the 1930s contributed the "social history" meant to be elicited when the history of an illness is obtained from a patient. (This is the aspect of the patient's history that includes habits such as alcohol or smoking, the medical history of the family, marital circumstances, and occupational exposures.) Third-party insurers such as "the Blues" had their origin in that era as did the group health movement. The Health Insurance Plan (HIP) of New York, one of the earliest such groups in the United States, was founded at that time. An enduring belief on the part of many physicians—that medicine had a basic part to play in social progress beyond the mere treatment of individual illnesses—can be seen in the development of some academic departments of public health and preventive medicine. The role of medical schools in these activities, however, was probably not central. Indeed, it would be an error to suggest that the profession was of one mind about extending medicine's functions to include social melioration. Battles erupted, as each step in the direction of health insurance or group medicine was opposed by "organized" medicine (largely composed of local medical societies and the American Medical Association). The rallying theme of the opposition was the specter of "socialized" medicine and the intervention of the federal government (22).

Many of these new trends seemed to disappear, defeated by the Great Depression and the all-consuming effort subsequently required by the Second World War. But then again in the turbulent era of the 1960s the idea of medicine's social responsibility burst forth with a fervor that may be difficult to remember in these quieter times. Medical student activism—itself unusual—focused on demands that medical school curricula become "relevant" to the needs of the poor and the "oppressed" (23). Medical schools were urged to become involved in the health problems of their communities. As a result, in many schools, Departments of Community Medicine replaced what had been departments of Public Health or Preventive Medicine. Money for all of these efforts was abundant as part of the federal government's commitment to a "war on poverty"—a war in which medicine played a major part.

The money ran out, preempted by the Vietnam War. By the mid 1970s the fervor again subsided. The relationship of Americans to doctors and medical care changed, not to return to where it had been when the activism died down. But what did *not* die—and what was an inevitable outcome of the ferment within and in opposition to the social medicine movement through all these decades—was the growing belief that *sickness could not be completely understood apart from personal lifestyle and the social setting in which it occurred.* If the poor have more sickness than the comfortable, if their illnesses are more severe—both well-known phenomena—then the social setting in which disease occurs must influence its origins, course, and treatment. While this conclusion may be obvious, and may well have influenced the behavior of most physicians throughout history, the facts make it difficult to still believe that diseases are simply entities that occupy a body. After all, if diseases are simply entities—things that get into the body—why should they be worse in the poor? After the successes and failures of the war on poverty and community medicine "outreach" programs were tallied up, it was apparent that the increased prevalence of disease among the poor could not be seen in simple terms—poor housing, lack of education, inadequate medical care, breakdowns in family structure, and other features of poverty all seemed to play their part in a complex manner. Indeed, it is possible to view these factors associated with ill health as part of the dynamic interplay of other social and economic components that determine the "health" of (say) the urban social unit in a larger sense (24). Unfortunately, in the present era of conservatism, the failures of the aggressive approach of the 1960s and 1970s to solve the associated problems of poverty and sickness have been taken as a warrant for the retrogressive and simplistic notion that it does no good to directly help the weak in society—the poor, the aged, and the sick. It has been possible to identify several intellectual trends that have been crucial to the emergence, during this century, of the ideas on which this book is based. First, the conflict between the physiological and the ontological view of disease and the gradual replacement of the latter by the former. Second, the conflict of the ideas of the social medicine movement with those whose understanding of medicine and medicine's mission were narrower. And, third, the conflict between the ecological viewpoint, in which disease is believed to arise from the interaction of organism and environment, and the perspective that sees a disease as complete in itself. These sets of oppositions seem clearly related, with their differences being primarily ones of setting and scale. In each instance, the contrast is between understanding diseases as fixed entities, almost static forms, or understanding them as processes that unfold, with their toll being the human malfunction by which individuals know themselves or are known by others to be unhealthy. In the ontological versus the physiological view, the setting of the contrast is the body or person; in the social medicine conflict the setting of the contrast is the society; in the ecological outlook, the setting of the contrast is the environment, physical as well as social. The historical progression seems to be from a structural to more process oriented understanding. It would seem to be more accurate, however, to say that, in the last fifty years, the dynamic viewpoint became prominent, only to recede again into the background. I suggested earlier that these dynamic ideas in medicine seemed well on their way in the 1930s, only to drift into obscurity until the 1950s when they re-emerged.

This is written at a time when fundamentalism seems dominant in the world and the United States has turned toward conservative views. The prevailing values in medicine are commercial, with medical care viewed as a commodity and physicians like other marketplace purveyors. The ideals discussed here are difficult to discern. To some, examining the conflict between the two views of disease, the ontological versus the physiological, may seem strangely inappropriate. But the ideas are of real and lasting importance because they influence the scientific study of disease as well as its treatment. More important, they are part of a larger change in the manner in which humanity views itself and its relationship to nature. The history of this century tells us that the force of this change in fundamental beliefs may be temporarily obscured, but will not be denied.

Ideas and theories in medicine come to life in the actions of physicians. In the next chapter we see the effect that changes in theory, science, and technology have on our ideas about physicians.

References

1. Hudson, Robert P. *Disease and Its Control: The Shaping of Modern Thought.* 1983. Westport, Conn., Greenwood Press, Chap. 4 and 6.

2. Taylor, F. Kraupl. *Concepts of Illness, Disease, and Morbus.* 1979. New York, Cambridge University Press, Chap. 2.

3. Coulter, Harris L. *Divided Legacy: A History of the Schism in Medical Thought.* 1975. Washington, D.C., Weehawken Book, Vol I, Introduction.

4. Cassell, Eric J. The Conflict Between the Need to Know and the Need to Care for the Patient. *Medicine and Metaphysics.* 1978. Boston, D. Reidel.

5. Popper, Karl R. and Eccles, John C. *The Self and Its Brain.* 1977. New York, Springer International, p. 45.

6. Cassell, Eric J. *Talking with Patients: The Theory of Doctor-Patient Communication.* 1985. Cambridge, Mass.: MIT Press, p. 157.

7. Coulter, Harris L. *Op. cit.* Vol. I, p. 506.

8. Faber, Knud, *Nosography.* 2nd ed. Revised. 1930. New York, Haber, p. 210ff.

9. Hertzler, Arthur E. *The Horse and Buggy Doctor.* 1938. New York, Harper Brothers.

10. Spinelli, Anthony. Personal communication.

11. Lewandowsky, 1912. Quoted in Faber, op. cit., p. 183.

12. Galdston, Iago. *Social and Historical Foundations of Modern Medicine.* 1981. New York, Brunner/Mazel, p. 115.

13. Peabody, Francis W. The Care of the Patient. *JAMA* 1927; 88:877–82.

14. Deuschle, Kurt. *Daedalus* Vol. 115, No. 2, Spring 1986.

15. Wellin, Edward. Water Boiling in a Peruvian Town. In *Health Culture and Community.* Ed. by Paul, Benjamin. 1955. New York, Russell Sage Foundation.

16. McDermott, W., Deuschle, K., and Barnett, C. Health Care Experiment at Many Farms. *Science* 1972; 175:23–31.

17. Dubos, Rene. *The Mirage of Health.* 1959. New York, Harpers, p. 85ff.

18. Dubos, Rene. *Man Adapting.* 1965. New Haven, Yale University Press.

19. Dubos, Rene. *So Human an Animal.* 1968. New York, Scribner.

20. Hayes, D., ed. *Earth Day—The Beginning.* 1970. New York, Bantam Books.

21. Cassell, E. J. 19th and 20th Century Environmental Movements. *Archives of Environmental Health* 1971, 22:35–40.

22. Starr, Paul. *The Social Transformation of American Medicine.* 1982. New York, Basic Books, p. 271ff.

23. Ebert, Robert. *Daedalus* Vol. 115, No. 2, Spring 1986.

24. Forrester, Jay W. *Urban Dynamics.* 1969. Cambridge, Mass., MIT Press, Chap. 7.

2

The Changing Concept of the Ideal Physician

ONE DAY ABOUT ten years ago, I got a call from the Chief of Neurosurgery of an excellent upstate medical center to tell me about one of my patients who had fractured her skull in a skiing accident. He wanted to discuss not only her injury but also the behavior of her family and friends. She was unconscious and in danger of dying because of the swelling in her brain that followed the fracture. There was then no method of proven effectiveness for dealing with that common and life-threatening complication. Because her circumstance was so grave, he had proposed to her family that she be given a new and experimental treatment. Rather than signing the consent, the parents and particularly my patient's friends attacked him for "using her as a guinea pig." Following the call, the issues that concerned them were resolved, they gave permission, and she did very well.

He and I talked about the episode later. He was accustomed to having his judgment accepted as in the best interest of his patients and was shocked by the obvious lack of trust. Nothing like that had ever happened to him. I assured him that he would not have to wait long before it happened again, because in New York City such episodes had already become commonplace.

This incident exemplifies a striking change in the public image of doctors and the relationship between physicians and patients. Where previously physicians' decisions were rarely questioned, now patients are frequently sceptical and may doubt both the physician's motives and judgment. The bioethics movement is another force concerned with respect for patients and their protection from physicians in medical care and research. Concurrently, there is a strengthened interest in teaching physicians how to be doctors, as opposed to merely teaching them the scientific basis of medical practice. Walsh McDermott called this Samaritanism, the human dimension of the physician–patient relationship.

Sorting out those factors that have contributed to the transformation of the doctor–patient relationship is a complex process. First and foremost, medicine's total embrace of science had profound effects. Doctors trained in the last two generations have difficulty in dissociating medicine and science, but their historical ideals are distinctly different. Science is based on a belief that it and its methods are value free—anything that happens in nature is neither good nor bad, it simply *is*. On the other hand, medicine has a tradition in which a hierarchy of values—the patient comes first, doctors must above all do no harm, the good of the patient is intended—is firmly established. In addition to being value free, a scientific description does not ascribe *qualities* to things; adjectives like warm, tall, swollen, or painful exist only for persons but, ideally science deals only with measurable quantities like temperature, vertical dimensions, diameters. It is obvious that medicine could not exist without reference to qualities and their meanings to humans. Moreover, science does not deal with individuals, it deals with—and its methods are only suited to—generalities. Medicine has to do with individuals, period. As Richard Zaner has made clear, this tension resonates back to ancient medicine as a conflict between emphasizing theoretical knowledge and the actual experience of the doctor with *this* sick person (1). Science and medicine are inextricably bound, but the paradoxes and strains produced by believing they are the *same* led to a conception that could not last—that of the ideal physician as a scientist.

My second point is that the effect of technology, in its general sense, has altered the character of physicianship in these last fifty years. Technology's impact is not fully comprehended because of the mistaken idea that the effects of science and technology on the thinking and behavior of physicians are the same. Because of this confusion, no discussion of the changing concept of doctors can be complete without reference to the special effect that the disarming simplicity and certainty of technology has had on physicians. It is the burden of doctors to have great responsibility in a sea of doubt and uncertainty. The intrinsic promise of technology—that it will relieve uncertainty and lighten doubt—is virtually irresistible given the special circumstances of medical practice. However, despite the uncountable benefits of technology, uncertainty and doubt remain, although often shifted or concealed.

My third point is that the effect of these factors on the character of physicians took place over sufficient time so that the usual forces acting in the affairs of humans—politics and the succession of generations—could combine to alter the dominant group of physicians in the United States from the role models of the past, the academically minded practicing clinicians (and their organizations) to the full-time medical research scientists of the academic medical centers who embraced and exemplified the new values and who became the new model for the ideal physician.

The fourth point is that, since World War II, the meaning of the words "person" and "individual"—central to American beliefs—have been undergoing profound alterations. Since physicians are persons and treat persons, it was inevitable that this social turmoil result in a new understanding of the nature of doctors, patients, and their relationship. Among the changes in the social climate have been the well-known distrust of science and the rise of the bioethics movement in which preeminence of patients and their protection are stressed. The redefinition of patienthood (following from the redefinition of personhood) and its expectations has been sharpened by the fact that the present generation of Americans, raised on mass communications in the midst of technical and scientific complexity, have become so knowledgeable that (it is commonly believed) physicians can no longer lay sole claim to medical knowledge.

The Effect of Science on the Ideal of the Doctor

Perhaps apocryphally, it was said in the 1950s that in a display case in the Department of Radiology of the Massachussets General Hospital a stethoscope was shown as an obsolete instrument. That display case is symbolic of the belief commonly held then that scientific medicine and its attendant technology would render obsolete the individualism and subjectivism that had so hindered medical progress. The time of great clinicians, doctors who primarily practiced medicine—some of whom were my teachers and their contemporaries—was believed over. I remember attending a luncheon when I started my fellowship in which these issues were being discussed. It was the general belief that no one would ever again rise to prominence as a clinician as a sole result of expertise in the case of patients. How different from the end of the nineteenth and in the beginning of this century, when doctors aspired to greatness because of their abilities with the sick. During the decades that followed World War II, such individualism came to be viewed negatively—science became the physician, although necessarily working through the hands of individuals. Similarly, the term "anecdotal medicine" came to be seen as the equivalent of subjective contamination and to stand for sloppy, unscientific medicine. Since individual experience is inevitably anecdotal (one can have no other kind) and individual clinical judgments contain subjective elements (they are the product of a subject), banishing the subjective and anecdotal from medicine necessarily demotes the individuality of the physician to the level of a contaminant.

The philosophical basis of the early twentieth-century science that medicine embraced could have it no other way. As we saw in Chapter 1, medical science is based on several postulates that allow no divergence. Science attends to objects that are free of value and quality, separate from one another, divorced from the context and times in which they would occur naturally, and whose workings can be known by the analysis of their parts. The ability to predict is a central test of the adequacy of scientific theory and knowledge, but scientific prediction does not deal with the future in quite the same way that prediction does in daily life or medical prognosis. Scientific prediction is performative—given certain conditions, such and such will happen without regard to clock and calender time. For medical science, the basis of all function is structure, and any alteration in function must be related to a change in structure. Everything about the human condition will ultimately be explained in physicochemical terms—things like mind and soul, for example, are illusions or at best epiphenomena (1)(2). (The reader will recognize that current concepts of science have softened some of these stances, albeit without satisfactory alternatives.) Because of these postulates, medical science could not deal effectively with individuals, value-laden objects, things that change through time, or wholes that are greater than the sum of their parts. Since that list contains the characteristics of persons (be they patients or doctors), medical science could not handle persons—but disease lay clearly within its purview. The phenomenal success of medical science in showing how the body works in health and disease requires no comment.

*The Promise of Science: To Know the Disease Is To Know the Illness and Its Treatment**

Knowing about disease was what counted. The history of the era of scientific medicine really starts with the "discovery" of diseases by the French school of physicians in the 1830s, the first to provide clinicopathological correlation. The enormous success of modern medicine appears to rest completely on the combination of disease theory and science. Thus, physicians came to believe that to know the disease and its treatment is to know the illness and the treatment of the ill person. This provided further basis for the idea that individual physicians count for little *as individuals;* it is their knowledge of disease and medical science that cares for the patient. In this thinking, a disembodied knowledge connected to some sort of mechanical doctoring machine would do as well and so one should not be surprised at the numerous attempts to formulate computer diagnosticians or therapists. That they have all failed should have brought into question the underlying conception, but this has not yet happened.

The uncomfortable fact remains that doctors cannot get at diseases without dealing with patients—*doctors do not treat diseases, they treat patients.* Further, the same disease in different individuals may have a different presentation, course, treatment, and outcome depending on individual and group differences among patients—from personal idiosyncrasies to genetic or anatomic variations. The scientific basis of medicine does not recognize nor provide a methodology to deal with such individual variations on the level of patient-doctor interactions. Such issues were relegated to the "art" of medicine or to individual judgment.

*There is a distinction between disease and illness. Disease is primarily defined in terms of the body and its systems. Illness is the entire complex that involves not only the sick person's body parts, but the person and the group. Illness, one might say, is what you have on the way to the doctor, disease is what you have on the way home. One can feel or be ill in the absence of disease and one can have a disease (hypertension, for example) and not be ill.

Science has solved only half the problem—a systematic basis has been provided for understanding the body and its ills—but the other half, that having to do with sick persons, remains "art." Art is, by definition, based on individual skills so that medical practice remains shackled to the problem presented by the differences among individuals—both patients and doctors—and to subjectivism. Attempts to get around this by establishing a scientific basis for dealing with values and human qualities, such as Feinstein's proposal for "clinimetrics," are doomed because science cannot deal with what it does not recognize as existing (2).

Instead, each physician must solve the problem internally. The academic physicians who were my teachers, such as Walsh McDermott, William Tillet, and Paul Beeson, had been trained by the clinicians of the previous era. While they may have passed on to their students the ideals of scientific medicine, they contained within themselves the values of the Samaritan functions of the personal-encounter system and other important aspects of the art of medicine. Dr. McDermott noted that the change in hospital architecture from large open wards to small rooms effectively moved the human support functions of the professor making rounds from the public to the private arena so that the students did not learn them. Whereas previously every act of the attending physician was open for all to see, it became common to demonstrate physical findings or discuss the patient's disease before students and house officers, but then to ask them to leave the private or semi-private room as the attending physician turned to more personal matters in support of the sick person. But hospital architecture alone cannot be blamed. I remember, in the 1950s, an attending physician teaching students in the outpatient clinic about the care of patients with congestive heart failure. The discussion was couched in terms of the pathophysiology of the failing heart, and neglected entirely such issues as the need to acquire some understanding of who the patient was, empathy, support, and the understanding of everyday life and function necessary to ensure that the patient followed the prescribed diet, took medications as ordered, and in general lived a life that would maximally enhance the function that his or her failing heart might support.

The Impact of Technology as Distinct from Science

Physicians have a reputation for conservativism, at least politically, that is generally attributed to their economic standing. But anybody who has ever tried to get them to alter their ways in medicine itself would be happy to tell you that their resistance to change (a characteristic usually associated with being conservative) is as great in medicine as in other aspects of their lives. That resistance appears to be related to the uncertainty and direful responsibility that are dominant elements of the physician's life. The simple fact is that it is frequently difficult to be certain of the best thing to do in the face of serious illness. In response, physicians may become set in their ways, dependent on recipes for diagnosis and treatment rather than on the thoughtful examination of alternatives.

Objective clinical techniques such as X rays—indeed, the whole panoply of modern medical technology—seem to offer the possibility of banishing the uncertainties of subjectivisim. It is not clear why we forget that the X ray may be objective but the physician's assessment is subjective and varies from individual to individual, but that is indeed the case (3). Call to mind an intensive care unit with monitors blinking and beeping and remember how all eyes (even family members') go to the machine—and away from the patient. It requires effort *not* to watch the monitors. Technology—machines, instruments, drug treatments—like blinkers on a horse, restrict and define and thus simplify the viewpoint. But unlike blinkers, technology also defines the values that represent good or bad, success or failure. The values of technology are unambiguous and nonmetaphorical, unlike other things in the clinical world. Numerical readouts seem certain; they do not announce their fallibility. Watch a cinearteriogram of the heart and you believe you are watching the patient's heart instead of a movie of one representation of a heart (which, because of the possibility of mislabeling, may not even be the films of the patient's study). The existence of antibiotics provides the pressure to find an infection to treat—even if infection, while perhaps present, is not making the patient sick. Endless examples could be provided to document the well-known statement "technology is sweet." Its power to oversimplify the inherently complex and produce certainty where doubt is necessarily present has proven irresistible not only to medicine but to the whole culture.

The Shift of Power in the Medical Establishment: Scientific Knowledge as Medical Power

Related to the changes wrought by science and technology was the manner in which the rise of scientific medicine undermined the status and power of medical authorities whose eminence was based primarily on expertise in the care of the sick—clinical achievement. Since many of these elite clinicians were private practitioners as well as members of the faculties of medical colleges and hospitals, the increasing prominence of scientific medicine accelerated the shift of power in medicine toward the full-time faculty of the medical schools. These changes in relative power are reflected in the changing authorship of Cecil's *Textbook of Medicine.* Originally, Cecil, an academic private practitioner, realized that one individual could no longer stand as an authority in all of internal medicine (as had Sir William Osler, also a practicing physician, when he wrote his single-authored textbook of medicine), so Cecil's textbook was written by specialists in the diseases about which they wrote. With the passage of time and the rise of scientific medicine, Cecil invited Loeb, a full-time academic, to join him as editor. Ultimately, the editorship of the book passed entirely into the hands of full-time academic physicians because by mid-century only they had the prestige necessary to be recognized as authorities. Concomitantly, what constituted the medical "establishment" changed so that the American Medical Association, which in the first half of the century was seen as monolithic when it spoke in the name of doctors, gave way to medical schools and the academic elite. Before World War II, doctors were concerned lest they offend or be expelled from their state or local medical society and lose their hospital privileges. By the time I entered practice in 1961 the medical societies had lost their sting, and in recent years they have been working to regain membership among younger physicians. It must be understood that these shifts in the relative power of clinicians and the new breed of medical scientists were not occurring in a cultural vacuum. During the same period that saw a transition in power within medicine from the clinician—the practicing physician—to the medical scientist, the American public was according medicine increasing prestige and power based on a growing respect for science (4). Thus, as is so often the case, the change in what was beheld as the ideal physician arose from a complex of reasons related to beliefs about science, the superiority of scientific medicine, the impact of technology in the doctors' world of uncertainty and doubt, and, last but not least, to matters of power in the profession.

Medical Power Spreads to the Laity

It is not surprising that a generation of physicians should have come to power for whom the scientific and technologic aspects of physicianship represented not *part* of being a doctor, but all of medicine and its practice incarnate. The American public embraced the wonders of medical science and technology, further enhancing the reputation of medicine as a science and of doctors as medical scientists. Funds for research poured in and the enterprise of modern technologic medicine grew. Americans not only supported medicine's expansion, they became knowledgeable partners. For hundreds of years the power of physicians had come from their specialized knowledge and their status. During this last generation the scientific knowledge of medicine has become increasingly accessible to laypersons and the public has shown a voracious appetite for scientific information. Obviously, some knowledge of medical science does not make a person a doctor. And while physicians enjoy stressing that fact, they miss the point. *The promise of scientific medicine is that the knowledge does the work.*

Knowledgeable patients do not believe that they are doctors; the belief is that a piece of knowledge the same as their doctors' will do the same work in their hands as in their doctors'. Witness the phenomenon of the *Physician's Desk Reference.* The patient calls the doctor after arriving home and looking up the prescribed drug in the *PDR*. The patient is upset that a drug with such side effects was suggested. Wasn't the doctor aware? The physician knew what the side effects were, but believed their occurrence so unlikely that they were of no consequence. Further, the doctor is upset that the patient was not trusting. Trust is not the issue (at least not the entire issue); a fact is a fact—as true for the patient, it would seem, as for the doctor. With the doctor as an individual of trained judgment left out of the picture, a fact *is* a fact. Another fact is that no piece of knowledge floats free. All are connected to other facts and to underlying beliefs and all are applied only on the basis of individual judgment. Individual physicians may argue that they do not believe that *they* are insignificant and that only medical science does the work. Individual doctors may not hold such beliefs, but the system of medical education of the last several decades is clearly based on that belief. That is the basis of the current practice whereby the intern serves as the patient's doctor and attending physicians are excluded from writing orders on their own patients. Science, this practice implies, makes all of us equal before the mysteries of disease, and technology is the great therapeutic equalizer. Those who know best what nonsense this is and who pay the heaviest price for it are, of course, the patients and, to a lesser extent, the interns (5). If it were not believed that the scientific facts about disease do the work, physicians would be manifestly trained about how to be doctors, how to make judgments, how to use their own individuality as part of their medical skills. If the doctor and not medical science is the agent of cure, why have physicians not been trained in that belief? Only in the past few years has systematic attention been given to such training (6)(7).

Social Turmoil and the Change in the Concept of Person

It does not seem reasonable that simply owning a piece of knowledge would embolden patients in its use. Something has happened to displace physicians from their previous preeminent status, something powerful enough to allow patients to commonly express the belief that "doctors aren't gods" (8). In fact, the fall of doctors from absolute authority on matters of health occurred at a time when all authority found itself challenged. So much confusion attended the changes of the 1960s that it will require decades for historians to sort it all out. The anti-Vietnam War movement muddles the issue, because that makes it possible to view the period as primarily concerned with the war. However, at the same time, the authority of the Catholic Church was crumbling, German students were on the barricades, and the French were in turmoil. These aspects of the social disturbances of the times cannot be blamed on the Vietnam War. It would seem (in retrospect) that a new wave of individualism was breaking over the Western world—most marked and most advanced in the United States. The old political individualism of the United States found itself being succeeded not merely by the individualism of effort considered such a national trait but rather by a personalized—me, myself, and I—individualism that stressed differences and newly discovered the importance of the interior of the person. Have individuals in any culture ever revealed so much of their private lives? There is some irony if we consider that physicians were the bastion of individualism from the 1930s through the 1950s, when American society was dealing with the problem of anomie created by advancing industrialization [see Chaplin's *Modern Times*] and the growth of the modern corporation. And then, when individualism was again becoming a vital force in the culture, physicians became almost faceless.

Changes in the Doctor-Patient Relationship

During the last thirty years the belief that "doctor knows best" has virtually disappeared. From being seen as effectively passive in relation to the physician (except that patients have always been expected to be active in the sense of "fighting to get well"), patients currently frequently believe themselves to be active partners in their care. They want to take part in decisions formerly reserved for the doctor; they demand choice in therapy and have high expectations as to outcome. These expectations have been nourished by the media and the exploitation of medical achievements by medicine itself in its quest for public support.

The force of these changes can be demonstrated by examining the change in treatment of cancer of the breast. The radical mastectomy of Halsted remained the treatment of choice from the early part of this century until this last decade. When I entered practice in 1961 it would not have been uncommon to tell a patient who had awakened after surgery for a mass in the breast that "We had to remove the breast because there were some suspicious cells." The patient would not be informed that she had carcinoma of the breast. Telling patients the truth about their malignancies was considered bad for them—a potential cause of severe depression or suicide. It is essential to realize that these deceptions were not something "done to" unsuspecting patients. McIntosh has documented the attitude of patients and doctors in this regard in Great Britain, where ideas about truth-telling lag behind the United States. There, doctors do not believe patients should be told the painful truth, and neither do patients (who generally know the truth nonetheless) (9). To understand how both physicians and patients have changed, it should be remembered that thirty years ago personal sufferings, unhappiness, and even doubts were largely kept private, whereas presently such matters are much more likely to be ventilated. Doctors were not believed to be interested in patients' personal problems (except out of mere kindness), confining themselves to the "medical" aspects of a case—that is, the physical. In the United States, it is now virtually impossible to conceal the diagnosis of malignancy under euphemisms such as "suspicious cells." A doctor who does not understand this or is insensitive to the unhappiness of his or her patients is now considered merely a technician. Many women have definite ideas about proper treatment for breast cancer and, further, they may feel that the surgeon is as much their enemy as the tumor. I believe these beliefs have forced surgeons away from the Halsted radical mastectomy as much or more than developing scientific evidence that followed the changing attitude of patients. Changes in patients' attitudes are manifest throughout the range of medical services and are matched by the rise of commercialism, free-standing for-profit emergency care centers, advertising, medical marketing, and other evidences of the demystification of physicians and medicine.

The Concurrent Rise of Interest in Medical Ethics

In 1966, Henry Beecher demonstrated the failure of investigators to protect the interests of their research subjects in several major projects (10). His work is frequently cited as a landmark denoting the start of the present interest in bioethics. Catholic ethicists had always addressed specifically Catholic concerns in medical care, and theologian Joseph Fletcher published a work in the 1950s discussing ethical issues in medicine, but not until Beecher's paper did concern become widespread. In 1966, for the first time, prior review for protection of human subjects was required of all United States Public Health Service grants. In 1969, The Institute of Society, Ethics, and the Life Sciences (The Hastings Center) was formed specifically to address moral problems raised by biomedical advances. In 1973, the Department of Health, Education and Welfare (now the Department of Human Services) published its first set of proposed regulations on the protection of human subjects. In 1974, investigators were presented with final regulations that specifically discussed the nature and duties of institutional review boards. In 1981, the requirement was widened so that all institutions receiving federal research monies had to establish institutional review boards to ensure the inclusion of ethical standards in research. Concern for the rights of research subjects and patients has become an established fact of medical life.

Central to any moral understanding is the concept of person. Ethical standards; rules about good and bad, right and wrong; rights and their corollary obligations; matters of custom and conscience that guide the moral aspects of life are always in terms of persons (even though they may be directed toward nonhuman matters, such as animals or the environment). It follows that all understandings of the moral and morality are based on some idea of the nature of persons, whether manifest or latent. In the United States, the individual most often embodied by the bioethics movement is free-standing and autonomous, with freedom and independence the highest values. The impact of this picture of persons on medicine and its distance from older American concepts (still embodied in Europe) can be found in a paper by Pedro Lain-Entralgo on the subject of the good patient, and the commentary on that paper by Childress. For Lain-Entralgo, just as the physician has obligations to the patient, the patient has obligations to the physician and to the work of getting better. Both are embedded in a social matrix, and their obligations stem not only from themselves, but from the fact of their relationship and its ineluctably social character (11). For Childress, who represents a stance much more common among American writers on bioethics, the disease, the doctor, the relationship with the doctor, and the social setting pall in importance next to the patient's rights as an autonomous being. Freedom and self-determination represent values more important than recovery from illness (12).

Clearly, autonomy is threatened by sickness. Most physicians believe that the patient's independence and freedom of choice are removed by the effects of disease—by the uncertainties and impediments to understanding and action that inevitably accompany serious illness. In fact, helping patients regain autonomy would seem to be a prime function of medicine (13). Often, in the current scene, physicians are perceived to threaten the patient's autonomy—they are seen as paternalistic, authoritarian, and too concerned with profit to be reliable servants or partners in care. In the same manner, modern drugs are often viewed with the suspicion that their side effects are more prominent than their benefits. During their convalescence from serious infection, for example, patients may attribute their fatigue to the effects of the antibiotics rather than to the illness from which they are recovering.

There is some evidence that a single-minded concern with autonomy is beginning to pass from the bioethics scene (14). Ethicists are focusing more on the relationship between doctor and patient as a relationship, and broadening their interests to include understandings of not only rights but corollary obligations as well (15). The study of ethics in medicine is maturing and becoming more concerned with moral problems in medicine than with moral philosophy *per se* (16). Richard Zaner's work stands well ahead in this regard (17). Stephen Toulmin has made it clear that the relationship between philosophy and medicine has been two-sided, that philosophy has benefited greatly from the infusion of real-world problems and the sense of urgency that always attends issues in clinical medicine (18).

From faint whisperings in the late 1950s, gathering strength in the 1960s, and emerging in force in the 1970s, bioethics has become an established presence in medicine. Very few American medical schools are without some program in ethics, institutional review boards are an accepted feature of the research scene, and both patients and physicians are very conscious of patients' rights to refuse treatment, of the need for informed consent, and, increasingly, the importance of patients' participation in their own care. These changes have occurred with the expansion of the notion of person to include as matters of public concern interior sources of happiness, suffering, achievement, and even illness—all previously held to be private—and the rise of a radical individualism as a political force.

Commercial Contradictions

Space permits only brief mention of the commercialism that has arisen over the same period during which the importance of the personal has permeated medicine. Both the shift to primarily monetary values and the phenomenal increase in malpractice suits and the size of their awards are having profound effects on medicine. It is almost as if patients are asking for a medicine that is at once intensively directed at their personal needs, desires, beliefs, concerns, and fears, employs the most up-to-date technological advances, while being inexpensive and sufficiently uniform so that fixed pricing for services makes sense.

These are mutually incompatible goals because a medicine intensively directed toward patients' personal goals is time consuming—thus expensive—and unavoidably nonuniform because of individual differences between patients. It may well be that the breakdown in authority and tradition that heralded the new directions of individualism also signaled other ruptures with the medical traditions that have held commercialism at bay during this century.

The Return to Ideals

The history of the last fifty years suggests the strong beginnings of change. The great physicians of the 1920s contained within themselves older humanitarian ideals of their profession as they reached toward science to provide a solid intellectual basis for medicine. In the course of what followed, the importance of the individual physician as an individual lost its warrant as science seemed to provide equality to all in the quest for nature's secrets and in the treatment of disease. Science became dominant in medicine and provided the basis for the values embodied in medical schools. In concert with surrounding society, however, the importance of the individual person and ethical issues has grown in medicine over the last decade. Once again the qualities of the individual physician have assumed importance, but they are now ineluctably married to science and technology.

Medicine is fundamentally a moral enterprise because it is devoted to the welfare of the persons it treats. Medicine is also primarily therapeutic, a matter of helping those who cannot help themselves and who are thereby critically vulnerable. Because of this, it is not at its roots a system of knowledge except as that knowledge advances therapy. Science and morality are not opposed—they are joined in medicine. Science cannot be the dominant force in medicine because it is in the service of something larger than itself. Science, properly understood, must be conceived as being as fully responsive to human needs as possible. Caring for the sick cannot be done without the kind of controlled rigorous research and disciplined thinking that science brings to its understanding of nature. A systematic basis for a return to ideals of physicianship in medicine, on the other hand, cannot be created without a deeper understanding of the goals of medicine. It is a knowledge of the nature of suffering and the full implications of what is required for its relief—what kind of understanding of the human condition, what new theory in medicine, what kind of training of physicians—that can lead us there.

References

1. Zaner, Richard. *Ethics and the Clinical Encounter.* 1988. Englewood Cliffs, N.J., Prentice-Hall, p. 138.

2. Feinstein, Alvin R. An Additional Basic Science for Clinical Medicine: III. The Challenges of Comparison and Measurement. *Ann. Intern. Med.* 1983; 99:705–12.

3. McDermott, Walsh. Evaluating the Physician and His Technology. *J. Amer. Acad. Arts and Sci. (Daedalus)* 1977; 106:135–57.

4. Starr, Paul. *The Social Transformation of American Medicine.* 1982. New York, Basic Books, p. 338ff.

5. Cassell, E. J. Conflict Between Attending Physicians and House Officers: Theory Verus Practice in Medicine. *Bulletin of the New York Academy of Medicine.* Vol. 60, No. 3, pp. 297–308, April 1984.

6. Cassell, Eric. *Talking to Patients.* Volume II. Clinical Technique. 1985. Cambridge, Mass., MIT Press, Introduction.

7. Lipkin, M., Jr., Quill, T. E., and Napodano, R. J. The Medical Interview: A Core Curriculum for Residencies in Internal Medicine. *Ann. Intern. Med.* 1984; 100:277–84.

8. Mechanic, David. The Public Perception of Medicine. *NEJM* 1985; 312:181–83.

9. McIntosh, Jim. *Communication and Awareness on a Cancer Ward.* 1977. New York, Prodist.

10. Beecher, Henry. *NEJM* 1966; 274:1354–60.

11. Lain-Entralgo, Pedro. What Does the Word *Good* Mean in *Good Patient?* In *Changing Values in Medicine.* Ed. Cassell, Eric J. and Siegler, Mark. 1985. Washington, D.C., University Publications of America.

12. Childress, James. Rights and Responsibilities of Patients. In *Changing Values in Medicine. Op. cit.*

13. Cassell, Eric. The Function of Medicine. *Hastings Center Reports* 1977; 7:16–19.

14. Gaylin, Willard. Introduction to Autonomy-Paternalism-Community: A Symposium. *Hastings Center Report* 1984; 14:5.

15. May, William. *The Physician's Covenant.* 1983. Philadelphia, The Westminster Press.

16. Jonsen, Albert R., Siegler, Mark, and Winslade, William J. *Clinical Ethics.* 1982. New York, Macmillan.

17. Zaner, Richard. *Ethics and the Clinical Encounter.* 1988. Englewood Cliffs, N.J., Prentice-Hall.

18. Toulmin, Stephen. How Medicine Saved the Life of Philosophy. *Perspectives in Biology and Medicine* 1982; 24:736–50.

3

The Nature of Suffering

THE OBLIGATION OF physicians to relieve human suffering stretches back into antiquity. Despite this fact, little attention is explicitly given to the problem of suffering in medical education, research, or practice. I will begin by focusing on a modern paradox: that even in the best settings and with the best physicians it is not uncommon for suffering to occur not only during the course of a disease but as a result of its treatment. To understand this paradox and its solution requires an understanding of what suffering is and how it relates to medical care.

Consider this case (occurring a number of years ago): A thirty-five-year-old sculptor with cancer of the breast that had spread widely was treated by competent physicians employing advanced knowledge and technology and acting out of kindness and true concern. At every stage, the treatment as well as the disease was a source of suffering to her. She was frightened and uncertain about her future but could get little information from her physicians, and what she was told was not always the truth. She was unaware, for example, that the radiation therapy to the breast (in lieu of a mastectomy) would be so disfiguring. After her ovaries were removed and a regimen of medications that were masculinizing, she became obese, grew facial and body hair of a male type, and her libido disappeared. When tumor invaded the nerves near her shoulder, she lost strength in the hand she used in sculpting and became profoundly depressed. At one time she had watery diarrhea that would occur unexpectedly and often cause incontinence, sometimes when visitors were present. She could not get her physicians to give her medication to stop the diarrhea because they were afraid of possible disease-related side effects (although she was not told the reason). She had a pathologic fracture of her thigh resulting from an area of cancer in the bone. Treatment was delayed while her physicians openly disagreed about pinning her hip. The view that it was wrong to operate on someone with such a poor prognosis prevailed. She remained in traction but her severe pain could not be relieved. She changed hospitals and physicians and the fracture was repaired. Because of the extent of metastatic disease in the unrepaired leg, she was advised not to bear weight on it for fear that it might also break—a possibility that haunted her.

She had come to believe that it was her desire to live that would end each remission, because every time that her cancer would respond to treatment and her hope rekindle, a new manifestation would appear. Thus, when a new course of chemotherapy was started, she was torn between her desire to live and her fear that allowing hope to emerge again would merely expose her to misery if the treatment failed. The nausea and vomiting of the chemotherapy were distressing, but no more so than the anticipation of hair loss (but the hair loss itself was not as distressing as she had thought and she never wore the wig that had been made in advance). In common with most patients with similar illnesses, she was constantly tortured by fears of what tomorrow would bring. Each tomorrow was seen as worse than today, as heralding increased sickness, pain, or disability—never as the beginning of better times. Despite the distress caused by such thoughts, she could not think otherwise. She felt isolated because she was not like other people and could not do what other people did. She feared that her friends would stop visiting her. She was sure she would die.

This young woman had severe pain and other physical symptoms that caused her suffering. But she also suffered from threats that were social and others that were personal and private. She suffered from the effects of the disease and its treatment on her appearance and her abilities. She also suffered unremittingly from her perception of the future.

What can this case tell us about the ends of medicine and the relief of suffering? Three facts stand out: The first is that this woman's suffering was not confined to physical symptoms. The second is that she suffered not only from her disease but also from its treatment. The third fact is that one could not anticipate what she would describe as a source of suffering; like other patients, she had to be asked. Some features of her condition she would call painful, upsetting, uncomfortable, distressing, but not a source of suffering. In these characteristics her case is ordinary. When I asked sick patients whether they were suffering, they were often quizzical—not sure what I meant. One patient, who said he was not suffering, had metastatic cancer of the stomach from which he knew he would shortly die. On the other hand, a woman who felt her suffering bitterly was waiting in the hospital for her blood count to return to normal after it had been long depressed by chemotherapy. Aside from some weakness, she was otherwise well and would remain so. Another patient, someone who had been operated on for a minor problem, in little pain and not seemingly distressed, said that even coming into the hospital had been a source of suffering. When I discussed the problem of suffering with laypersons, I learned that they were shocked to discover that it was not directly addressed in medical education. My colleagues of a contemplative nature were surprised at how little they knew about the problem and how little thought they had given it, whereas medical students were not sure of the relevance of the issue of suffering to their work.

The relief of suffering, it would appear, is considered one of the primary ends of medicine by patients and the general public, but not by the medical profession, judging by medical education and the responses of students and colleagues. As in the care of the dying, patients and their friends and families do not divide up suffering into its physical and nonphysical sources the way doctors do, who are primarily concerned with the physical (1). A search of the medical and social science literature did not help in understanding what suffering is; the word "suffering" was most often coupled with the word "pain" as in "pain and suffering." (The sources used were *Psychological Abstracts,* the *Citation Index,* and the *Index Medicus.*)

While pain and suffering are not synonymous, physical pain remains a major cause of human suffering and is the primary image formed by people when they think about suffering. However, no one disputes that pain is only one among many sources of human suffering. With the notable exception of the work of David Bakan (2), the medical literature did not bring me closer to understanding medicine's relationship to suffering because the topic is rarely discussed. Indeed, a recent issue of *The Journal of Medicine and Philosophy* subtitled "Suffering, Empathy, and Compassion" hardly mentions the issue of suffering at all except in an opening "editorial fragment" that takes philosophy to task for not addressing suffering (3).

In their fight against scourges such as cancer and heart disease (and in former times the infectious plagues), doctors and their patients share a common goal and dedication to eliminating the causes of suffering. In view of the long history of medicine's concern with the relief of sources of suffering, it is paradoxical that patients often suffer from their treatment as well as their disease. The answer seems to lie in a historically constrained and presently inadequate view of the ends of medicine. Medicine's traditional concern primarily for the body and for physical disease is well known. In addition, the widespread effects of the mind-body dichotomy on medical theory and practice are also known. Indeed, I hope to show that the dichotomy itself is one of the sources of the paradox of doctors causing suffering in their attempts to relieve it.

Today, as ideas about the separation of mind and body are changing, physicians are concerning themselves with new aspects of the human condition. One critic, Illich, complains of an overbearing medicalization of humanity (4). For him, any concern of the medical profession that does not have to do with the body enters the domain of the spiritual. While many may share his concern, the fact remains that the profession of medicine is being pushed and pulled into new areas (sometimes contradictorily) both by its technology and by the demands of its patients. Attempting to understand what suffering is and how physicians might truly be devoted to its relief will require that medicine and its critics overcome the traditional dichotomy between mind and body, subjective and objective, and person and object.

The remainder of this chapter will be devoted to three points. The first is that suffering is experienced by persons. In the separation between mind and body, the concept of person, or personhood, has been associated with mind, spirit, and the subjective. However, as I will show, person is not merely mind, merely spiritual, nor only subjectively knowable. Person has many facets, and it is ignorance of them that actively contributes to patients' suffering. The understanding of the place of person in human illness requires a rejection of the historical dualism of mind and body.

The second point derives from my interpretation of clinical observations: Suffering occurs when an impending destruction of the person is perceived; it continues until the threat of disintegration has passed or until the integrity of the person can be restored in some other manner. It follows, then, that although it often occurs in the presence of acute pain, shortness of breath or other bodily symptoms, suffering extends beyond the physical. Most generally, suffering can be defined as the state of severe distress associated with events that threaten the intactness of person.

The third point is that suffering can occur in relation to any aspect of the person. To demonstrate this, I will present a very simple topography of a person that I think will be useful in understanding both suffering and the relationship between suffering and the goals of medicine.

"Person" Is Not "Mind"

The concept of person is not the same as the concept of mind. The idea of person is not static; it has gradually changed over history. The split between mind and body that has so deeply influenced our intellectual history and our approach to medical care was proposed by Rene Descartes to resolve certain philosophical issues. There is some reason to believe that Descartes' proposal, whatever other origins it may have had, was a successful political solution that allowed science to escape the smothering control of the Church.* However, Descartes lived in a religious era in which one might justly claim that what is non-body is within the spiritual domain. In such eras, which include every social period until the recent past, spiritually derived rules govern virtually every aspect of life. But the general concept of the person has broadened over time, and the spiritual realm has diminished. The decline of the spiritual includes two simultaneous changes: an enlarged belief in a self as a legitimate entity apart from God and a decline in the power of belief. Changes in the meaning of concepts like person occur with changes in society while the words for the concepts remain the same. This fact tends to obscure the depth of the transformations that have occurred in the meaning of person. People simply are "persons" in this time, as in past times, and have difficulty imagining what it might be like to be a person in an earlier period when the concept was more restrictive. For example, the uniquely individual nature of persons is some-

*Richard Zaner argues convincingly that in regard to the mind-body dichotomy, Descartes has been treated unfairly by history—he knew full well that no such separation is possible. (*Ethics and the Clinical Encounter.* 1988. Englewood Cliffs, N.J. Prentice-Hall. p. 106ff.)

thing we take for granted (currently the words "individual" and "person" are often used interchangeably); yet the idea of individuality (in our sense) did not appear in Western tradition until around the twelfth century (5). One can see this best in the face as portrayed in painting and sculpture. In earlier art faces are similar and lack distinguishing characteristics. As the centuries pass, the faces acquire the unmistakable aspect of unique individuals. The facade of the Cathedral of Notre Dame in Paris is a striking illustration, because there the earlier statuary lacks individuality while the later sculptures show individual differences.

Political individualism is fundamental to our national heritage, yet its origins are in the seventeenth century and only in the last century has it come to stand for the unprecedented degree of personal freedom we enjoy. The recent stress on individual differences rather than on political equality is a predictable new direction of self-image. The key word is "self." What the last few decades have witnessed is an enlargement of that aspect of the person called the self. The contemporary identification of self (or self-awareness) and person is a case of mistaken identity, like the confusion of mind for person. In its contemporary usage, my self is one aspect of my person that may be known to me and may even be a condition of personhood. But there are parts of my person that can only be known to others just as there are parts of my self that can only be known to me. Self is that aspect of person concerned primarily with relations with oneself. Other parts of a person involve relations with others and with the surrounding world. Self is only one part of person, included in but not synonymous with personhood (6). Similarly, one cannot divorce the concept of person from the notion of mind, but the two are not interchangeable.

If the mind-body dichotomy underlies the assigning of body to medicine, and person is not in that category, then the only remaining place for person is in the category of mind. Where the mind is problematic (not identifiable in objective terms), its very reality diminishes for science, and so too does that of person. The concept of person then becomes identified with mind, the spiritual, and the subjective, for lack of an alternative place in medicine's objective categories. Therefore, as long as the mind-body dichotomy is accepted, suffering is either subjective and thus not truly "real"—not within medicine's domain—or identified exclusively with bodily pain. Not only is the identification of suffering with bodily pain misleading and distorting, for it depersonalizes the sick patient, but it is itself a source of suffering. Finally, that bodily pain causes personal suffering cannot itself be understood until the dichotomy between mind and body is rejected. It is not possible to treat sickness as something that happens solely to the body without risking damage to the person. An anachronistic division of the human condition into what is medical (having to do with the body) and what is nonmedical (the remainder) has given medicine too narrow a notion of its calling. Because of this division, physicians may, in concentrating on the cure of bodily disease, do things that cause the patient as a person to suffer.

An Impending Destruction of Person

Suffering is ultimately a personal matter—something whose presence and extent can only be known to the sufferer. Patients sometimes report suffering when one does not expect it or do not report suffering when it can be expected. Further, people often say that they know another is suffering greatly, and then ask and find that the other person does not consider himself or herself suffering. Finally, a person can suffer enormously at the distress of another, especially if the other is a loved one. But, as will become clear later, suffering exists, and often can only be understood, in the context of others.

Suffering itself must be distinguished from its uses. In some theologies, especially the Christian, suffering has been seen as presenting the opportunity of bringing the sufferer closer to God. This "function" of suffering is at once its glorification and relief. If, through great pain or deprivation, someone is brought closer to a cherished goal, that person may have no sense of having suffered but, instead, may feel enormous triumph. To an observer, the only thing apparent may be the deprivation. This cautionary note is especially important because people are often said to have suffered greatly, in a religious context, when we know only that they were injured, tortured, or in pain, not whether they suffered.

Although pain and suffering are closely identified in the minds of most people and in the medical literature, they are phenomenologically distinct. The difficulty of understanding pain and the problems of physicians in providing adequate relief are well known (7)(8)(9).

The greater the pain, the more it is believed to cause suffering. However, some pains, like those of childbirth, can be extremely severe and yet considered uplifting. The differences in methods used to control the pain of childbirth in the United States cannot be explained on their efficacy in relieving pain alone. In some hospitals in Denver, at one time, only conduction anesthesia was employed, while at others natural childbirth was the predominant method. During the same period in San Francisco, epidural anesthesia was favored, but in New York City it was almost never used. This issue seemed to be more the woman's desire to exercise control over the process of childbirth than merely to eliminate pain. This explanation is consonant with other recent trends that give women greater say in pregnancy and childbirth. The perceived meaning of pain influences the amount of medication required to control it. For example, a patient reported that she had initially believed that the pain in her leg was sciatica and that she could control it with small doses of codeine, but when she discovered that it was due to the spread of malignant disease, much greater amounts of medication were required for relief. Patients can writhe in pain from kidney stones and not be suffering (by their own statement) because they "know what it is." In contrast, people may report considerable suffering from apparently little pain when they do not know its source.

There are three other times when suffering in close relation to pain is commonly reported: First, when the pain is so severe that it is virtually overwhelming—the pain of a dissecting aortic aneurysm is of that type. The second is when the patient does not believe that the pain can be controlled. The suffering of patients with terminal cancer can often be relieved by demonstrating that their pain truly *can* be controlled. They will then often tolerate the same pain without any medication, preferring the pain to the side effects of their analgesics. Another type of pain that can be a source of suffering is pain that is not overwhelming but continues for a very long time so that it seems that the pain is endless. Physicians commonly tell patients that they will "get used to the pain" but that rarely happens. What patients learn is both how little tolerance other people have for their continued report of pain and how pain becomes less bearable the longer it continues. Patients with recurrent pain even suffer in the absence of their pain, merely anticipating its return as do people with severe frequent migraine headaches who constantly worry whether it will reappear to ruin yet another important occasion.

In sum, people in pain frequently report suffering from pain when they feel out of control, when the pain is overwhelming, when the source of the pain is unknown, when the meaning of the pain is dire, or when the pain is apparently without end.

In these situations, persons perceive pain as a threat to their continued existence—not merely to their lives but their integrity as persons. That this is the relation of pain to suffering is strongly suggested by the fact that suffering can often be relieved *in the presence of continued pain,* by making the source of the pain known, changing its meaning, and demonstrating that it can be controlled and that an end is in sight. These same facts apply to other physical sources of suffering such as shortness of breath.

It follows, then, that suffering has a temporal element. For a situation to be a source of suffering, it must influence the person's perception of future events. "If the pain continues like this, *I will be overwhelmed,*" "If the pain comes from cancer, *I will die,*" "If the pain cannot be controlled, *I will not be able to take it.*" Note that at the moment the individual is saying "If the pain continues like this, I will be overwhelmed" he or she is *not* overwhelmed. At that moment the person is intact. Fear itself always involves the future.

In the case that began this chapter, the patient cannot give up her fears; she cannot relinquish her sense of future, despite the agony they cause her. Because of its temporal nature, suffering can frequently be relieved in the face of continued distress by causing the sufferers to root themselves in the absolute present—"This moment and only this moment." Unfortunately, that is difficult to accomplish. It is noteworthy, however, that some Eastern theologies suggest that desire is the source of human suffering. To end suffering one must give up desire. To give up desire one must surrender the enchantment of the future. As suffering is discussed in the other dimensions of person, note how suffering would not exist in the absence of the future. To move from the body as a source of suffering to suffering that arises from the other dimensions of person, two other aspects of pain that cause suffering should be mentioned. The first is when physicians do not validate the patient's pain. If no disease is found, physicians may suggest that the patient is "imagining" the pain, that it is "psychological" (in the sense that it is not real), or that he or she is "faking." Somewhat similar is that aspect of the suffering of patients with chronic pain who discover that they can no longer talk to others about their distress. In the former case the person comes to distrust his or her perceptions of self, and in both instances the social isolation adds to the person's suffering.

Another aspect essential to understanding suffering is the relation of meaning to the way in which illness is experienced. The word "meaning" is used here in two senses. In the first to mean is to signify. Pain in the chest may imply heart disease. We also say we know what something means when we know how important it is. The importance of things is always personal and individual, even though meaning in this sense may be shared by others or by society as a whole. The significance of something and its importance together constitute the personal meaning of the thing.

"Belief" is another word for that aspect of meaning concerned with implications, and "values" concerns the degree of importance to a particular person. The personal meanings of things do not consist exclusively of values and beliefs that are held intellectually; they include other dimensions. For the same word, event, object, or relationship, a person may simultaneously have a cognitive meaning, an affective or emotional meaning, a bodily meaning, and a transcendant or spiritual meaning (10). And there may be contradictions in the different levels of meaning. For example, in a patient who was receiving chemotherapy, the word chemotherapy could be shown to elicit simultaneously a cognitive meaning that included his beliefs about the cellular mechanism of drug action, the emotion of fear, the body sensation of nausea, and the transcendent feeling that God would protect him. Normally, all those levels of meaning are jumbled, but together they constituted the meaning for that patient of the word chemotherapy (11). The nuances of personal meaning are too complex to be captured in a few sentences, but it should be remembered that when I speak of personal meanings I am implying that complexity in all its depth—known and unknown. Personal meaning enters this discussion because it is a fundamental dimension of person that cannot be divorced from any other; no understanding of human illness or suffering will be possible without taking it into account.

A Simplified Description of the Person

Unlike other objects of science, persons cannot be reduced to their parts in order to better understand them. But a simple topology of person may be useful in understanding the relation between suffering and the goals of medicine. The features identified should also apply to ourselves and thus be confirmable on the basis of our own life experiences. They should also point the way to further study and to the possibility of specific action by individual physicians. Persons have personality and character. All parents know that personality traits appear within the first few weeks to months of life and are remarkably durable over time. Some personalities handle some illnesses better than others. What may be destructive for one person is easily tolerated by another, but some stresses that may accompany illness, such as loss of control, are universally difficult to bear. Individuals vary in character as well as personality. During the heyday of psychoanalysis in the 1950s, all behavior was attributed to unconscious determinants laid down early in life. No one was bad or good; they were merely sick or well. Fortunately, such a simplistic view of human character is passing from popularity. Some people do, in fact, have "stronger" character than others and bear adversity better. Some are good, kind, and tolerant under the stress of terminal illness, while others become mean and strike out when even mildly ill.

A person has a past. Things done and places visited. Accomplishments and failures. The lived past is a story that has taken place over time, in many places, and involving countless others. The experiences gathered during living one's life are a part of today as well as yesterday. Events of the present can be checked against the past, and events of the past contribute to the meanings assigned to present happenings. It would be an error to think that the past is simply memories stored in some old mental filing cabinet. Rather, the constant flow of happenings reinforces some past experiences and dilutes others. Memory exists in the nostrils and the hands as well as in other body parts. A fragrance drifts by and an old memory is evoked. My feet have not forgotten how to roller skate and my hands remember skills I was hardly aware I had learned. When these memories and past experiences involve sickness and medical care, they can influence present illness and medical care. They can stimulate fear or confidence, bodily symptoms, and even anguish. It damages people to rob them of their past, deny the truth of their memories, or mock their fears and worries. A person without a past is incomplete.

Life experiences—previous illness, experiences with doctors, hospitals, medications, deformities and disabilities, pleasures and successes, or miseries and failures—form the background for illness. The personal meaning of the disease and its treatment arise from the past as well as the present. If cancer occurs in a patient with self-confidence resulting from many past achievements, it may give rise to optimism and a resurgence of strength. Even if fatal, the disease may produce not the destruction of the person but rather reaffirm his or her indomitability. The outcome would be different in a person for whom life had been a succession of failures. Some time ago I reviewed an examination meant to test the interpersonal skills of medical students by having them interview an actress playing the part of a patient. The "patient" was a woman who had just discovered a lump in her breast. Her past history is given. Her father died when she was very young and her mother was an alcoholic. The patient's first marriage ended in disaster, leaving her with a brain-damaged child. She has been unable to hold a job. She has finally made a liaison with a man and is about to go off with him when she discovers the breast mass. The students' job is to convince her of the need for surgery. The examination sheet that provides this history ends with, "The patient was very optimistic about her future." That is not true to life—nobody with her history could be optimistic. She "knows" that the mass will be cancer, and it does not matter whether it is or not. Nothing good has ever happened to her, and this tumor is just another piece of her that is rotten. Her suffering, one might postulate, would start before her operation, when she became aware again of how much less whole she is than other people. Like an old wound that aches when it rains, one can suffer again the injuries of yesterday. The lived past provides other occasions for suffering. It may simply be lost, as in the case of amnesia, leaving the person less whole. Or its truth may be denied by the events of today, as in "All my life I believed in . . . , and now, when it is too late to change, it turns out not to be true."

A person has a family. The intensity of family ties cannot be overemphasized; people frequently behave as though they were physical extensions of their parents. Things that might cause suffering in others may be borne without complaint by someone who believes that the disease is part of the family identity and thus inevitable. I remember a man with polycystic kidney disease who was quite proud of his ultimately fatal disease because he was finally "one of them," like his mother and sister. Many diseases where no heritable basis is known are also acceptable to an individual because others in the family have been similarly affliected. What seems to count is the connection of the individual to the family. One of my patients, dying of cancer of the lung, literally shrugged his shoulders over his impending death from the disease that killed his father and two brothers. His children suffered at his bedside. He was fulfilling his destiny while they were losing a father. Just as a person's past experiences give meaning to the present, so do the past experiences of the person's family. They are part of the person.

A person has a cultural background. It is well known that socially determined factors, such as diet, environment, and social behaviors, contribute to disease patterns. Because culture also contributes to beliefs and values, cultural factors play a part in the effects of disease on a person. Culture defines what is meant by masculine or feminine, what clothes are worn, attitudes toward the dying and the sick, mating behavior, the height of chairs and steps, attitudes toward odors and excreta, where typewriters sit and who uses them, bus stops and bedclothes, how the aged and the disabled are treated. These things, mostly invisible to the well, have an enormous impact on the sick and can be a source of untold suffering. They influence the behavior of others toward the sick person and that of the sick toward themselves. Cultural norms and social rules regulate whether someone can be among others or will be isolated, whether the sick will be considered foul or acceptable, and whether they are to be pitied or censured.

Returning to the sculptor described earlier, we know why that young woman suffered. She was housebound and bedbound, her face was changed by steroids, and she was masculinized by her treatment, one breast was twisted and scarred, and she had almost no hair. The degree of importance attached to these losses—that aspect of their personal meaning—is determined to a great degree by cultural priorities.

With this in mind, we can see how someone devoid of physical pain, perhaps even devoid of "symptoms," can suffer. People can suffer from what they have lost of themselves in relation to the world of objects, events, and relationships. Such suffering occurs because our intactness as persons, our coherence and integrity, come not only from intactness of the body but from the wholeness of the web of relationships with self and others. We realize, too, that although medical care can reduce the impact of sickness, inattentive care can increase its disruption.

A person has roles. I am a father, a physician, a teacher, a husband, a brother, an orphaned son, an uncle, and a friend. People are their roles (whatever else they may be), and each role has rules. Together the rules that guide the performance of roles make up a complex set of entitlements and limitations of responsibility and privilege. By middle age the roles may be so firmly set that disease can lead to the virtual destruction of a person by making the performance of his or her roles impossible. Whether it is a doctor who cannot doctor, or a parent who cannot parent, the individual is unquestionably diminished by the loss of function. I am aware that the "sick role" allows patients to be excused from their usual role requirements but, in practice, the concept of the sick role has not been very useful (although it offers some insight into illness behavior). Here, as in each facet of person, the degree of suffering caused by the loss varies from person to person.

There is no self without others, there is no consciousness without a consciousness of others, no speaker without a hearer, no dreamer who does not dream in relation to others, no act or object or thought that does not somehow encompass others. There is no behavior that is not, was not, or will not be involved with others, even if only in memory or reverie. The degree to which human interactions are literally physically synchronized is amazing (12). Take away others, remove sight or hearing, let the ability to synchronize activities be injured, and the person begins to be diminished. Everyone dreads becoming blind or deaf, but these are only the most obvious injuries to human interaction. There is almost no limit to the ways in which humans can be cut off from others and then suffer the loss.

It is in relationships with others that sexuality, giving and receiving love, and expressing happiness, gratitude, anger, and the full range of human emotionality find expression. Therefore, in this dimension of the person illness may injure the ability to express emotion. Furthermore, the extent and nature of a sick person's relationships strongly influence the degree of suffering that a disease may produce. There is a vast difference between going home to an empty apartment or returning to a network of friends and family after hospitalization. Illness may occur in one partner of a long and strongly bound marriage, or it may be the last straw in a union that was falling apart. Suffering caused by the loss of sexual function associated with some diseases depends not only on the importance of sexual performance to the sick person but its importance in his or her relationships. The impact of the relationships a patient has was brought home to me as I sat at the bedside of a dying man who wanted to stop the futile treatments being given for his malignancy. His wife sat stunned after hearing him speak and then screamed, "*Damn you, you're just trying to get out and leave me like you always have.*"

A person has a relationship with himself or herself. Self-esteem, self-approval, self-love (and their opposites) are emotional expressions of the relationship of a self to itself. To behave well in the face of pain or sickness brings gratification just as to behave poorly in these situations may leave lifelong disappointment in its wake. The old-fashioned words honor and cowardice stand for states that are much more with us than their lack of currency would suggest. In our times we have been more concerned with relationships with others than with ourselves (13). Nonetheless, suffering may follow on failing oneself, if the failure is profound enough.

A person is a political being. A person is, in the larger sense of political, equal to other individuals, with rights, obligations, and the ability to redress injury by others and by the state. Sickness can interfere here, producing the feeling of political powerlessness and lack of representation. The recent drive to restore the disabled to parity is notable in this regard. All relationships between people, in addition to whatever else they may be, are relationships of power; of subordinance, dominance, or equipotence. The powerlessness of the sick person's body and the ability of others to control the person by controlling the body are part of the political dimension of illness. The change in the relationship of doctor and patient previously described represents a change in their relative power. However, the fundamental political loss and source of suffering in this dimension of person derives less from the actions of others as from disease itself. In the Book of Job, Job in the extreme of his suffering, which he feels is undeserved, wants to plead his case directly with God. But his bodily affliction and fear have undermined his being—"There is no umpire between us, who might lay his hand upon us both. Let him take his rod away from me, and let not dread of him terrify me. Then I would speak without fear of him, for I am not so in myself" (9:33–35) (14). The actions of others can increase the fears of the sick.

Persons do things. They act, create, make, take apart, put together, wind, unwind, cause to be, and cause to vanish. They know themselves and are known by these acts. More than the requirements of a role, more than is necessary in a relationship, more than they know themselves, and some more (or less) than others, things come out of their mouths, or are done by their hands, feet, or entire bodies that express themselves. When illness makes it impossible for people to do these things, they are not themselves.

Persons are often, to one degree or another, unaware of much that happens to them and why. Thus some things in the mind cannot be brought to awareness by ordinary reflection, memory, or introspection. Where some have behaved, in recent times, as though a person was only a political being, others have acted as if the only important part of a person was solely his or her unconscious mind. The structure of the unconscious is pictured quite differently by different scholars, but most students of human behavior accept that such an interior world exists. People can behave in ways that seem inexplicable and strange even to themselves, and the sense of powerlessness the person may feel in the face of such behavior can be a source of great distress.

Persons have regular behaviors. In health, we take for granted the details of our day-to-day behavior. From the moment of awakening in the morning to the manner of sleep at night, a person's behavior follows a customary pattern. Persons know themselves to be well as much by whether they behave as usual as by any other set of facts. If they cannot do the things they identify with the fact of their being, they are not whole.

Every person has a body. The relation with one's body may vary from identification with it to admiration, loathing, or constant fear. There are some who act as though their body's only purpose was to carry their heads about. The body may even be a representation of one parent, so that when something happens to that person's body it is as though an injury was done to a parent. Into this relationship with the body every illness must fit. Disease can so alter the relationship that the body is no longer seen as a friend but an untrustworthy enemy. This is intensified if the illness occurs without warning so that the person comes to distrust his or her perceptions of the body. As illness deepens, the person may feel increasingly vulnerable or damaged. Much was made a few years back of the concept of body image and the suffering caused by disease-induced alterations of that image. The body does not actually have to be altered to cause damage to the wholeness of the person—damage to the person's relationship with the body is sufficient. Just as many people have recently developed an expanded awareness of self as a result of the changes in their bodies from exercise, so the potential always exists for a contraction of self through injury to the body.

Everyone has a secret life. Sometimes it takes the form of fantasies and dreams of glory, and sometimes it has a real existence known to only a few. Within that secret life are fears and desires, love affairs of the past and present, hopes or fantasies, and ways of solving the problems of everyday life known to only the person. It is proper that they remain secret, because they arise from a discrete part of human existence—a separate, private life that cannot be predicted from what is known of the public person. Modesty is not merely a behavior that hides one from public view; it hides the parts of a person that are none of the public's business. There are cultures where women have their pubic hair removed. It is no surprise that in those societies privacy is not allowed. Disease may not only destroy the public person but the secret person as well. A secret beloved friend may be lost to a sick person because he or she has no legitimate place by the sickbed. When that happens, the sick person may have lost that part of life that made tolerable an otherwise embittered existence. The loss may be of only the dream—the wish or fantasy (however improbable) that one day might have come true. Such loss can be a source of great distress and intensely private pain.

Every person has a perceived future. Events that one expects to come to pass vary from expectations for one's children to a belief in one's creative ability. Intense unhappiness results from a loss of that future—the future of the individual person, of children, and of other loved ones. It is in this dimension of existence that hope dwells. Hope is one of the necessary traits of a successful life. Alisdair MacIntyre's definition is unsurpassed: "Hope is in place precisely in the face of evil that tempts us to despair, and more especially that evil that belongs specifically to our own age and condition. . . . The presupposition of hope is, therefore, belief in a reality that transcends what is available as evidence" (15). No one has ever questioned the suffering that attends the loss of hope.

Everyone has a transcendent dimension—a life of the spirit, however expressed or known. Considering the amount of thought devoted to it through the ages, the common wisdom contains very little about transcendence, which is all the more remarkable given its central place in the relief of suffering. It is most directly dealt with in mysticism and in the mystic traditions both within and outside formal religions. But it seems evident that the frequency with which people have intense feelings of bonding with groups, with ideals, or with anything larger and more enduring than the person—of which patriotism is one example—is evidence of the universality of human transcendence. The quality of being greater and more lasting than an individual life gives this aspect of persons its timeless dimension. However, the profession of medicine appears to ignore the human spirit. When I see patients in nursing homes who seem to go on forever, existing only for their bodily needs, I wonder whether it is not their transcendent dimension that they have lost.

The Nature of Suffering

For purposes of explanation I have outlined various parts that make up a person. However, persons cannot be reduced to their parts so that they can be better understood. Reductionist scientific methods, so successful in other areas of human biology, are not as useful for the comprehension of whole persons. My intent was to suggest the complexity of persons and the potential for injury and suffering that exists in each of us. Consequently, any suggestion of mechanical simplicity should disappear from my definition of suffering. All the aspects of personhood—the lived past, the family's lived past, culture and society, roles, the instrumental dimension, associations and relationships, the body, the unconscious mind, the political being, the secret life, the perceived future, and the transcendent-being dimension—are susceptible to damage and loss.

Injuries may be expressed by sadness, anger, loneliness, depression, grief, unhappiness, melancholy, rage, withdrawal, or yearning. We acknowledge the individual's right to have and give voice to such feelings. But we often forget that the affect is merely the outward expression of the injury, much as speech is of thought, and is not the injury itself. We know much less about the nature of the injuries themselves, and what we know has been learned largely from literature and the other arts, not from medicine.

If the injury is sufficient, the person suffers. The only way to learn whether suffering is present is to ask the sufferer. We all recognize certain injuries that almost invariably cause suffering: the death or suffering of loved ones, powerlessness, helplessness, hopelessness, torture, the loss of a life's work, deep betrayal, physical agony, isolation, homelessness, memory failure, and unremitting fear. Each is both universal and individual. Each touches features common to us all, yet each contains features that must be defined in terms of a specific person at a specific time. With the relief of suffering in mind, however, reflect on how remarkably little is known of these injuries.

The Melioration of Suffering

One might ask why everybody is not suffering all the time. In a busy life, almost no day goes by that a little chip is not knocked off one or another of the parts of a person. Obviously, one does not suffer merely at the loss of a piece of oneself but instead when intactness cannot be maintained or restored. Yet I suspect more suffering exists than is known. Just as people with chronic pain learn to keep it to themselves because others lose interest, so may those with chronic suffering.

There is another reason why each injury—even large assaults—may not cause suffering. Persons are able to enlarge themselves in response to damage, so that rather than being reduced by injury, they may indeed grow. This response to suffering has led to the belief that suffering is good for people. To some degree, and in some individuals, this may be so. We would not have such a belief, however, were it not equally common knowledge that persons can also be destroyed by suffering. If the leg is injured so that the athlete can never run again, the athlete may compensate by learning another sport, or skill, or mode of expression. And so it is with the loss of relationships, loves, roles, physical strength, dreams, and power. The human body may not have the capacity to grow another part when one is lost, but the person has.

The ability to recover from loss without succumbing to suffering is sometimes called resiliency, as though merely elastic rebound is involved. But it seems more as if an inner force is withdrawn from one manifestation of person and redirected to another. If a child dies and the parent makes a successful recovery, the person is said to have "rebuilt" his or her life. The verb suggests, correctly I think, that the parts of the person are assembled in a new manner allowing renewed expression in different dimensions. If a previously active person is confined to a wheelchair, intellectual or artistic pursuits may occupy more time and energy. Total involvement in some political or social goal may use the energy previously given to physical activity. We see an aged scholar, for whom all activity is restricted by disease and infirmity, continue to pursue the goals of a lifetime of study and we marvel at the strength of "the life of the mind."

Recovery from suffering often involves borrowing the strength of others as though persons who have lost parts of themselves can be sustained by the personhood of others until their own recovers. This is one of the latent functions of physicians: lending strength. A group, too, may lend strength: Consider the success of groups of the similarly afflicted in easing the burden of illness (e.g., women who have had a mastectomy, people with ostomies, fellow sufferers from a rare sickness, or even the parents or family members of the diseased).

Meaning and transcendence offer two additional ways by which the destruction of a part of personhood or threat to its integrity are meliorated. The search for the meaning of human suffering has occupied humanity on an individual and cultural level throughout history. Assigning meaning to the injurious condition often reduces or even resolves the suffering associated with it. Most often a cause for the injury is sought within past behaviors or beliefs. Thus, the pain or threat that causes suffering is seen as not destroying a part of the person because *it is* part of the person by virtue of its origin within the self. The concept of Karma, in Eastern theologies, is a complex form of that defense against suffering, because suffering is seen to result from behaviors of the individual in previous incarnations. In our culture, taking the blame for harm that comes to oneself because of the unconscious mind reduces suffering by locating it within a coherent set of meanings. Physicians are familiar with the question: "Did I do something to make this happen?" A striking example of this mechanism is when a woman takes the blame for rape, as though she had done something to invite it. It is more tolerable for a terrible thing to happen because of something one has done—and even suffer the guilt—than that it be simply a stroke of fate; a random, chance event. Like Job's friends warding off the possibility of an unjust God, others around the victim often encourage self-blame.

Transcendence is probably the most powerful way in which one is restored to wholeness after an injury to personhood. When experienced, transcendence locates the person in a far larger landscape. The sufferer is not isolated by pain but is brought closer to a transpersonal source of meaning and to the human community that shares that meaning. Such an experience need not involve religion in any formal sense; however, in its transpersonal dimension it is deeply spiritual.

In Judaism, as in virtually all theologies, the issue of suffering is central. The book of Job presents the perplexing puzzle of humankind; not only do the righteous suffer, but the best may suffer the worst fate. Other biblical passages suggest that personal suffering offers a means for self-transcendence and a concern for the suffering of others. Acting virtuously necessarily entails suffering. As Rabbi Jack Bemporad has said, "In standing for justice and righteousness the righteous and the Godly suffer, as did God's obedient servants, the prophets. . . . This is the dilemma of the prophet—obedience brings suffering instead of joy" (16). But transcendence brings relief to the pain and deprivation—to the suffering itself—by giving it a meaning larger than the person.

Pain or loss offers the Christian the chance, through suffering, to identify with the suffering of Christ. On the cover of a magazine article about Christian retirement homes can be read "The best motivation for providing loving care is knowing Christians don't die; they merely pass from human care to God's care." But if there were no Christ with whom to bond, no God to give the suffering meaning, would the agony then be uplifting? I think not. Christian suffering (in this sense) is not suffering precisely because of the occasion for transcendence it offers. Patriotism is a secular example of transcendence as a means for relieving personal agony, as in Nathan Hale's last words, "I only regret that I have but one life to lose for my country."

When Suffering Continues

But what happens when suffering is not relieved? If suffering occurs when there is a threat to the integrity of the person or a loss of a part of the person, then suffering will continue if the person cannot be made whole again. Little is known about this aspect of suffering. Is much of what we call depression merely unrelieved suffering? Considering that depression commonly follows the loss of loved ones, business reversals, prolonged illness, profound injuries to self-esteem, and other damages to person, the possibility is real. In many chronic or serious diseases, persons who "recover" or who are seemingly successfully treated do not return to normal function. Despite a physical cure, they may never again be employed, recover sexual function, pursue career goals, re-establish family relationships, or re-enter the social world. Such patients may not have recovered from the nonphysical changes that occur with life-threatening illness. Consider the dimensions of person described above and it is difficult to think of one that is not threatened or damaged in profound illness. It should come as no surprise to discover that chronic suffering frequently follows in the wake of disease.

The paradox with which this chapter began—that suffering is often caused by the treatment of the sick—no longer seems puzzling. How could it be otherwise, when medicine has concerned itself so little with the nature and causes of suffering? This lack is not a failure of good intentions. None are more concerned about the relief of pain or the restoration of lost function than physicians. Instead, it is a failure of knowledge and understanding. We lack knowledge because, in working within the constraints of a dichotomy contrived in a historical context far removed from our own, we have artificially circumscribed our task in caring for the sick.

Problems of staggering complexity arise when we attempt to understand all the known dimensions of person and their relationship to illness and suffering. These problems are no greater than those initially posed in trying to find out how the body worked. The difficulty is not how to finish solving the problems—it's how to start. But if the ends of medicine are once again to be directed toward the relief of human suffering, the need is clear.

References

1. Cassell, Eric J. Being and Becoming Dead. *Social Research* (August) 1972, 39:528–542.

2. Bakan, David. *Disease, Pain, and Sacrifice.* 1968. Boston, Beacon Press.

3. Natanson, Maurice, Ed. Suffering, Empathy, and Compassion. *The Journal of Medicine and Philosophy.* (February) 1981; Vol. 6, No. 1.

4. Illich, Ivan. *Medical Nemesis: The Expropriation of Health.* 1976. New York, Bantam Books.

5. Morris, Colin. *The Discovery of the Individual.* 1973. New York, Harper Torchbook.

6. Zaner, Richard. *The Context of Self.* 1981. Athens, Ohio University Press.

7. Marks, Richard, and Sacher, Edwin. Undertreatment of Medical Patients. *Ann. Intern. Med.* 1973; 78:173–81.

8. Kammer, Ron M., and Foley, Kathleen M. Patterns of Narcotic Drug Use in Canada. *Annals of New York Academy of Science* 1981; 362:161–72.

9. Goodwin, J. S. et al. *Ann. Intern. Med.* 1979; 91:106–10.

10. Cassell, Eric J. *Talking with Patients: Volume I. The Theory of Doctor-Patient Communication.* 1985. Cambridge, MIT Press, Chap. 5.

11. Ibid., p. 179ff.

12. Condon, W. S., and Ogston, W. D. *J. Psychiat. Res.* 1967; 5:221.

13. Storr, Anthony. *A Return to the Self.* 1988. New York, Ballantine Books.

14. Bemporad, Jack. Job. In *A Modern Jew in Search of a Soul.* Edited by Spiegelman, J. Marvin and Jacobson, Abraham. 1986. Phoenix, Arizona, Falcon Press.

15. MacIntyre, Alisdair. Seven Traits for Designing Our Descendants. *The Hastings Center Report* 1979; 9:5–7.

16. Bemporad, Jack. *Op. cit.*

4

Suffering in Chronic Illness

SUFFERING THAT OCCURS during acute illness seems to arise largely from sources external to the person—from the injury or the disease. This appears true to those who suffer, even though the factors that convert even severe pain into suffering depend on the particular nature of the individual, and although painful sensations may arise from deep inside the body. Thus, if suffering results from the pain of cancer, both the pain and the cancer are not considered part of the suffering person. The cancer is a "thing" that afflicts the patient and the pain arises from that distinct alien thing. In fact, the cancer is not so easily separable from the tissues of the patient, and the factors that have promoted its growth are part of the patient's physiology. Similarly, the pain is the pain it is and the suffering takes the form it does in part because of the contribution of meanings of the patient. Same disease, different patient—different illness, pain, and suffering.

Examination of suffering in chronic illness extends our understanding of this phenomenon. When suffering occurs in the course of acute disease, medical understandings of the body and categories of disease seem adequate to explain why the threat to the integrity of person exists. This is not so in chronic illness. Here, disease theory or even organ or molecular pathophysiology are inadequate to predict suffering or provide a basis for its relief. Worse, these mainstays of medical thinking are a source of confusion when considering suffering in chronic illness. Long-standing or constant sources of distress are not only symptoms in themselves but become part of the chain of causation responsible for the illness. Further, in acute illness the threat is perceived as distinct and limited, whereas in chronic illness the threat is ongoing, long-lasting, global (encompassing all aspects of the person's life), and incapable of direct resolution. Suffering in chronic illness may also arise because the integrity of the person is threatened by internally generated dissension between different aspects of the patient, despite the continuing perception that the threat is external. For example, a destructive conflict may occur between other parts of the person and the body and its needs, or between the social demands of everyday existence and the private needs of the individual.

Chronic Illness Defined

Chronic illness and chronic disease are distinct from one another. Diseases, for our discussion, are specific entities characterized by disturbances in structure or function of any part, organ, or system of the body. Illnesses, on the other hand, afflict whole persons and are the set of disordered functions, body sensations, and feelings by which persons know themselves to be unwell. Diseases should be understood as category names that include only one in the series of events that is chronic illness. Disease, as defined by scientific medicine, is that dimension of the process that takes place within parts of the body (whether organs or molecules). While diseases, as they have been conceived of classically, are confined to the body and its parts, the illness of one person may be accompanied by disorder in that person's extended system—for example, associates, the family, or even the community.

It does not follow that if a chronic disease is present so too is chronic illness, or vice versa. Thus, diabetes, hypertension, hyperlipedemia, or osteoarthritis are chronic: however, persons who have these diseases often do not perceive themselves as ill. When persons *do* know themselves to be ill, the degree to which they believe themselves disabled or disordered is often poorly predicted by knowledge of their disease. There are instances when the severity of illness *can* often be surmised from knowledge of the disease, as in active rheumatoid arthritis where joint swelling and inflammation are inevitably accompanied by pain or active ulcerative colitis where diarrhea is always present. But whether the person with these afflictions is also suffering is more difficult to predict.

The inadequacy of scientific understandings of disease in explaining suffering in chronic illness (or explaining chronic illness itself) is seen from the occurrence of chronic illness in the absence of disease. For example, persons who have had paralytic poliomyelitis may still consider themselves to have a debilitating illness years after the disease, acute poliomyelitis, has disappeared. Some may develop a new illness years later as a consequence of their initial paralyzing episode of disease. A recent article in *The New York Times Magazine* cited the opinion of some physicians who held that these symptoms arose from the continued presence of the disease. Other doctors believed that the patients were not plagued by a continuing disease but rather by the accumulating difficulties associated with years of impaired function. The first idea—that the disease is still present—is an attempt to contain the problem within disease thinking. Persons with congenital deformities may also develop chronic illness in their adult years when, again, no disease is present. A more common example is the suffering that may arise from obesity or other eating disorders, in the absence of disease.

A final example is a state called the chronic pain syndrome. Here persons may be disabled by pain in the absence of any disease that would account for the symptoms. A man in his late fifties has done heavy labor in steel mills all his working life. From time to time his back may have been strained or injured, but it always got better and he continued working. As the years went on, his back became increasingly painful. It is now stiff and hurts when he awakens. With a few aspirins and the heat of the mill, the pain eases early in the day, only to return as the day wears on. Finally, it is too painful for him to work. He goes to physicians who assure him that there is nothing wrong: "It's only muscular." The condition does not really improve and he goes on disability. Repeated X rays and tests demonstrate no disease. If his doctors are experienced enough, they help him get his disability payments despite the absence of objectively confirmable disease criteria. (See the discussion in Chapter 7.) If not, they continue to deny the existence of any objective basis for his complaints. His behavior at home and in the outer world begins to organize itself around his pain until he has been transformed in all dimensions of his existence from a productive member of society to an invalid.

This example should make it clear that the absence of disease does not mean the absence of abnormalities, disturbances, or alterations in body functions. In the steel worker, the worn-out back no longer functions normally, and soon neither does the rest of him. If the illness started in some other level of human existence—within the person or socially—there would soon be abnormality or alteration in body functioning. We are all of a piece. If one part of us is altered in its function, so too will other parts be changed. In each instance cited, there is either some abnormality of performance in relation to everyday life and function or a deformity compared to the person's or the culture's ideal. The deformity does not have to be outwardly apparent or important; it is both in the eyes of the deformed.

It might be said that I have raised a false issue in arguing that classical understanding of disease does not help us solve the problem of suffering in chronic disease. It is true that in recent years physicians have increasingly abandoned classical disease theory in favor of a pathophysiological basis for medical practice. Pathophysiology emphasizes the dynamic nature of the normal and abnormal workings of the body. Unfortunately, as it is studied and taught, it starts at the molecular level of human malfunction and proceeds to the organ level. It does not go far enough to be a science of chronic illness. The dimensions of chronic illness extend to virtually all levels of human existence from the molecular to the social.

Symptoms as Causes in Chronic Illness

At the risk of being repetitive, it is important to remember, in thinking about the self-sustaining nature of chronic illness, that the illness involves all aspects of the person, not merely the body. The symptoms and abnormal functioning in chronic illness lead inevitably to compensatory abnormalities of function or behavior. These counteractive mechanisms then become active parts of the illness. One group of compensatory mechanisms serves the purpose of avoiding unpleasant symptoms. For example, simple guarding of a joint to avoid pain reduces the activity of the joint, which leads to increasing involuntary immobility (and increased pain when it is moved)—the origin of the common condition called frozen shoulder. Similarly, simple reduction in physical activity begins to reduce effective muscle mass, which, in turn, makes physical activity more difficult. On another level, the sick person may develop reclusive behaviors that further exaggerate the social loss when symptoms such as abnormalities of speech, gait, or physical appearance make social intercourse painful. On occasion the sick person may unintentionally exaggerate some symptom—such as a speech defect—to have an excuse to avoid social relations.

Other compensatory mechanisms serve the function of attempting to maintain normalcy. One such group consists of the so-called overuse syndromes, where alternate muscle groups or joints employed to restore the lost function (e.g., walking) sustain too much activity and show the damage of wear and tear. Such measures are probably the basis of much of the current troubles old polio patients are experiencing. It is not uncommon for patients with chronic diseases to become obsessive competitors who must win at any cost. Their lives become unidimensional attempts to make up for losses induced by their illness. Recall the young man memorialized in the movie *The Terry March Story* who lost his leg to a malignancy and then attempted to run across Canada on his prosthesis. Other examples are the disabled persons who become the life of the party or develop extreme sexual acting-out behaviors.

In all these symptoms, drawing sharp distinctions among physical, psychological, and social factors prevents understanding. This is because all social behaviors involve body motions, whether it be shaking hands, kissing, sexual intercourse, eating, or sitting. All interferences with function at the whole-body level have psychological consequences. All body actions have social meanings and ramifications. To reiterate, symptom avoidance and compensatory mechanisms, at whatever level of the human condition they occur, frequently aggravate the illness and produce further losses. Further, more than one counteractive measure may be taking place at the same time, and they may even be in conflict with one another.

A Changed World Perception

One of the alterations produced by chronic illness is changing perception of the world. Every sensation, percept, or experience is now interpreted in the light of and from the history of the illness. As a consequence, perceived reality begins to change for the chronically ill person. At the moment of acceptance of the diagnosis of chronic disease, the person perceives himself or herself to be a "diseased person." This should not be understood as a compensatory mechanism, since each of us sees the world in the light of our unique history as well as our shared knowledge and values.

The Mental Life

The usual picture of the mental life encompasses conscious behaviors, including reasoning; unconscious determinants of behavior; automatic, instinctual, or habitual behaviors; and a physical body (often seen as a self-regulating machine that is, in many respects, passive to the mind). As a culture we value consciousness highly. *My* voice represents *me, my* actions are under *my* control, *I* think *my* thoughts. The "me, myself, and I" of this view of consciousness is unitary. However, many people also believe that unconscious determinants of behavior exist largely inaccessible to awareness. In most psychological schools of thought, these unconscious factors are considered conflicts, negative influences on behavior that have been formed in childhood as a result of emotionally traumatic events. Behavioral schools of psychology, often denying the existence of unconscious determinants, have emphasized the place of learned and subsequently automatic control of even complex behaviors.

The body has received more attention in the United States in the last two decades as a result of the increasing interest in physical fitness. As part of this trend, the contribution of physical health to mental health has been emphasized. Despite this, the body remains largely conceived of as a machine, albeit wondrously complex. In this century, belief in the influence of the mind on the body has received special prominence. Merely sketching the various current conceptions of the relationship between mind and body, and what each is, could be a thesis in itself.

Convincing evidence has not been advanced to indicate that acutely or chronically physically ill persons are best understood in terms of traditional psychodynamics, although these are frequently employed in treating the largely self-defined malfunctions that bring individuals to psychiatrists and psychotherapists. Such things as ego, superego, id, unconscious, and similar entities are often discussed as though they were actual structures. They are better conceptualized as words that allow conversation about dynamic mental functions or processes that are difficult to capture in static concepts. Speakers who use these words may mean concepts different in important respects from the ideas of their listeners. Instead of being held to artificial categories of mental processes, it is better to examine those functions, interactions, or relationships relevant to a particular issue. In understanding chronic illness we will find it more helpful to look at two separate aspects of the human condition: first, the interaction of the person with the social world; second, the relationship of the person with himself or herself.

The Relation with the Social World

Western emphasis on the individual and individualism has left our knowledge of the connections, interactions, and relations among people stunted. If we existed by ourselves and unto ourselves, suffering from illness would be less common—given that to suffer is to be diminished or threatened in one's personhood. Even though suffering is an essentially private matter, the notion of privacy supposes a public world. Much suffering arises from disturbances between the sick person and the public existence. Arthur Lovejoy, in *Reflections on Human Nature,* discusses the human characteristics that, in the eighteenth century (and continuing to the present), were considered universal and vital in understanding human behavior: self-esteem, approbativeness (the desire to be approved of), and emulativeness (the desire to be considered superior) (1). Related to these characteristics is the desire to be like those one admires. I believe these internal and external forces act on us every single moment. The print media, television and radio, the clothes in the closet, the paint on the house, the stories of friends constantly portray these social forces and their exemplifying standards.

The same forces operate within and on the sick person. Unfortunately, the chronically ill are unable to meet most of the standards that would allow them to experience approbativeness or emulativeness. Self-esteem and the desire to be like those they admire are often also inaccessible because of the behavior enforced by sickness. Our culture does not approve of people who take many medications, but this is frequently necessary for these patients. The use of strong painkillers has particularly negative connotations, but in order to move to a wheelchair, much less wash or dress themselves, many patients must use narcotic analgesics. They often attend to their bodily functions in public; their weaknesses are on display; they require the help of others; they are frequently the subject of prurient curiosity. I saw a huge graffito sprayed on one of the concrete columns of the Henry Hudson Parkway: **M128—THE WORLD WILL KNOW OF ME.** People who walk with two canes do not paint such bold slogans.

The cripple's hands may not be able to hold a spray can, but the cripple's mind cannot turn off the characteristics described by Lovejoy. While most chronically ill individuals cannot play the game, they rarely stop wanting to. Thus, the chronically ill person whose disability interferes with the satisfaction of approbativeness or emulativeness (and who cannot turn these social forces aside to attend to other aspects of life) will be in powerful conflict. It is common to locate the source of the conflict outside the person. The chronically ill person is attempting to comply with social standards that appear to be *external*—the "demands of society." In fact, however, *the social standards are internal* but continually reinforced and reinterpreted externally. The social requirements, rules for behavior, and expectations of the world of others are contained within verbal categories—the meaning of words such as "patient," "cripple," "pain," "disabled," "mother," "teacher," "doctor," "arthritis," "polio," "lover," "leader," "success." Behavior or expectations contrary to the notions contained within the concepts these words stand for are conflict filled. Otherwise there would be no need for the changes in language that have accompanied the move to obtain equal status for the disabled. We now have "someone with a handicap," not "a handicapped person"—and certainly not "a cripple." The implication is that the meanings of terms such as these are larger than merely the words. One has merely to think of terms like "love" or "mother" to confirm the number of dimensions included in the meaning of a word. One might argue that it is not the term "mother" but rather the category "mother" that carries all the baggage. For everyday usage, I find them the same.

The contents of the meanings of these verbal categories are contained *within* the chronically ill person. It is also true that these words and their meanings are contained within others in the group, from family members to doctors. That they are shared provides the illusion that the standards of daily action, rules for behavior, requirements of dress and deportment are external. This is a fabrication of the mind, however. Because the ideas and beliefs—indeed, all the content of social categories—are contained within the person, it follows that the conflict for the chronically ill person evoked by the social forces epitomized by self-esteem, approbativeness, and emulativeness is in large part self-conflict.

Self-Conflict

Ill persons rail against the unfairness and prejudicial nature of everyday rules, standards, and expectations even while they try to meet them. These standards are expressed in the height of street curbs, chairs, toilet enclosures, and subway steps and also in the length of concerts, hand-shaking customs, rules for sexual encounters, and countless other behaviors of dailiness that to normal indiviudals represent no barriers. Despite frequent anger and bitterness, occasional expressions of unfairness, and attempts to hide, withdraw, or pretend indifference, sick persons try to stick it out in the world. They must remain part of the community; they need friends and associates, to have conversations, to achieve—they need all the things the rest of us require from group life. Chronic illness may put major obstacles in the way of achieving these goals. Not only may the standards and expectations of dailiness require abilities that the sick person has lost, but actual physical distress may be produced by the attempts to live in the communal world. Watch a person with helpless legs using crutches in an attempt to get on a bus and comprehend the price paid for living "like everybody else." Not only are the physical exertions strenuous, but the rhythm and duration of the act ensure that everyone on the bus watches the effort—and notes the delay in moving on. The person has committed two breaches of the social rules: attracting stares and slowing everybody down.

It is little wonder that, when chronically ill persons are exposed to such situations, part of them will want to withdraw to the safety of a private world to avoid the physical and emotional pain and humiliation. Attempts to accommodate to the social world continue, however, because the social aspect of the person desires to keep trying, driven by the ineluctable forces of human society. Because social standards, rules, and expectations are actually internal, conflict between the desire to live in society and the need to retreat continues even in the privacy of the person's thoughts. The more intransigent the conflict between these competing needs, the more the conflict becomes a source of suffering as it threatens to tear the person apart or, at the very least, cause constant unresolvable unhappiness. Family, friends, and acquaintances reinforce the conflict by continually urging the ill person to "try and be like everyone else." It is precisely that urge coming from inside the person that has provoked the suffering, because it is *impossible* for the sick person to be like everyone else. What is needed instead is a way of teaching disabled persons how to be themselves to the fullest extent possible—to rewrite the standards and rules for behavior in the light of their capacities as well as in the expectations of others.

In describing suffering that arises from internally generated conflict with social norms, I do not mean to minimize the suffering that arises from losses that are fundamentally personal, such as thwarted opportunities and progressive inability to do things (e.g., reading), whether or not they are also social losses.

Disharmony and Disorder

Social interactions can also be measured in aesthetic terms. The relation of individuals and their actions to others and to the world are usually harmonious, rhythmic, and orderly. Observe people walking in large groups: they walk in an orderly fashion, like flocks of birds flying in formation. Our everyday experience of people on the street may not seem to support the notion of harmony yet one has merely to recall a riot or social disorder to realize how rhythmically coordinated our everyday motions are.

Disorder, discord, and disharmony are painful experiences and individuals go to considerable lengths to avoid them. The chronically ill person may be unavoidably out of harmony with his or her world and other persons—the walking motions of those with spastic or disabled legs are the most obvious examples. There are disorders of dress produced by deformity (itself aesthetically displeasing), and disorders of facial appearance that result from scars, congenital diseases, or the manifestations of disease. The hand of rheumatoid arthritis may be ugly; it is difficult to match the slow pace of the speech of Parkinson's disease; the wait while a disabled person gets into a seat may seem interminable; even the aged person may be aware of no longer matching the rhythm of the surrounding world. All of these are aesthetically disjunctive experiences for the normal bystander. The chronically ill person is also aware of the discomfort arising from the disharmony. Unless the discomfort can be set aside, it can become an intolerable barrier between the ill person and the surrounding society, a source of suffering that remains until internal harmony is restored in a manner that makes the external rhythm and texture of life irrelevant. This is a difficult accomplishment.

The Conflict of Self with Self

I argued earlier that, in part, the conflict of the sick person with the external world becomes, by internalization, self-conflict. This is because the movement from external reality to an internal world forms a continuum. A world of persons, objects, and relationships exists—stubborn facts shared by all. Then come the symbolic and linguistic categories that make possible the sharing of these facts of existence. It is these, contained within each person, that set the stage for internal conflict which may appear to be external conflict.

A primarily internal world exists as well, in which conflicts arising from illness can threaten to destroy the integrity of the person. Here, confrontation between the person and his or her body may occur, as well as dissension within the various aspects of the self.

Self Versus Body

Let us examine the situation that occurs when the needs or demands of the body conflict with other needs of the person. Here, the body is often seen as being separate from other aspects of the person. Frequently, sick individuals behave as though their body were their enemy. This seems also to be true for victims of torture, as Elaine Scarry makes clear in her book, *The Body in Pain.* Tortured persons suffer not only from the pain, but from the conflict of their principles with the weakness of their bodies. Their principles—their determination not to reveal what is demanded—make them go on, while it is their bodies that command that they give in (2).

Attempts to resolve what is seen as the conflict between the needs of the body and the spiritual dimension of humankind are present in all modern religions. Reaching toward Christ through sharing the bodily suffering of others or through punishment imposed on one's own body are familiar aspects of early Christianity. Denials of bodily needs, tolerance of awful afflictions, and self-inflicted tortures are commonplace in the history of the saints. In at least that part of the legacy derived from the Greek heritage of Christianity, the body was believed to both stand in the way of spiritual fulfillment and provide a means of punishment for its own weaknesses. The manner in which it is spoken about in this tradition suggests that the body has its own intentions—that one of its purposes is to tempt, to lead the penitent astray. Our beliefs about individual suffering are framed by this Christian heritage. There is a vital difference, however, between the behavior of those who experience great pain or hardship in order to experience Christ and those who suffer as a part of illness.

Suffering occurs not merely in the presence of great pain but also when the intactness of the person is threatened or sundered, and remains until the threat is gone or the intactness can be restored. The key to understanding suffering is the realization that it takes place when the person is diminished by the experience. If the experience is enlarging, the suffering is resolved, although the pain may remain. Suffering is good *only to the extent that it provides one with the engine that drives toward enrichment*—toward fulfillment in dimensions of the human condition other than those closed by the illness or toward attainment of some transcendental goal. If the saints had experienced their terrible afflictions and privation only to lose their belief in Christ, then they would have suffered.

The chronically ill person may be in conflict with the body in several ways, none of which is unique to illness. What is special about the sick person's experience is that he or she may be unable to resolve the internal dissension with the body. For example, the body is frequently seen as an untrustworthy other. Like a mother who can never be depended on, the body fails the sick person when needed most. Persons with active arthritis never know when the pain will destroy an event, a day, a week. They go to bed feeling fine, perhaps looking forward to some celebration the next day, and awaken impaired. They look for reasons in their diet, emotional state, or the weather, but no consistent explanations present themselves. The body is so untrustworthy that it does not even misbehave consistently. As with arthritis, so it is with severe asthma, ulcerative colitis, multiple sclerosis, and other chronic illnesses. The person can become so angry with the body that he or she will punish it—inflict pain on it, deny it medicine, not bathe it, overwork it. With each punishment inflicted on the body, the person is also punished.

The body may not only be untrustworthy but also a source of humiliation. Control of the bowels and the bladder can be problematic in chronic illness, particularly in neurological conditions, exposing the sick person to embarrassment. The possibility of odor, the fear of loss of control, preoccupation with performance—matters of concern to all at some time or other—may come to dominate the sick person's life. A woman with emphysema was admitted to the hospital because she could no longer perform her daily tasks without severe shortness of breath. She seemed to be suffering greatly, more than could be explained by her difficult breathing. When she was first examined, there were strange callouses on her thighs, just above her knees. The explanation became clear. As her illness progressed, she had begun to dribble urine with her very frequent coughing. The symptom was impossible for her fastidious self to accept. She was so humiliated that she stopped going out and then no longer allowed others to visit her. She spent her time sitting on the toilet (resting her elbows on her knees) to keep her bladder empty, lest urine spill to the floor when she walked. Her suffering was a result of the destruction to her life and the isolation resulting from this symptom, not the problems with her breathing. An indwelling catheter stopped her suffering.

Body urges may constantly force the person to behaviors that inevitably lead to social failures. Sexual desire is an obvious example, but much simpler events, such as the need to laugh, may precipitate a publicly humiliating loss of physical control in a chronically ill person. The healthy have such experiences from time to time; the chronically ill may not be able to avoid them.

Many other examples could be cited, but the point is that conflict between self and body is possible; it may be produced by the illness and it may exacerbate the illness. But why do some suffer from these struggles while others do not?

I believe the answer is to be found in the understanding that *suffering always involves self-conflict*—conflict within the person. Even in the acute circumstances of overwhelming pain, dissension exists. There are always alternatives (although the sick person usually perceives no other possibilities); the sufferer, overwhelmed by the pain, might simply give up or die. But dying is not so easy—one wants to live, not die. To give up seems cowardly. On the other hand, to struggle seems inevitably to invite more pain. After the event, the person can relive it in ways that make it seem better than what actually occurred. In recalling the suffering, dissension continues. If the suffering was severe or lasted long enough, it never leaves the memory. There must have been other ways to have done things, the sufferer thinks; excuses are searched for, but no wholly satisfactory answers appear to meliorate the dreadful fact of the suffering that has been endured. This is true even in the acute situation and still more pronounced in all others, especially in chronic illness, where the suffering can go on and on.

Strategies for Reducing Suffering

The nature of the inner conflict that is an inevitable accompaniment of suffering is further illuminated by examining four strategies that can prevent, relieve, or reduce suffering. The first is living entirely in the present because suffering requires anticipating a feared future. Remember, suffering occurs when the integrity of the person is lost and cannot be restored. With this in mind, we must distinguish the suffering of acute and chronic illness. With acute symptoms the injury is of limited duration, and thus—except perhaps with overwhelming pain or loss—at any precise moment the person is intact—at least in some fashion, and sufficiently to speak to his or her self. The very act of stopping to reflect or reassure oneself, however briefly or minimally, creates a whole person for that moment—a community of self. Generally, however, people are continually tumbling into the future of the coming moment, a future landscaped by fear. When they do speak to themselves it is more often to tell themselves that if the pain keeps up they will not be able to stand it. At that moment, however, their integrity is intact. The person must maintain the understanding that the symptom is not the enemy, no matter how severe; the *real* enemy is fear, because the fear of impending dissolution is the root of the suffering. The suffering will continue after the immediate event—the reconstitution of the person that is required cannot take place—if the sufferer either continues to dwell on the awful happening or fears its return (the two often go hand in hand). (In the best of circumstances, however, if the distress was sufficiently severe or long-lasting, regaining intactness may take a long time.)

In chronic illness, just as in acute illness, the immediate onslaught of distress—physical, emotional, or social—may evoke suffering, but the temporal reasons for its continuing are different. Suffering may persist because the person will not relinquish the past. For such individuals the present, whatever its pleasures or achievements, always fails in comparison with the past. "You should have seen what I used to be able to do." "A life without reading is no life at all; I used to love to read." The person cannot become whole again, because he or she defines wholeness solely in the past tense. Sometimes the sufferer will not give up the anger or resentment associated with the onset of the illness or, perhaps, its treatment. As a consequence he or she is forced to dwell on what might have been instead of what can be. On the other hand, since the reason for the recurrent episodes of acute distress never goes away, the chronically ill person anticipates the future with such dread that he or she cannot become whole again. The person may say, "I will never, never go back to classes. I will never, never be stared at like that again. I can't take it again, I just can't." At the moment of telling it would seem that there is no one staring and there is no humiliation (and she *did* in fact, tolerate it), so why is she suffering now? Because as long as she dreads returning the *inner conflict* is as active out of the painful circumstance as it was in it. She wants to go to school, she wants to *be* somebody. But going to school means exposing herself to those stares again and again and to the terrible aloneness. Once again, the inner conflict is ignited because a painful future is constructed out of the hurts of the past. The inner voice is speaking not of reassurance but of fears of a future whose distress is experienced again and again in anticipation.

When suffering occurs because people are humiliated by events in the body, their words to themselves generally do not provide comfort. They do not say, "This humiliation of myself soiled by my own excretions is unendurable only because my eyes are representing the gaze of others. Feces are a natural aspect of the human condition and soiling occurring in circumstances like this is not a cause for humiliation." Instead, they view their soiled selves from the perspectives of early childhood training and repelled onlookers (imagined or real). They more readily take the viewpoint of others than a viewpoint by which they might protect themselves from humiliation. They could say to themselves, "I don't care what anybody thinks." But this statement is so often heard in circumstances that deny its truth that one doubts it is a useful source of support.

Alternatively, it is possible for persons to hold their own personal time still for a moment of awareness of the actual events—*prior* to the interpretation that brings feelings of shame. In this state the person has the opportunity of choosing a perspective from which to view the timeless instant as well as subsequent events. The person's choice of interpretation is central to how that person experiences the events—it is the interpretation that determines whether suffering or merely distress is experienced. Maintaining oneself entirely in the present moment, exempt from the rush of interpretations, is a difficult skill at any time, more so under stress. In the example of incontinence, one might question how awareness of the actual moment would be helpful as opposed to humiliating interpretations. One answer is that soiling itself is a disgusting smelly mess that demands doing something *now.* As awful as that may be, it is nothing more than that. Shame is a destructive emotion that robs individuals of their wits and their sense of humor at a time when they most need them both.

The second way that suffering can be altered is by the development of total indifference to what is happening. In the situation of acute pain, this means assuming a stance of absolute unconcern to the fate of the body part or the self; one allows the physical distress to roll over oneself as a wave on the beach rolls over a pebble. This strategy relieves suffering for two reasons. The first is that to be indifferent to the fate of the self is to remove the basis for suffering, which is the loss of the person's integrity. One may become indifferent for different reasons. One may not care about oneself because of an act of will (which must be difficult in the extreme). Alternatively, someone may be completely indifferent to his or her immediate fate because of total indifference to bodily existence or through achievement of a sense of complete union with God. Further, whether a body part or the whole person is threatened, the person's resistance to the pain or threat heightens the severity of distress. It is interesting that patients with severe pain who become delirious frequently stop complaining of the pain. They ramble on in their confusion or actively hallucinate but their pain ceases to trouble them. If a rational patient can be induced to completely relax and not attempt to move, withdraw, or guard the painful part, the pain is greatly lessened. Remember, the issue at hand is not why people have pain but why they suffer, and why some suffer more than others. Most people are unable to stop fighting their pain; indeed, the more it hurts the more they struggle (and vice versa). As they continue (and if the pain or distress continues), their struggles become increasingly exhausting. As exhaustion approaches, they face the certainty (to them) that their pain will overwhelm them, and they begin to suffer. The same is true for other symptoms. It is common for people with difficulty breathing to *increase* their activities, as they begin to run out of breath, from fear that they will be unable to finish their task or find a place to sit down. Often they will start functioning again before they are adequately rested. So the cycle continues, with periods in which there is adequate breath for effort becoming ever shorter, providing such persons with the evidence that they will soon be able to do nothing *except* rest, which to some is the equivalent of nonexistence. Learning to give in to symptoms so as to live a more productive life is not a simple task and, as in other aspects of their lives, some persons are more open to mastery than others.

The same strategy for the avoidance of suffering expresses itself differently in chronic illness. There the suffering results from the conflict between the person's desires and expectations—whether of social origin or from the character of the individual—and the limitations imposed by the illness. People do not want to see themselves as limited; they want to prove (to themselves as well as others) that they can achieve everything they strive for. Giving in further diminishes self-esteem because the restrictions of the body are dealt with as though the whole person is limited. The desire to be admired, to be like those one admires and to be superior are powerful forces that must be put aside for the strategy of unconcern to be effective. It is difficult and rare for those who are healthy and advantaged to achieve such self-confidence that they no longer care what others think of them; how much more so, it would seem, for someone whose every day is crowded with threat and injury. But sick persons can frequently accomplish what the healthy cannot because the sick are strongly motivated and they *know what is important* beyond the superficialities of the everyday world.

Denial is a third strategy that permits people not to suffer in circumstances where they might otherwise live in misery. It is more commonly seen in chronic illness, where disabled individuals may become habitually oblivious to the stares of onlookers. They may no longer be aware that they have a bad odor, that they appear strange, that each motion takes them palpably longer than normal persons (thus delaying everybody else). Unless some degree of oblivion attends the day-to-day activities of persons who have long-term illnesses, then acute awareness of their difference is constantly with them and they will be driven into isolation. Either alternative is unbearable—to always be aware that one is irremediably different or to be driven into isolation. Denial would seem to be a simple answer to the problem of suffering in chronic illness, but it has a price. Selective obliviousness is an unusual skill. When one is no longer aware of the looks, comments, and behaviors of others in respect to one's differences, then one also loses an appreciation of the activities, language, and emotions of others in respect to things other than oneself. For some persons (myself, for example) such a loss would, in itself, be intolerable. Thus, denial (in its various forms) is another manner by which suffering can be relieved in both acute and chronic illness, but it is more available, in its various forms, to some than to others.

Flexibility, a fourth and final way in which suffering can be relieved or prevented, also highlights how individual differences in the nature of persons are crucial in determining whether suffering will occur. The threat to the intactness that initiates suffering may occur in relation to any aspect of an individual. Similarly, suffering is relieved when the threatened or destroyed part of the person is replaced in importance by another aspect. Thus the lifelong athlete who suffers paraplegia may reduce the terrible burden of the loss by (say) becoming totally involved in helping others. Unfortunately, in severe chronic illness, the loss of an aspect of the person is commonly followed by another loss. First the person can no longer walk. Next, crutches become useless. Then fine hand motions are impossible, then it becomes increasingly difficult to move about even in a wheelchair. Then pain effectively removes half the days of the month. The new interests in life that compensated for the first loss must be replaced, and then replaced again. Such flexibility is difficult to achieve. Chronically ill persons must arrive at the ultimate knowledge that it is not what they do that counts but who they are. For some it is difficult to conceive of what is left when the self is defined apart from its roles or projects. Such mastery must contend with widespread counteractive social values—values that reside *within* (as well as around) the sick person.

The forces that (1) prevent the sick person from remaining within the immediate moment of experience (and free from interpretations that pull toward the future), (2) keep the person from achieving indifference to distress, (3) overwhelm denial, and (4) reduce the flexibility that might make up for the personal losses caused by the illness are internal to the person. These personal forces are different, however, in each instance. This suggests again that the self is not unitary. As there can be conflicts between the self and the body, dissension can exist within the self. This struggle between parts of the self can make the illness more severe and be a source of suffering. More simply stated, in complex circumstances we are rarely "of one mind." Such internal disagreement does not arise, *de novo,* at the moment of illness or even during its progression. Rather, there has been a history of internal dissension (of varying degrees) from which it is possible to predict future internal conflict. Such self-conflict in acute illness may produce anxiety, great fear, or even paralysis of action. For example, a married teacher in her fifties (whose daughter is a physician) has always rushed to physicians for each little ache or pain, proclaiming herself a hypochondriac. On one occasion she demanded an immediate appointment with the doctor because blood had appeared in her stool that morning. Looking into her bowel, the physician told her that the blood was probably from something more serious than hemorrhoids. She said, "Well, I'm embarrassed to say, but it really started a couple of weeks ago." As her doctor was writing out the name of the specialist she was to see for the next test, she said, "You know how I am about these things—symptoms and all. The blood really started three months, maybe even longer, ago." She had a cancer of the colon. It is common to ascribe such behavior to fear or denial. When most of us do things like that, one voice tells us to act and another voice says, "Not yet." If we ask further questions of such patients, they tell us they were afraid it would be cancer. However, it is not cancer, the thing, that they are afraid of, but all the multiple meanings played out into the future associated with the diagnosis of cancer. They have created a cancer scenario that one part of them lives out in anticipation. Another part has another scenario with a different sequence of events. The two are in contest with one another until (in this instance) the continued bleeding tilts the issue toward the more "realistic" part of the person.

I have illustrated a number of situations where there is internal personal conflict in illness. In these situations, the illness sparks the conflict and the conflict frequently worsens the impact of the illness. This characteristic of internal conflict shares in the processual nature of all aspects of chronic illness.

I noted earlier that the usual views of the mental life are of little help in understanding the problems of chronic illness or the reasons why it may lead to suffering. There is an alternative way of viewing mental life that does illuminate the difficulties of chronic illness and provides a basis for understanding how suffering arises primarily from self-conflict, even when the actual cause of the distress may be external to the person. One aspect of the self is involved in interacting with the social world. This is the "self" described by George Herbert Mead.* It is constantly meeting the expectations of others in all the multitude of possible ways in which such demands are placed. This aspect of the person must also control the urges of the individual that seem to threaten self-consistency and social existence—hardly the nefarious urges so often pictured in descriptions of the unconscious. They may be something as simple as the desire to express emotion in an exuberant fashion—love, joy, anger, humor—in a society that frowns on personal expressiveness, or the wish to express artistic creativity in a group that values businesslike industry. In a different social group, businesslike industry must be restrained or innate taciturnity overcome. The point is that our inner selves are not always a perfect match for the social world in which we live. Yet we must get along.

This is the opposite face of the *need* to live among others, the undeniable requirement for a social existence discussed earlier. People do not merely exist among others, as one pebble among a pile of stones. They live by the rules, and the rules for social participation override the inner needs of the individual except in unusual instances. Unfortunately, for the chronically ill, the rules are often problematic. They demand behaviors that sick persons may not be able to achieve, except at great cost. Acutely ill patients are often relieved of these social burdens because of the state of sickness, but chronically ill persons are not. And if society does treat the chronically ill person more like a patient than a person, that too has a high price. Compliance with societal demands may require so much energy of the chronically ill that little is left for other pursuits. The chronically ill, in common with everyone else, have inner needs, goals, desires, even beliefs, at variance with the social self. But their opportunities for expression may be reduced by sickness. Thus the conflict between the social and inner parts of the person may be heightened—even to the point of dissension so severe as to threaten to tear the person apart. Much "depression" of chronic illness may be of this nature. It is not depression but suffering that goes on and on, as the integrity of the person remains threatened by an inner struggle seemingly unresolvable.

In the United States, we tend to treat the self required by and presented to

*This use of the word self is somewhat different from its contemporary usage. For George Herbert Mead the "self" was created in the interaction with others and primarily by language. His work was done early in this century prior to the dissemination of the work of Freud and other psychoanalysts and the interiority of person that is widely accepted today was not a part of his thinking. The word self as generally employed today stands for a unitary conception of person—everything that is me is part of myself. I use the word person to stand for all the aspects of person described in the previous chapter. As such it is a broader concept than self. As a simple example, others know things about me as a person that I do not and cannot know. These things are not part of my self, but they are part of my person. So too are the conflicts with (say) my mother arising in infancy and which remain buried within me unaccessible to me without special effort, still determining my day-to-day behavior.

the world as the only legitimate voice of the person. Any self-conflicts that present themselves are often seen as neurotic difficulties to be "treated away" so that the person can live better in the world. This may be appropriate for the well, but it poorly serves the sick, who must learn, above all, to live with themselves. Thus, problems of the chronically ill are particularly difficult in a culture that has no language for the conflict or even the suffering.

Summary

Chronic illness is a thing apart from chronic disease, with which it may or may not be associated. In fact, classical disease understandings or even modern organ-based pathophysiology are inadequate for understanding chronic illness. This is because the illness is generated not only in the body but exists at every level of the human condition, from the molecular to the communal. Chronic illness is a process in which the symptoms arise from the illness and then contribute to the continuation of the illness. This is so much the case that, with long-established chronic states, even being restored to physical normality would not alone be sufficent to end the illness.

Suffering arises in chronic illness because of the conflicts within the person that are generated by the simultaneous need to respond to the demands and limitations of the body and to the forces of society and group life. These struggles to meet opposing needs become internalized, and suffering occurs as the integrity of the person is threatened by the dissension. The suffering is exacerbated by conflicts of the self with the body and by dissension within the various parts, or aspects, of the person. Such struggles, and the suffering they cause, illustrate the way in which an attempt to understand suffering in chronic illness requires major changes in the goals of medicine that have arisen from and for the study of acute illness. Exploring these problems would not only help us relieve the suffering of the chronically ill but would also illuminate the care of all the sick.

The mandate for the existence of a profession of medicine in society is its obligation to relieve the suffering caused by human sickness. In the past two chapters we examined the nature of suffering and its origins within our being as persons. It has been clear that where the primary concern of physicians is the diagnosis and treatment of disease, they may fail to prevent or treat suffering adequately or even inadvertently cause it as a result of treatment. In part this is because physicians have basic concepts about sickness and the nature of sick persons that are inadequate to the causes of suffering, and in part because doctors are not trained to the belief that one of their primary tasks is the relief of suffering.

But before we can explore the solution to these problems, it is necessary to better understand two fundamental aspects of medicine: the relationship between patients and doctors and the nature of diseases. These are the concern of the next two chapters.

References

1. Lovejoy, Arthur O. *Reflections on Human Nature*. 1961. Baltimore, Johns Hopkins Press.

2. Scarry, Elaine. *The Body in Pain*. 1985. New York, Oxford University Press, Chap. One.

5

The Mysterious Relationship Between Doctor and Patient

SUFFERING IS PERSONAL and medicine is a personal profession—one doctor and one patient, each incomplete without the other. All medicine—all care and caregivers, all medical science and technology—rests on that special relationship, without which this book would be meaningless. Doctors could not know about sick persons or their diseases if not for this unique relationship because patients would not otherwise permit the invasion of their physical or personal privacy. Patients could not receive the extra margin of effort expected of physicians if it were not for their relationship. Current depictions of physician and patient as adversaries struggling over a commodity called medical care bear no relation to the actual care of sick persons because of this special connection. The nature of sickness and the bond between patient and doctor also renders false those views of the relationship in which autonomous sick people are seen as exercising their rights against paternalistic doctors (1, 2). The relationship does not require a doctor; nurse, shaman, or anyone in the role of healer can be substituted. In our culture that role is called doctor.

So often invoked, like a totem, the doctor-patient relationship has become a bland omnipresence in discussions about medicine; however, how it works and its relevance to patient or doctor remains obscure. My claim, therefore, that the *whole* in medicine (as in "holistic") is not merely a whole patient but rather patient plus doctor, requires an examination of the glue that binds them. Doctors and patients may have an economic relationship, a political relationship, a community relationship, a social (in the everyday sense of the term) relationship, a personal (involving merely two persons), or even an intensely private relationship. In fact, parents and their children can also have each of these relationships. When we refer to the parent-child relationship, however, we generally mean something more basic than the economic, political, community, social, personal, or private relationships into which they, as a parent and child, may enter. In this chapter, when I speak of the doctor-patient relationship, I am referring to the central and basic relationship between doctor and patient which rests solely on the fact that one is a patient and the other a doctor. All the other possible relationships between doctors and their patients derive from this foundation. Because this subject can generate heated discussions, I ask that as you read this chapter, you keep these distinctions in mind.

Let me start with some anecdotes.

Some years ago, a patient of mine was operated on for an early cancer of the ovary. At that time such patients were given a chemotherapy drug called melphalan (Alkeran) for a period after their surgery. Unfortunately, when I gave her the melphalan it destroyed her bone marrow—her body was unable to make red or white blood cells or platelets. Aplastic anemia of such severity is almost always fatal. One administers transfusions of blood, white blood cells, and platelets and hopes that the marrow will ultimately recover. In effect, in treating her, I had endangered her life. Yet our relationship was as close as any I had had with a sick patient. She remained in the hospital for many weeks receiving transfusions. One day I asked her why she let me take care of her since I was the one who had caused what we believed to be her impending death. "Oh," she said, "you didn't mean to do it." I thought that was remarkable. (Remarkably, also, she recovered and remains well.)

A physician I know told me about the treatment for his asthma. He was taken care of by a wonderful chest physician whose skills he had seen demonstrated many times before and since. He was on high doses of prednisone (a cortisone-like drug) and other medications for many months but he could not seem to get off the drugs without getting sick again. He would meet his doctor in the hospital corridor and ask what to do next. The doctor-patient did what was suggested but to no avail. His own knowledge of asthma was not inconsiderable but that was no help either. He told me that he could not get his friend and colleague to treat him like a patient. Finally, desperate, he went to another doctor whose speciality was asthma. The new physician promptly made my informant into a patient. He told him what to do (what he said seemed the same as what had been previously tried), scheduled office visits frequently and regularly, and within six months my friend was off all medication. What was the difference? It was not the medications or their schedule—they were the same (at least at the start). The difference, I believe, was that the second physician made him become a patient. Once that happened, the new doctor was able to begin "pulling strings" inside his doctor-patient's body. No one knows how this comes about or how the physician is able to have an influence on a patient's illness apart from explicit medical or surgical treatments, but this is the process involved. Current research is increasingly revealing the influence of mind on immunity and other body functions, so there should be little surprise that doctors are also able to affect the patient's physiological process. No one doubts that doctors have an influence on their patients' states of mind—we are of a piece, affecting one part alters the whole.

Another odd thing about the relationship is that you can meet a stranger (the doctor) and ten minutes later all your clothing is off and he or she has a finger in an uncomfortable place—and then you say thank you!

The relationship affects not only the patient. When I was an intern at Bellevue, an old derelict was admitted to the emergency ward under my care with the diagnosis, "sick old man." What a nothing diagnosis, I thought. I asked the patient what his trouble was and he said, "athlete's foot." But, as it turned out, the admitting resident knew a lot more than I did. The man was filthy and covered with lice, so I asked that he be cleaned up so that I could examine him. He went into his bath filthy, pink, and alive and he came out clean, white, and dead! I tried desperately to revive him, but could not. I cannot describe how shocked and horrified I was. I was not dismayed by fear of criticism; such deaths were commonplace. It was as if something terribly wounding—but impossible to identify—had happened to me.

The longer I take care of a patient the more responsible I feel for the welfare of that person—regardless of whether I "like" or "dislike" him or her. Traditionally, when physicians send a consultation letter, it ends with a phrase such as "Thank you for sending me this nice patient." What does it matter if the patient is nice or not? Because, even if the patient is not nice, the consultant has become involved. One should avoid getting too romantic about the doctor-patient relationship, which also exists and does its work with hookers, bums, crooks, junkies, murderers, the mean, dirty and down-and-out, and the worst and nastiest of humanity.

As a medical resident I was sometimes responsible for the medical care of patients in Bellevue's psychiatric wards. One time the police brought in a disoriented, screaming, struggling man in handcuffs who also had a high fever. I asked them to remove the handcuffs, stop restraining him, and leave us alone in the examining room. They reluctantly left and the man quieted down immediately. He had meningitis. On another occasion I had to examine a violently psychotic man with a fever who was confined to a room empty of everything except wall padding and a mattress on the floor. The attendants wanted to accompany me for my protection, but I went in alone. As I started to examine him (we were both standing), he suddenly raised both fists above my head. I almost perished from fear. But then he put both hands down and I completed the examination. In both instances I disdained protection because I had learned, as doctors often do in municipal hospitals like Bellevue, that I was shielded by the fact of being a doctor.

The relationship exists even if or when the doctor is burned out, nasty, callous, mean, cruel, and ignorant—and even when the doctor does not believe in the relationship. The doctor-patient relationship can be employed, exploited, badly used, or sabotaged, but it cannot be disowned; it is there whether a doctor wants it to be or not.

To make the whole thing even stranger, the relationship starts its work within moments of the beginning of the interaction—before there can be a true relationship. The sicker the patient, the more this is so. It occurs between people who do not share a spoken language or cultures, and has occurred throughout the history of the profession. I do not mean to imply that the doctor-patient relationship and its effects are equal in all circumstances. Clearly, it can be better or worse, improved or destroyed. Observation of current hospital medicine suggests that its therapeutic power is largely rejected, untapped, undervalued, or merely neglected with resultant impoverishment of medical care. Further, I believe that the therapeutic power of the doctor-patient relationship *grows* in importance as the technology of cure becomes more powerful. It is unfortunately common for a patient to become caught up in a parade of tests, treatments, and subspecialists with no physician clearly responsible for the whole problem. Patients find themselves required to be their own physicians, making lonely decisions about high technology matters that doctors have trouble figuring out. On occasion the patient is cared for by a "team" and cannot figure out the politics of responsibility and leadership—with the result that despite so many caregivers, the patient may be essentially alone at critical junctures. In these increasingly common circumstances the disregard and derogation of the patient-doctor relationship may be even more sad. *It is a healing relationship.* It has been one of the most basic errors of the modern era in medicine to believe that patients cured of their diseases—cancer removed, coronary arteries opened, infection resolved, walking again, talking again, or back home again—are also healed; are whole again. Through the relationship it is possible, given the awareness of the necessity, the acceptance of the moral responsibility, the understanding of the problem and mastery of the skills, to heal the sick; to make whole the cured, to to bring the chronically ill back within the fold, to relieve suffering, and to lift the burdens of illness.

Some things the doctor-patient relationship is not: *pace* my psychiatric colleagues, it is not a transference relationship in the usual sense of that phrase. Although a transference relationship may be formed so that the patient's reactions to the physician mirror the patient's earlier reactions to a parent, the power of the relationship is not transferred from the relationship with a parent. To put it another way, the doctor-patient relationship does not do its job because the doctor is seen as a parent. When my daughter was nine we went camping across the United States and she became quite ill with acute tonsillitis. I gave her penicillin in the usual oral doses, but she did not get better. After three or four days, my worried wife asked me to take her to a doctor. Chagrined, I drove down off the mountain to a small town and found a doctor. He was wonderful with her, and after his examination gave her a shot of penicillin. The next morning she was much better. (Physicians will know that injectable penicillin is not more effective than oral in these circumstances and that she had already had sufficient time to get better prior to the doctor's examination and treatment.) My daughter's father may be a physician, but he is primarily her father. Therefore, her behavior when ill and being treated by her father is more likely to be determined by factors in her relations with the father part of him than the doctor part. Of course, the two become conflated, which is why doctors are so careful when they treat even an adult who is a doctor's child. They want to tap into the doctor-patient relationship, not the father-child relationship. Another anecdote may illustrate. When she was a teenager, my daughter developed a symptom, just before leaving on a trip, that could not be disregarded. The X ray was normal. As she and I were leaving the X-ray suite, the young woman radiologist (a doctor's child) said to me, "Perhaps if her father spent more time with her she would not get sick."

The doctor-patient relationship is different from the psychotherapist-patient relationship. I believe this is because the body is involved in sickness. When a psychotherapy patient becomes ill, although the patient's loyalty to the therapist remains intact, the therapist does not automatically acquire the power of the doctor-patient relationship. A terminally ill patient may have a superb relationship with a psychiatrist, but the power of hope is invested in the physician or surgeon. It may be simply that the psychotherapist is not prepared by social convention or training to deal with physical illness.

The impact of the doctor-patient relationship is not simply psychosomatic in the common usage of the term—the effect of the mind on the body. It has gained that reputation partly because of things like the placebo effect and the fact that pains often disappear after a doctor's reassurance. I believe the relationship is poorly understood, in part because of the inadequacies of the distinction between physical and pyschological. As Otto Guttentag pointed out years ago, mind and body are best considered as polar terms, like North and South. One extreme is pure mind and the other is pure body, but anyplace else is a variable mixture. For example, we do not usually consider learning to ride a bicycle a psychological process, although there may be psychological (as well as physical) limitations to be overcome. If you continue to believe that the doctor-patient relationship works because the mind works on the body, try to define precisely what is working on what (in more than geographic terms). Ask yourself what you *mean* by mind and what you *mean* by body. Rather than squeezing the relationship into narrow ideas about mind-body, it is better to let its realities expand those categories.

That the doctor-patient relationship must have a social or cultural dimension is evidenced by its immediate effect during emergencies in which doctor and patient have never met before. A doctor who is a stranger can make pain ease, panic subside, and breathing improve within moments (3). The same doctor can make pain increase, worsen breathing, and exacerbate panic by doing the wrong thing—the relationship works both ways. Physicianhood is a role—a set of performances, duties, obligations, entitlements, and limitations connected to a function or status. The socialization of the medical student includes learning about the content of the doctor's role so that he or she emerges as both a physician and in the role of a physician. Like a lock and key, the role must have its counterpart in the patient. Where, in the patient, does the role reside? Not merely in the intellect, because it works when the patient is too sick to think straight. Not merely in the emotions, because it also works (although not as well) when the patient is very angry at the doctor. I believe it also works in the body, although you may properly ask how a role can have effects that reside in a body.

To answer I must go off on a brief tangent about meanings to demonstrate that meanings are not merely intellectual, but affective (emotional), physical, and transcendent (spiritual) as well. It is possible to direct a hypnotized subject to respond to a word *only* in one or another of these four dimensions. Thus, the subject can provide separate and distinct cognitive, affective, and spiritual segments of meaning. An example was provided by a hypnotized patient with cancer of the stomach who was receiving chemotherapy. To the word chemotherapy he gave a complex cognitive definition involving ideas about DNA, an affective definition that included fear and a transcendant definition that involved hope. When presented with the word solely in its aspect of body sensation, he did not merely think of nausea, he *became* nauseated. [The phenomenon is described at length in Volume One of *Talking with Patients* (4).] Meaning is not something that resides solely in words. Mom, apple pie, and the American flag are not only things in their own right, but also symbols that carry all the above stated dimensions of meaning, which in turn bring with them expectations—apple pie accompanied by its taste, for example. Expectations also produce effects on the body. We have known since Pavlov's experiments with his dogs that learned meanings can have effects on the body. One might object that his demonstrations were of conditioned reflexes; however, when Pavlov rang a bell at the same time that food was presented to the dogs, did he not give the bell a new meaning? (We use the term conditioned reflex rather than acquired meaning because we both artificially separate mind and body and hold a prejudicial belief that meaning can be perceived only by humans and not by dogs.)

Given this understanding about words, it seems reasonable that roles also have meanings that include bodily effects. These do not include merely the fear, with its physiological consequences, experienced by some people when they enter a physician's office. It is common to speak of the same words as having different effects when spoken by different people. The lover's words may produce profound physical effects—blushes, raised pulse rates, and a thrill in the chest (or, conversely, draining of blood from the partner's face and squeezing chest discomfort). We explain these differences by variations in receptivity to the words of another.

Thus, the doctor's role offers the opportunity to cause change in the patient's body in two distinct ways: first, by the direct action of the role itself and, second, by the special access to the patient that the role provides for the doctor's words. All sick people know how much better they begin to feel when a competent physician comforts and reassures them (and how much worse when an inept doctor tries to do the same). Again and again I hear, "He'd stop smoking if you told him to," "You may be the only person he listens to." "Doctor, you tell her, she'll listen to you," "I stopped smoking right after I saw you the last time," or "I can't tell you how important our last conversation was." The corollary of this is that doctors learn how important and special their words are. (See Chapter 9 on rhetoric.)

At least in part, the effect of the doctor-patient relationship depends on how words do their work and the socially mediated influence of role on whose words do what. The meaning of "The Doctor" is complex in that it not only affects the functions of words, but provides a basis for the interpretation of events. Many of the things that physicians do would, in other circumstances, be considered prying, seductive, or cruel, but when done by physicians are thought of as concerned, supportive, and, although painful, necessary for recovery. Generally, the presence of the doctor creates an expectation of benefit and improvement.

I have, or course, portrayed an idealized version of the possibilities afforded by the doctor-patient relationship. However, for every opportunity for making the sick better through the vehicle of the relationship, an equal opportunity exists for damage. And yet, even here the relationship survives and can work effectively for patients. How can we account for its hardiness? Unfortunately, our knowledge of the extent and types of bonding between individuals is deficient. In the case of the sick, our knowledge of their openness and need to make connections to the well is equally lacking. As the sick get sicker, their need to bond—to be a part of others—increases. The doctor, for all the reasons discussed above, is the person to whom they may be the most open. The origin of the attachment in the human condition is invisible—sick persons do not know that what they are feeling about their doctor arose because of something called the doctor-patient relationship; it feels to them simply like affection—sometimes very strong affection, which may become possessive. The doctor's achievements become theirs, their doctor's worries become their worries, they may, like lovers, become jealous of other patients, acting as if (despite all evidence to the contrary) each is the doctor's only patient. The doctor's smile elates them, the doctor's frown casts them down, and they become desperately afraid the doctor will abandon them. As they become sicker the connection deepens. Not surprisingly, patients, feeling their attachment to the doctor become stronger, may believe it is reciprocal and related to them as persons independently of the illness. Thus they may feel hurt when they get better after long illnesses and their doctors do not pay as much attention as when they were ill. Once, in such circumstances, I explained to a patient that I was not really her friend, I was her doctor. She became angry and hurt at what seemed to her to be sudden, inexplicable coldness. I will not do that again.

But in reality the attachment is always reciprocal. Victory for one is victory for the other, and when one is defeated so is the other. Physicians may remain objective; they may (in fact, must) retain their boundaries in order to remain private persons. But, as the sick are in bondage to them, they are in bondage to the sick, who provide the basis of their power and the source of personal reward and status. Physicians are also bound to their patients in another way, for it is from their patients that they learn, understand, and improve what they are and what they know. Even the worst physicians respond to this indebtedness, the most unfeeling are moved, and almost every doctor holds jealously to his or her patients. Medical students begin to experience this bonding when they are first exposed to patients. Despite the "us versus them" mentality so common in the arenas of medical training and the virtual denial of emotionalism in all of medicine, the potential intensity and depth of the connection between doctor and patient emerge and begin to exert their influence on students. The extraordinary power of sickness to make patients susceptible to change at all levels of the human condition is matched by the equal power of this benevolent relationship with its unseen but powerful connection to induce physicians to extend themselves at all levels of the human condition. The bond between doctor and patient shares aspects of the bond between teacher and student (in its best sense) and is a facilitator of learning and changing (all learning requires personal change). This is the basis, I believe, of the fact that the word 'doctor" derives from the Latin, *docere,* to teach. The bond between patient and doctor is like the bond between parent and child in that actions of a parent may cause changes within the child, including changes in the child's body.

The nature of the bond requires further comment. Some people are more emotional and demonstrative than others; they make obvious their connections or attachments to others. Other people seem more distant, impassive, indifferent, or even unfeeling. Their connection to others, including physicians, may be unapparent. There are also cultural determinants of the surface display of emotion and attachment to others. Public interactions can be learned behaviors that do not accurately reflect the actual nature of the relationship. The words "connection," "attachment," or "bond" in this description of the doctor-patient relationship should not be confused with the surface phenomena shown in displays of relatedness to another. These evidences and effects of the bond may be present in the absence of any overt display of emotion.

Remember that bonds can extend in both directions. As the doctor can pull strings inside the patient, the patient can pull strings inside the doctor. As part of learning their role doctors must learn to protect themselves from the effects of bonding with dozens of sick patients, attachments that can allow access to the doctors' interior emotional and physical life. The self-protection can be so great that it effectively nullifies the doctor's ability to use the bond to accomplish the work of doctoring. Freud pointed out the tension in physicians between empathy and objectivity, but a kindred tension exists between empathy and self-protection. Moreover, the constraints inherent in the role itself provide deep-seated protection; no matter how much loving feeling may flow between patient and doctor, somewhere in both is the awareness that it is a doctor being loved, not a man or a woman. Physicians who do not attend to the boundaries of their role learn this the hard way. A cartoon showed one doctor asking another about his black eye. "I mistook asthma for passion," said the first doctor. On the other hand, older physicians frequently take care of seriously ill long-term friends with whom they share deep affection or love. As a result of the emotional discipline that comes with long experience, they become the doctor the friend requires, subordinating those aspects of affection that might interfere with meeting the friend's needs—including, where necessary, ceding to another doctor. It is clear that the issue of the doctor's feelings is not simple. Doctors require awareness of their feelings in order to empathically experience the patient's feelings (see Chapter 12), they must discipline their feelings in the presence of the strong feelings of their patients, they must subordinate their feelings so that they can reason clearly and make difficult decisions, and they must reawaken their feelings with their family and friends in order to have a rewarding emotional life!

The closeness and bilaterality of the bond between healer and patient are acknowledged by the healing myths of some cultures that depict the healer assuming the patient's disease. This is symbolized by "extraction cures" wherein the healer searched for the diseased part of the patient's body and sucks out the disease, which may then be displayed for all to see. Sometimes it is a little bit of feather previously hidden in the healer's mouth and then bloodied from the healer's bitten cheek. The peril to the shaman is acknowledged but he is presumed to have the power to withstand what endangers the sick person. In Western medicine, a similar belief is evident in the familiar myth—if it is a myth—that specialists frequently die of the disease of their speciality. The same conception may underlie the hypochondriasis of second-year medical students—they develop symptoms of many of the worst diseases they study—which is virtually universal and a source of amusement to their faculty. Young physical therapists and third-year medical students also develop sympathetic pains in concert with their patients. By contrast, like the shaman with the bloodied feather in his mouth, senior house officers and attending physicians, in their frequent failure to wash their hands and disregard of other infection precautions, often act as if they were immune to disease. The contempt that many older physicians have for doctors afraid to take care of patients with AIDS seems to have a similar origin. Behaviors such as these are often considered to represent psychological defenses against the fears of acquiring diseases from patients—not merely infectious diseases, but all types.

The painful paradox of the relationship between doctor and patient is that for it to be employed to the fullest in the care of the patient, maximum possible openness to the patient must be present—but to be open is to be physically and emotionally endangered. If physicians are closed to their patients, on the other hand, they fail their patients—and fail themselves.

The Physician as a Person

Discussions of the relationship between patient and physician are prone to concentrate on the essential humanity of the patient and portray the physician as a stick figure. There are two persons in the relationship. It is true that to some degree the doctor can be defined by the role, but so can the patient. The doctor within that role is a person also; do physicians not also have "hands, organs, dimensions, senses, affections, passions" (5)? Fortunately, in the last fifteen years greater attention has been paid to the individual development of physicians. Concentration on the physician as a unique individual whose actions *as an individual* make a difference in the patient's care is directly derivative from the social trends discussed in Chapter 2. It is interesting to see the increased notice given to the individual development of student and physician in the Prefaces and Introductions to the Beeson-McDermott editions of the *Cecil-Loeb Textbook of Medicine.* This is a natural extension of Walsh McDermott's interest in person-encounter medicine and seems to stem in part from an effort to counter a recent public belief that the health status of a society has nothing to do with the work of individual physicians (6). It has become clear in recent years that medical training—particularly in the postgraduate years—is strongly directed to the moral development of physicians, not only the technical. This point has been well documented by Charles Bosk in his study of surgeons in training (7). But while many have stressed the importance of the moral values implied in the relationship between physician and patient, what is most important but has been of less concern are those aspects of the behavior of individual physicians that would both undergird the scientific and technological tools of the modern physician and be *teachable.* The difficulties involved in teaching virtue have engaged humankind since Hellenic Greece. Too often the problem is written off by saying that virtue is unteachable—students either have the propensity or they do not. But it has once again become apparent that the tools of modern medicine, with what seem to be their enormous power, must be directed by human faculties whose guiding precepts in the use of the technology will be moral as much as technical. In fact, it is too often forgotten that technology itself has *no* power—humans acquire power by employing the technology. Wherever power is present, it is the case both that responsibility exists that may or may not be accepted and that it is as logically possible that the power be used for ill as for good. It seems inadequate to stop at the notion that virtue in medicine is unteachable. What is necessary is some idea of what to include in the idea of the good physician that might provide a basis for the beginnings of systematic understanding and disciplined training.

What Defines a Good Physician

Walsh McDermott believed that one could define a good physician as one who is trustworthy, and a trustworthy physician as one who has self-discipline (8). With remarkably few wasted motions, he gets to the center of physicianship—trustworthiness and self-discipline. That good doctors are worthy of trust does not tell us why the care of the sick requires that trait. Doctors are persons who apply a specialized body of knowledge to the care of vulnerable sick persons. The sicker one is, the more knowledge that is accurate is absolutely necessary, and the more inadequate it often is. Because of both the inadequacies of knowledge and the fact that knowledge cannot act on its own, sick persons require doctors. Even if, as is often the case these days, the sick have the knowledge, they still require doctors because of the nature of sickness (9). Further, sickness always contains a threat to existence (real or imagined) and is always filled with uncertainties that impede or even paralyze effective action.

Uncertainty is intolerable at all times but more so in the ill because their existence seems threatened, yet they are required to make decisions about themselves. Unfortunately, as they perceive themselves to be increasingly endangered there is an increased urgency to act. But decisions and actions that are seen as having to do with one's very life require levels of certainty that are not available to the sick person—they simply do not have enough information, as no one does in such circumstances. Trust in others is one of the central human solutions to the paralysis of unbearable uncertainty. For these reasons the sick put their trust in doctors. The requirement for trust adds to the relationship between doctor and patient.

Sick persons, then, are people who are forced to trust. The better the doctor, the more trustworthy and the stronger the relationship. But doctors are also faced with uncertainties and are also threatened. Let physician readers remember their training days and how scared they always were that something untoward might happen to one of their patients; they were not merely concerned lest they fail—as anyone might be who tries to do a good job—but frightened in the same sense as when a loved one is endangered.

One important element of the threat to the doctor inherent in the patient's illness is the physician's responsibility for the patient. The doctor acquires the power to act on the patient's behalf because of the patient's trust. (In a complex society such as ours, cultural and legal factors have come to play a part in insuring that the doctor is responsible, but these factors are derived, I believe, from the basic need of the sick person to trust the doctor.) Wherever power is present, there is always the communal demand for responsible action—power always implies responsibility (10). It is true that the physician is not threatened unless responsibility is accepted. But society acknowledges the responsibility that physicians acquire because of their power by holding them accountable morally and legally in certain situations when they do not fulfill their responsibilities. The equation is complete. Doctors are people who, because of their special knowledge, are empowered to act by virtue of the trust given by patients, and who acquire responsibility thereby. In their actions on behalf of the sick person, endangered by the possibility of failing their responsibility, doctors become threatened by what threatens the patient. *Doctor and patient are bound in a reciprocal relationship*—failure to understand that is failure to comprehend clinical medicine.

In the light of this understanding it is possible to examine trustworthiness and self-discipline. The sick person bestows trust on a doctor in the context of sickness, the practice of medicine, and medical science. Patients always have at least social or cultural knowledge of medicine, and nowadays very much more than that. In these contexts, knowledge and competence are givens. That often-heard question "Would you rather have a technically competent doctor or one who is humane?" is beside the point. A doctor without technical competence would be inadequate and unworthy of trust. Knowledge by itself cannot indicate which patient it is to be used on and how. To be effective, physicians must be adept at working with patients—taking histories, establishing rapport, achieving compliance with regimens that may be extremely unpleasant, being sensitive to unspoken needs, providing empathetic support, and communicating effectively. Doctors who cannot do these things are neither adequate nor entirely trustworthy.

The Relation Between Trust and Altruism

Altruism, which seems important in physicians, is a concept muddied by the unfortunate history of the word. In the eighteenth century the idea was much debated in black-or-white terms. One was either altruistic or acted out of self-interest. Because many actions on behalf of others were seen to have an element of self-interest, altruism was denied. This all-or-none idea of altruism has, unhappily, been continued by sociobiologists who apply the term when an animal sacrifices itself to the continuation of the group. One would hope that sophistication about human behavior has increased enough in the last 200 years so that we can be free to accept the idea that when humans act in behalf of others the central question is not whether they also gain, but what it means to act in behalf of another. In keeping with modern usage, altruism here denotes actions on *behalf* of another.

It should be clear from the above that altruism is implied when a physician acts on the responsibility to care for a patient based on the sick person's trust. (Responsibility alone is not sufficient to demand altruism; a prison doctor may be responsible because of his or her duties, not because of the sick prisoner's trust.) It is quite clear that to act on behalf of another in medicine no longer means to act only on behalf of the other's body. The changes in the notions of person, of patienthood, and of the doctor-patient relationship that have occurred over these last decades emphasize that when the doctor acts for patients the action is meant to work toward the goals that the patients would choose if they could act on their own. What patients believe to be in their own best interests may well require the active participation of the physician to discover but can almost never be known without the patient's knowledgeable participation. Altruism in medicine requires more than knowledge of medical science; it also requires understanding illness—its causes, course, and outcome—from the patient's viewpoint, and then acting on the knowledge. Above all, it requires knowing about sick persons.

Self-Discipline

It is obvious that what threatens the sick is their diseases. Pneumonia is dangerous, but it generally responds to good care. Appendicitis is dangerous, but a relatively simple operation is curative. What gets in the way of good care for pneumonia or efficacious surgery for appendicitis is the wrong diagnosis. A diagnosis cannot simply be "pneumococcal pneumonia" or "appendicitis" but, as you will see in subsequent chapters, also must include appreciation of those factors—from the subcellular to the community—that underly the disease or affect the treatment. One wants to know all the answers: Is the pneumonia present because of underlying malignancy? Did the patient aspirate? Is the host malnourished or otherwise compromised? Will the patient follow the prescribed regimen? The question is not merely whether appendicitis is present but whether there is some hidden factor that increases the risk of surgery. The proper diagnosis results, above all, from thoroughness, from going through all the details—the dull, interminable details—that are involved in the treatment of the sick. Clearly, Walsh McDermott was correct in his belief that a trustworthy doctor is thorough and self-disciplined and that "*the deep belief in thoroughness is the most important element of medical education.*" (emphasis in the original) (11). It takes self-discipline to stay at the details. The internship is the place where the introduction to the details takes place. Alas, interns often believe that when they finish their internship, the details will be relegated to someone else—it certainly appears that way in modern training programs where the resident has often been elevated to the position of "advise and consent." But experienced physicians, when they are good, excel because of their mastery of the details as much as their mastery of medical knowledge. One of the signs of waning power in a surgeon is the loss of patience with the tiny moment-by-moment details of the operation.

Self-discipline and trustworthiness are involved in more than control of the details. Constancy to the patient is necessary. Constant attention and maintained presence are not difficult when things are going well. It requires self-discipline to maintain constancy when the case is going sour, when errors or failures have occurred, when the wrong diagnosis has been made, when the patient's personality or behavior is difficult or even repulsive, when impending death brings the danger of sorrow and loss because emotional closeness has been established. When constancy is absent or falters too frequently, patients lose that newfound part of themselves—the doctor—that promised stability in the uncertain world of sickness arising from their relationship.

With good reason, much has been made of the need for physicians to maintain their knowledge through constant educational effort, because it is evident that patients are threatened by physicians' ignorance. Good physicians admit their ignorance and call for help. It is true, but not self-evident, that over-referral is as bad as under-referral because it may reflect pandering, failure to take responsibility, or fear. Recognizing that a constant accompaniment of medical practice is fear that damage will be done to a patient through one's actions leads to the understanding that patients are also endangered by failure of the physician's nerve. This is something that most laypersons are fortunate not to know about. Whether it is not overdiagnosing serious illness, not starting or stopping treatment too soon, holding to a disputed diagnosis or course of action, or simply not turning and running when things get too bad, it takes nerve to care for the sick, and nerve requires self-discipline (both to be present and not to be converted to gunslinging). When doctors get old, the thing that probably goes first is not knowledge but nerve. Psychiatrists see suicide looming in every depression, surgeons feel cancer in every lump of fat in a breast, internists act as though every ache in the chest is a heart attack.

Self-discipline is necessary not only for thoroughness but for the maintenance of knowledge, constancy to patients, and nerve—all components of the trustworthy doctor and aspects of the relationship. When attributes of altruism and humaneness required to work with patients are added, it is obvious that technical competence is only the necessary beginning of a clinician. It seems clear that good physicians must not only command medical knowledge and comprehend sick persons, they must also understand doctors and, above all, have mastery over themselves. Perhaps in their best exemplification the virtues of a good doctor are unteachable. Perhaps in the same way it is not education that creates a Picasso. But just as even the inartistic can be taught to draw sufficiently to render a figure on paper, the basic attributes of these virtues are, I believe, both teachable and evaluable. Before the possibility is denied, it seems reasonable to ask who tried to do the teaching, how much time and money were spent, and how many people were committed to the task.

The relationship between physician and patient is a phenomenon as much a part of sickness and medicine as the diseases that make people sick. It makes a sick person into a patient and it makes a medical person into a doctor and a clinician. The most skillful practitioner raises the relationship to an art, not only encouraging its growth and promoting trust and faith on the part of the patient, but negotiating between intimacy and separateness, between empathy and objectivity. I remember reading, years ago, that one essential skill of the great racing driver, Juan Fangio, lay in coming as close to the coefficient of friction of his tires as humanly possible. Access to the patient is necessary for successful treatment. Intimacy makes that possible. One of the skills in the art of great clinicians lies in coming as close as ethically possible to intimacy—for the access to the patient that it provides—while maintaining independence of action. Therein lies the capacity for maximum therapeutic power in the patient's behalf.

References

1. Pellegrino, Edmund D. and Thomasma, David C. *For the Patient's Good. The Restoration of Beneficence in Health Care.* 1988. New York, Oxford University Press.

2. Pellegrino, Edmund D. and Thomasma, David C. *A Philosophical Basis of Medical Practice.* 1981. New York, Oxford University Press. Chap. 3.

3. Cassell, Eric J. *The Healer's Art.* 1985. Cambridge, Mass., MIT Press, p. 13.

4. Cassell, Eric J. *Talking With Patients: Volume 1. The Theory of Doctor-Patient Communication.* 1985. Cambridge, Mass., MIT Press, p. 175ff.

5. Shakespeare, William. *The Merchant of Venice.* III, i l.51–52.

6. McDermott, Walsh. Medicine: The Public's Good and One's Own. *Perspectives in Biology and Medicine.* 1978; 21:167–87.

7. Bosk, Charles. *Forgive and Remember.* 1979. Chicago, University of Chicago Press.

8. McDermott, Walsh. Education and General Medical Care. *Ann. Intern Med.* 1982; 96:512–17.

9. Cassell, Eric J. *The Healer's Art.* 1985. Cambridge, Mass., MIT Press, p. 35ff.

10. Jonas, Hans. *The Imperative of Responsibility.* 1984. Chicago, University of Chicago Press. Chap. 4.

11. McDermott, Walsh. Education and General Medical Care. *Ann. Intern. Med.* 1982; 96:512–17.

6

How To Understand Diseases

PREVIOUS CHAPTERS HAVE shown the difficulties that arise, first in the relief of suffering and then in understanding the chronically ill, when the primary focus of physicians is the disease. I have suggested that a shift is taking place in medicine away from a primary concern with diseases and toward a focus on sick persons. This chapter will begin to address the difficult issues that must be faced and solved before such a change in goals can be completed. First I would like to show why for clinicians—doctors who actually take care of patients—disease theory has been so necessary and successful. Clinicians have four fundamental tasks whenever they see a patient: (1) to find out what is the matter—diagnosis; (2) to find out how it happened—cause; (3) to decide what to do—treatment; (4) to predict the outcome—prognosis. Every aspect of dealing with a patient's complaints, from identification of a virus to reassurance, forms a part of these duties. So when practicing physicians—clinicians—attempt to find out what is wrong with someone, they seek something in that person which (with their specialized knowledge) will permit them to carry out their four fundamental tasks.

There have been many successes over the whole 2,500 years of medical history in the gathering of knowledge about disease. The essence of modern disease theory that developed in the early nineteenth century is contained in the beliefs that persons become sick because they have a disease; diseases are entities, each with a unique cause and a unique underlying structural or (nowadays) biochemical abnormality; and diseases can be discovered in the sick person by finding the characteristic structural or biochemical abnormality (Chapter 1). Not surprisingly, such ideas do not fit all the known afflictions of humankind—there are states of illness that seemed to be characterized by rather constant pathologic changes, but more than one cause can be found. These are usually called syndromes. There are other conditions that do not necessarily have any recognizable abnormalities of structure—that is, at autopsy a patient with one of these conditions is not found to have anything recognizably the matter with the body's organs. Hyperacidity of the stomach is one of these conditions; early hypertension is another. Originally they were known as functional disorders. These and many other words have entered medical terminology because no system of the classification of diseases is ever entirely satisfactory. The ills that afflict us are too diverse, our knowledge of them changes constantly, and our more fundamental ideas about diseases are also in a state of flux. In Chapter 1 I also discussed how theories of disease throughout the history of medicine have alternated, basically, between two concepts: physiological and ontological. The first viewpoint, the physiological (now most closely identified with the ecological perspective), is that diseases occur because of an altered balance in the inner relationships of the body and between the body and the environment. The founder of modern pathology, Rudolph Virchow, described that idea in 1847 when he was twenty-six years old: "Diseases have no independent or isolated existence; they are not autonomous organisms, not beings invading a body, nor parasites growing on it; they are only the manifestations of life processes under altered conditions" (1). The ontologic point of view is that diseases are *things,* entities with a separate existence from the person who has them. No one has described this concept better than the same Rudolph Virchow who, in 1895 at age seventy-four, *had completely reversed his position.* "In my view a disease entity is an altered part of the body. . . . In this sense I am a thorough-going ontologist and have always regarded it as a merit to have brought into harmony with genuine scientific knowledge the old and essentially justified assertion that disease is a living entity that leads a parasitic existence. Every diseased part of the body has indeed a parasitic relationship with the otherwise healthy body to which it belongs and at the expense of which it lives" (2). Virchow was so influential that his ideas prevailed long after he died.

I believe it would be useful to use three common diseases to show how the ideas contained in classic disease theory—diseases have unique structure and unique cause, can be discovered in sick people by discovering the characteristic abnormality, and are ontological versus physiological entities—are exemplified and used in the practice of medicine. At the same time I will be able to illustrate the practical consequences of the changes that have taken place in these axioms of disease theory over the last few decades. You will see how making a diagnosis is related to both the disease and prevailing ideas about it. Let us use cancer of the breast, pneumonia, and heart attacks (coronary heart disease) as examples.

Cancer of the breast is suspected if a woman (or rarely a man) has a lump in the breast. We only know with certainty that cancer is present if the tissue of the lump is examined under the microscope and its cells have the characteristic appearance (structural abnormality) of one of the several kinds of breast cancer. For this reason biopsies are done. Everything else—the way the lump feels to the fingers, mammograms, thermograms, or any other test—may be suggestive of cancer, but only the cells under a microscope tell the final story. The matter, however, does not end with simply finding the abnormal breast tissue. Even after a breast is removed because of cancer, a number of years later there may be evidence that the cancer is present somewhere else—that it has metastasized. If tissue is taken from the new place in which the cancer is found—a bone or the liver, for example—the cells will still (in most instances) be identifiable as breast cancer cells. As doctors we say that the person has breast cancer (in the present tense) even though the breast that had the cancer is gone. We speak in this fashion because, clearly, breast cancer is more than an abnormal breast, it is an entity with the capacity to spread to and grow in distant places even years after the original tumor. It has the potential for a number of different behaviors known to physicians (3). All that knowledge is organized around the entity that is defined by what its cells look like under the microscope. Cancer of the breast would seem to best fit the old ontological idea (restated by Virchow) that the tumor is a foreign entity, a parasitic thing separate from the body that spreads once it has taken hold, unless it can be removed before such spread has occurred. Indeed, that is the way people commonly speak of their own tumors, as an *it* (4). These beliefs are also the basis for the speed with which people want to have their cancer operated on, as well as for the common (but incorrect) fear that operating on it may disturb the cancer or dislodge its cells and stimulate it to spread.

Because cancer of the breast (and virtually every other kind of tumor) was considered a separate entity, it made sense that it should be completely removed surgically. The most common operation for breast cancer (until recently) was the radical mastectomy devised by the famous surgeon, William Stewart Halsted, in 1889. The reason for performing this operation was that it removed not only the breast but also the lymphatic tissue and adjacent muscle into which the cancer might have spread, thus maximizing the chance of "getting it all out"—removing the disease by removing the structural abnormalities. (I put the phrase in quotation marks because it is so commonly used in reference to cancer surgery.) The last two decades have witnessed a significant move away from radical mastectomy as the operation of choice for breast cancer. Controlled trials have demonstrated that patients with small tumors who merely have the tumor mass removed (lumpectomy) and then have radiation to the breast do not get recurrent cancer or die with any greater frequency than patients who have radical surgery. Further, there is a growing belief that the inherent biological behavior of any particular breast cancer (there is considerable variation) rather than the nature of the cancer of the breast in general is of greater importance in determining what will happen to a woman with the disease than (within limits) early diagnosis or the extent of the surgery. Clearly, hormonal and other factors influence what happens to a woman (or man) with breast cancer. The development of chemotherapy and hormonal therapy, the knowledge gained from their use, and newer insights into the molecular basis of malignant transformation have furthered the move away from the view that this and other cancers are merely foreign things that invade the body.

It is popularly believed that emotional factors play a part in the development, course, and outcome of breast and other cancers, but this has been, thus far, impossible to show conclusively. It is absolutely true, however, that emotional and social factors have an enormous impact on how the patient with breast cancer lives after the discovery of the tumor and, consequently, on the disease itself. Whether patients are operated on, what operation is chosen, whether an active sex life is resumed or persons return to work, whether chemotherapy is permitted and how it is tolerated, whether the remainder of the person's life is spent in active fear of the cancer's return or the matter is put behind her (or him) are all determined by the person. Presently, women frequently take an active part in the choice of operation or other treatment of breast cancer. It is mandated by law in New York State that physicians and surgeons present all the options for treatment to the patient. In addition, there is active concern (without much evidence of its utility) with the prevention of breast cancer through diet or the avoidance of certain medications. We are a long way from the old view of seeing cancer of the breast as solely a parasite in an otherwise healthy body or the patient as merely the helpless and hapless victim.

Pneumonia, as a disease, is, by definition, an inflammation of the alveoli, sacs in the lungs where oxygen and carbon dioxide are exchanged between the blood and the air. Normally, the lungs are light and spongy because of the innumerable air-filled alveoli. Where pneumonia is present, the lungs get heavy and feel thick, like liver, as the alveolar walls swell and they fill up with mucus, pus, and other products of inflammation. This inflammation is the structural abnormality characteristic of pneumonia. The air sacs no longer work as gas exchangers. Pneumonia, like cancer of the breast, was originally defined by the microscopic appearance of the lungs of people whom it killed. Because places in the lung where pneumonia is present are so dense, they appear distinctly abnormal on a chest X ray. They also sound different when a doctor listens with a stethoscope to air moving in and out of the lungs. We no longer require that the lungs be examined under a microscope to make a positive diagnosis of pneumonia; the characteristic appearance on an X ray is sufficient. Thus, the shadow that pneumonia casts on an X ray is now taken (for the purposes of caring for patients) as the equivalent of the thing itself. Although William Osler stated in his 1892 textbook, *The Principles and Practice of Medicine,* "An organism, the *Diplococcus pneumoniae* [the pneumococcus] is invariably found in the diseased lung," we now know that pneumonia can come from many different organisms—viruses, bacteria, fungi, or parasites—as well as many other causes, and sometimes pneumonia of different causes looks the same under the microscope—one cannot assume a specific cause. Doctors need to know what kind of pneumonia someone has before they can know what to treat it with or how it will behave. Often no definite identification of the organism or cause is made. Rather, the cause is inferred from other evidence—symptoms, how seriously ill the person is, what is found on examination and laboratory tests—with sufficient accuracy for effective treatment. Even though pnuemonia is a disease entity with a specific abnormality of the structure of the lung in the same manner as cancer of the breast is defined by specific changes in the structure of the breast, in everyday practice, doctors use substitutes (the X-ray picture) to stand for those changes in the structure of the lung. The substitution is possible because, over the years, criteria have been developed to help in deciding when there is enough other evidence to justify the inference that if one could actually look directly at the lungs, pneumonia would be found.

In the years since antibiotics entered medicine, attitudes toward pneumonia as well as the kinds of pneumonia have changed. When the little boy in *Mrs. Wiggs of the Cabbage Patch* developed pneumonia it was most probably caused by the pneumococcus. That is the classic type of pneumonia. Before antibiotics it was fatal in 20 to 35 percent of patients. Then, as now, the highest death rate occurred in the poor and in alcoholics. Its onset was dramatic—a robustly healthy young man had a common cold one day and the next day might be sick unto death, and one week later, dead! It commonly resolved by what was called a crisis—on the fifth, seventh, ninth, or eleventh day (usually in the morning) the fever fell precipitously to normal and the patient survived. Convalescence took weeks to months. There were "pneumonia doctors" who would sit by the patient's bedside through the worst of the illness. They knew how to read the signs of the illness and how to tell what was going to happen. My students are always amused when I tell them how much I admire the pneumococcus because it is an aristocratic bacterium and a noble enemy. It caused no smoldering, indolent infections of the kind so common these days; when the pneumococcus got a good hold, it killed quickly and cleanly—the kind of disease that reminds one of the romance of being a doctor. This is the pneumonia that is the classical model for the pathology and autopsy appearance of pneumonia that all doctors learn. Antibiotics changed all of that. Eighteen hours after the first dose of penicillin (and not much penicillin at that), the fever is gone. In a few days the patient feels well again. After the antibiotic is given, the lung does not show the same pathologic appearance.

Doctors do not see the autopsy appearance of pneumococcal pneumonia anymore. This is not because there are no deaths—many people still die of pneumococcal pneumonia, but they are mostly those with some underlying disease or who have had their spleen removed (adversely affecting their ability to resist the pneumococci). Rather, doctors hardly ever go to autopsies at all. The chest X ray or the CAT scan is the referee nowadays, not the autopsy. In addition, although there are important exceptions (Legionnaires' disease, for example), most pneumonias in otherwise healthy people are usually either trivially easy to treat or patients get better by themselves (despite the fear that the word itself still evokes). Pneumonia, however, has not ceased to be a problem. It may be one of the most common causes of death in patients with AIDS, cancer, chronic heart failure, Alzheimer's disease, stroke, and other afflictions that ultimately reduce the ability of the person to fight off infection. Since pneumococcal pneumonia is simple to treat, these people are saved from that infection by antibiotics. But since their basic problem ultimately gets worse, they almost inevitably get pneumonia again. But because of the antibiotics, the next pneumonia (or the one after that, or the third, or fourth, and so on) may be caused by a bacterium that is more resistant to treatment. Most often the causative organism is one that lives in the mouth or bowel of the patient and has become a cause of disease because the change in the person's resistance to infection has tipped in its favor the delicate balance all of us have with the billions of microorganisms that inhabit each of us. Sometimes the person acquires the infection in the hospital. Such bacteria are notoriously resistant to antibiotics. Because treatment requires more complex antibiotics that must usually be administered intravenously, there are more complications of treatment, including other infections (of the bladder or kidneys, for example), diarrhea, or fungus infections of the mouth. Each of these adds to the patients' difficulties and requires further treatment. In these circumstances, not surprisingly, the doctor is paying more attention to what bacteria can be grown out of the blood or sputum (since their identification and antibiotic sensitivities determine treatment) than to the pathologic appearance of the lung. In fact, pneumonia in these settings is not so much a disease in itself as a part of the process of the cancer, AIDS, chronic heart failure, or whatever is the patient's central problem. For the doctor, the fact that the infection is in the lungs, while obviously important (the person with lungs that are not working well requires a different kind of support from one whose kidneys are malfunctioning), is not the basic issue; the process of infection and its place in the compromised host are what must occupy decision making. And although each individual bacterium is surely the direct cause of the pneumonia, as in the original nineteenth century conception of the cause of disease, the fact of the patient's inability to fight infection is an even more important cause. Since, in many of these patients, a very important aspect of their care revolves around the ethical issues involved in treating people for pneumonia who will surely die in any case, even the bacteria do not get top billing in the minds of many clinicians. The issue is whether to treat at all—whether the patient should be allowed to die. Thus, like breast cancer, notions about pneumonia have changed in the last half-century. Currently, pnuemonia is conceived of more in terms of the relationship of the patient to his or her own bacteria and with the environment of medical care.

The way doctors think about the next disease we are going to consider, coronary heart disease and heart attacks, has moved even further away from being defined, in everyday practice, by abnormalities of structure. The disease in which heart attacks, also called myocardial infarction and (less often) coronary thrombosis, occur is formally known as arteriosclerotic heart disease—from the Greek for hardening of the artery. This name comes from the fact that when the blood vessels of the heart, the coronary arteries, are afflicted by the process known as atherosclerosis, they are changed from their normal uniform diameters into stiff, tortuous tubes whose muscular walls have deteriorated and become scarred, and whose normally smooth linings have proliferated in a manner that impedes the flow of blood, sometimes completely. The vessels may also be progressively closed down by plaques composed of fatty material that are attached to the lining. In those areas of the coronary arteries in which the disease (arteriosclerosis) has gone on long enough, the fatty plaques are converted into areas of scarlike tissue and bony hard material composed of calcium that further distort the architecture of the blood vessel, narrowing it even more. Ultimately the vessel closes down completely and deprives the heart muscle of blood from the artery. When the vessel has been getting narrow slowly, alternate blood vessels are formed, collectively called collateral circulation, to make up the deficiency in blood supply.

In circumstances where a blood clot forms in the abnormally narrow blood vessel, the blood is suddenly stopped from providing the muscle in that area with oxygen and nutrients (and removing CO_2 and waste products). The heart muscle in the area supplied by that vessel suddenly dies (becomes infarcted). In the process, the classic symptoms that have become known to virtually everyone are usually produced. The sudden onset of oppressive pain across the middle of the front of the chest sometimes accompanied by pain that radiates down the left arm in association with fear, cold sweat, and nausea, while by no means always present in heart attacks, are a signal of the heart's catastrophe. It is difficult to imagine a doctor (or even a layperson) alive who, on hearing of these symptoms, would not think first of myocardial infarction. The diagnosis is confirmed when either characteristic changes occur in the patient's electrocardiogram or blood tests reveal abnormally high levels of certain substances (enzymes) that are normally contained within the intact cells of normal heart muscle, but are released into the circulation as the cells lose their integrity because of the interference with the blood supply to that part of the heart.

Arteriosclerotic heart disease kills more Americans than any other disease, yet the diagnosis of heart attack was first made in a living person in 1912 by James B. Herrick of Chicago. Since that time, and until quite recently, doctors who made the diagnosis of myocardial infarction or coronary thrombosis (in the past interchangable terms) never actually saw the clot in the coronary artery or the damaged heart muscle. Both were *inferred,* in the earliest years, from the symptoms alone, then from the symptoms and the electrocardiogram, and subsequently from the symptoms, the electrocardiogram, and the blood tests for cardiac enzymes. As in the case of pneumonia, criteria have been established that state what degree of abnormality in electrocardiograms and blood tests are required before the diagnosis of myocardial infarction can be considered certain. When these criteria are not satisfied, the person will not be considered to have had a heart attack no matter what the symptoms may have been. I am sure many readers have spent a few days in hospital cardiac intensive-care units waiting to see if their tests "ruled out" (medical jargon) a myocardial infarction. Several years ago that process took a week, then five days, and now criteria can be met one way or the other after one to three days.

If at first symptoms alone were sufficient for the diagnosis, then (after its introduction) the electrocardiogram made the disease diagnosis in patients with or without classic symptoms, and now enzyme tests have been accepted as the final arbiters of the disease diagnosis no matter what the symptoms or the electrocardiogram suggest, then there are probably people who have symptoms but do not meet the criteria but do have heart disease. In medicine, we do not find out what is the matter (see Chapter 6), we make a diagnosis. One of the most important heritages of modern disease theory is that to be acceptable to doctors, a diagnosis must meet certain standards—match a previously agreed-upon pattern. It is not enough that I am satisfied that your Uncle Herbert had a heart attack and that Dr. Jones agrees; what we find on examining Uncle Herbert (and his electrocardiogram and blood tests) must satisfy criteria accepted by the profession or other doctors will not accept what Dr. Jones and I say. But heart attacks, like almost all things in nature, occur on a continuum—you may not be able to be a little bit pregnant, but you can have a little bit of a heart attack. Criteria for diagnosis, to be useful, must include the majority of instances of a disease (true positives) and exclude the majority of instances where *no* disease is present (true negatives). But it follows that there are people who have been told that they have had myocardial infarctions but have not (false positives), and people who have been told that they have not had a heart attack but have (false negatives), a concept introduced into medicine by Alvin R. Feinstein (5,6). Surprisingly, a study of people admitted to a cardiac intensive-care unit for chest pain showed that those who did *not* meet the criteria for heart attack (and thus were sent home under the assumption that they were without disease) had a death rate in the following year almost as high as those who did meet the criteria—were told that they had had a heart attack (7).

These facts show that heart attacks are not diseases in the same absolute manner as cancer of the breast or pneumonia. What would the disease be? Death of heart muscle (myocardial infarction)? The clot in the coronary artery (coronary thrombosis)? Neither is unique in structural change or cause. In fact, they are not diseases at all but rather incidents in the course of another disease—arteriosclerotic heart disease. Arteriosclerotic heart disease has certain characteristics that made the medical world think about all diseases somewhat differently. If diseases are *things* in the ontological sense—entities that parasitize or occupy the otherwise healthy organ or person—they ought to have a discrete beginning and end. That is one of the characteristics of entities and objects. But it is very difficult to determine when arteriosclerosis starts. The first hint of this was in the Korean War, when autopsies performed on soldiers killed in action—otherwise fit young men—showed unmistakable arteriosclerosis in the coronary arteries. The same discovery was made about young civilians who died in automobile accidents. By now, it is clear that the earliest signs of coronary artery arteriosclerosis (or atherosclerosis) can be found even in young children. As is well known, the disease never goes away, being discoverable in almost every very old person. When this information is combined with the widely accepted association among fat in the diet, cholesterol levels, and coronary artery disease, we begin to see that the previously accepted view of myocardial infarction as a disease in the classical, ontological sense does not work. Newer knowledge about the protective effects of exercise, the ability to reduce risk by altering lifestyle, and the benefit of stopping cigarette smoking (one of the most potent risk factors) increases the belief that most heart attacks come about because of the deleterious interaction of individuals with their environment as a result of how they choose to live their lives. The idea of choice is very much accepted at this time. People believe that individuals can choose to live a healthier life, that such choice is an important aspect of life, and that the healthier lifestyle will lead to a lower probability of heart attacks and other diseases.

When I was a medical student at New York University in the early 1950s and patients with heart disease were admitted to our wards, we were all eager to make a diagnosis. Our question was rarely whether the patient had heart disease—that was generally obvious because the poor did not go to a hospital until they were really sick—but what *kind* of heart disease? Was it rheumatic heart disease (still very common in those days), syphilitic heart disease (then becoming unusual), congenital heart disease, arteriosclerotic heart disease, or some other rare type? We listened to their hearts with great care and used every trick of physical examination that had been devised in the last century. Then we pored over the X rays that had been accumulated over the years (many of these patients had been followed for years in the famous IIIrd Division [Bellevue] Thursday Night Cardiac Clinic). Opinions were expressed and written in the chart in the formal manner devised by the New York Heart Association. When the patient died of the heart disease (a common occurence), we all went to the autopsy to see the truth revealed. Often the heart at autopsy looked exactly as had been predicted. Sometimes debates that had gone on for years among the senior attending physicians about exactly what heart valve was damaged were finally settled. At other times, to everyone's surprise, a different heart valve was involved than had been expected. If it turned out that the wrong diagnosis had been made when the patient was alive, no harm had been done (except to some expert's damaged ego) because the treatment was the same whatever the anatomical (structural) lesion of the heart.

What I have written may seem calloused, as though we did not care about treatment. Not true. We literally fought night and day to save their lives but, compared to current therapies, what we did was not very effective. (Physicians who are used to having death pull lives away from their hands find solace in the beauty of the ineluctable process of nature. For doctors, disease is merely nature working.) Cardiac surgery was still not an everyday matter, and cardiac catheterization—the technique of putting a fine tube inside the heart to measure its performance—although first perfected at our school, was sufficiently cumbersome so that it was not performed on everybody with heart disease. By the time of my residency (Bellevue Hospital, the IIIrd Medical Division), the emphasis had begun to change. Mitral valve surgery for rheumatic heart disease was becoming commonplace and other heart surgery was being increasingly perfected. The issue of importance had changed from *making the diagnosis* (to be confirmed at autopsy) to deciding who would benefit from surgery. The emphasis is decidedly different. If someone is to be operated on, two things must be true: what is wrong with them must be correctable by surgery, and the benefit must outweigh the risk. The wrong anatomical diagnosis was no longer tolerable. It would be terrible to send a patient for the repair of a damaged mitral valve only to discover at the operating table that the mitral valve was fine but the aortic valve was where the trouble lay. At the time, the only technique that afforded such precision of diagnosis was cardiac catheterization and angiography. These measured how the heart valves were working, provided an assessment of overall cardiac function, and produced X-ray motion pictures of the heart in action. Thus, cardiac catheterization became a routine procedure for the diagnosis of valvular (congenital, rheumatic, syphilitic, but not arteriosclerotic) heart disease. The question of risk versus benefit depended on some measure of the severity of the patient's condition, knowledge of the natural history of these kinds of disease (which medicine had accumulated for many years)—what would happen without treatment—in addition to an idea of how well the patient (not just the heart) was doing. After all, if an operation was very risky but the patient was able to function *in terms of his or her own lifestyle,* then the severity of the structural abnormality of the heart itself (how badly damaged the valve was) might not be sufficient reason to take the chance of an operation. (For many people who had become virtually bound to their chair or bed because they did not have enough breath to walk on the street, the risk of dying during the operation did not seem anything compared to the chance of being truly alive again. In those early days of heart operations, surgeons often seemed to have performed miracles. The patients were able to take part in an active life again in a fashion that had been closed to them for years.)

The importance of assessing the patient's function was not new. If one has no instruments to directly measure how well the heart performs, then what the patient is able to do (in which cardiac function is a limiting factor) must serve as a substitute. Carefully questioning someone about how many pillows are used at night, the ability to walk on a level, stair-climbing, lifting, carrying, haircombing, eating, and so on can give an estimate. For the patient's account to serve as a reliable measure of cardiac performance, however, the questioner must skillfully dissect the information away from the interpretations, additions, and subtractions that are part of every person's process of recounting (8). The great clinicians who taught themselves the fine art of asking about symptoms were primarily interested in what the *patient's function* told them about the *heart's structure.* Thus, if one can visualize the valvular anatomy of the heart as one is hearing symptoms, one can translate the patient's inabilities into the heart's abnormalities. In 1928, The New York Heart Association (then The Heart Committee of the New York Tuberculosis and Health Association) introduced its form of writing a cardiac diagnosis (9). These manuals, which were continuously updated and improved, contained the specific criteria that had to be met before a diagnosis of a particular kind of heart disease could be made. It cannot be stressed too strongly how important to medicine's progress it has been that the disease formulation started in the nineteenth century meant that when two doctors were speaking of arteriosclerotic heart disease, for example, *they were talking about the same thing!* The innovation (which was subsequently widely accepted) was not merely in entering the disease diagnosis (e.g., arteriosclerotic heart disease) or the anatomic abnormalities (e.g., coronary sclerosis), but rather that a diagnosis of heart disease was not considered complete unless it also contained both a physiological diagnosis (e.g., angina pectoris) and a statement of the patient's functional capacity (in terms of what the doctor thought the patient *should* do and what the patient *could* do). The book gave specific criteria for functional classes. The purpose of the New York Heart Association manuals was to standardize clinical practice and provide standardized measures of heart disease for research. However, it gave its blessing to an assessment of the patient's function as a formal part of clinical practice.

The effect of the newer technologies of cardiac assessment—cardiac catheterization and angiography—as with all that have followed (echocardiography, radionuclide cineangiography [RNCA], and exercise studies) and the electrocardiogram that preceded them was to provide means for directly determining the performance of the heart. This trend was given an enormous boost in the late 1960s when Americans began to take up exercise with their current zeal. I remember my excitement when I started to do exercise testing on a bicycle ergometer in 1968; the heart suddenly became for me a machine *in action.* All my previous examinations had been of the heart in persons at rest or engaged in some artificial exercise. It is not an exaggeration to say that I learned more about the heart's function in those first few months of exercise testing (and doing my own running) than I had in years before that. There is a vast conceptual difference between conceiving of the healthy or diseased body in static terms as opposed to dynamic ideas about something in motion. Static ideas about the body—the emphasis on structure—have occupied medicine for most of its history. My experience with exercise testing and its effect on my thinking have, I believe, been shared by many physicians.

The newer technologies of cardiac assessment have had major effects on medicine and medical practice. First, they markedly reduce uncertainty about what is the matter with the heart. Second, they displace the patient from the center of the assessment of function, focusing entirely on the organ. Third, they emphasize function and reduce the diagnostic importance of structural abnormality. The first and second effects are, as always, related. In medicine, whenever something reduces uncertainty, physicians (and laypersons) will follow the values inherent in and the dictates of the technology involved. Thus, although measurement methods such as cardiac catheterization or coronary angiography are brought into play because of patients' symptoms or dysfunction, they bring such certainty that doctors and patients begin to act as though reality were depicted on the X-ray movies of patients' coronary arteries. Thus patients begin to have coronary artery surgery because of the abnormalities found on their tests rather than because of their determined need for operation. While the two are often the same—what the patient needs and what the patient's coronary arteries require—they are frequently *not* identical.

The example of arteriosclerotic heart disease and heart attacks has also shown the change in these last decades from a concentration on diseases of the heart in terms of structural abnormalities characteristic of specific causes of heart disease—for example, rheumatic heart disease, arteriosclerotic heart disease, or syphilitic heart disease—toward a concern with the heart as a functioning machine. Now we can and do think of the heart as an electrical system necessary for the initiation of the heartbeat, a hydraulic system with valves that control flow, and a muscular pump required to move the blood. Treatment is similarly conceived. Physicians do not treat "causes," they use drugs and surgery to restore performance or relieve dysfunction in a manner specific to the problem. This way of thinking, which resulted from the study of pathophysiology, has become increasingly important in all fields of medicine supplementing and enriching the perspective of anatomical pathology. Further, heart disease has increasingly come to be seen as a disorder of lifestyle—a person can exercise considerable control over whether he or she will ever have a heart attack. The changes in diet and exercise considered "good for" the heart have become part of the American way of life. This, with the widespread decrease in cigarette smoking, may well be responsible for the considerable reduction in the incidence and prevalence of coronary heart disease. (The concentration on prevention is clearly an attack on basic causes, even if current therapies are not.) Because of the role played by persons in their own health and the concentration on pathophysiology and the performance aspects of the heart, one would have believed that a concurrent concentration on the *patients* who have heart disease would have occurred. However, that has not been the case. Once again, the specific effect of technology (not science) has been to maintain the focus of doctors on the object of the technology (here, the heart) and on the values of that technology—what is good or bad in terms of technology—rather than on the persons or the values of the persons whose hearts are the object of concern. It is apparent that the newer diagnostic and treatment technologies—for all their effectiveness—have moved the concerns of doctors (and laypersons) further from the arena of suffering than when physicians made their diagnoses primarily with their questions and their hands.

If I were to ask, after what you have read, what a disease is, you might have difficulty coming up with one definition that fits all the afflictions that befall persons. You can see that the structural definitions laid down in the nineteenth century, while enormously useful in bringing some order of classification to all those afflictions (and thus allowing science to enter medicine in a useful and important way), have real limitations. They are helpful friends for the clinicians (see the clinician's four fundamental tasks at the start of this chapter), but clinicians have gone beyond them as they pursue pathophysiology. In fact, I think you will be unable to come up with any definition that is not so vague as to be useless as a practical guide to action.

There is another possibility, and that is to refrain from creating any definition of disease at all, remaining content to focus the attention of medicine and doctors on the complaints of sick people. H. Tristram Engelhardt pointed out a number of years ago that disease nomenclature and medical practice tended to be responsive to the complaints of patients, and that disease nomenclature and medicine's high-minded concentration on science and diseases just covered up that fact (10). While Engelhardt knowingly exaggerated, the relationship of sick persons to their afflictions and through the sickness to doctors and medicine is not entirely clear. It is recognized universally that the relationship of patient and doctor is central to medical practice, but what has not been articulated is the nature of the sick person's association with the sickness. In the strict ontological view, when the disease is an entity, the patient is at best an unlucky and unhappy container of the sickness—it would not matter much who had it, the effect would be the same. But, as we have seen, ontological concepts are losing their grip on us, as we have come to believe the illness to be an integral aspect of the patient's life and environment. In this setting, how are the disease and the patient connected? As we will see in the next chapter, how that question is answered plays a fundamental role in ideas about medical care, notions of good doctoring, and the conception of the ideal physician.

References

1. Virchow, Rudolph. Quoted in R. Krupl Taylor. *The Concepts of Illness Disease and Morbus.* 1979. New York, Cambridge University Press. p. 11.

2. Virchow, Rudolph. Quoted in R. Krupl Taylor, op. cit., p. 12.

3. King, Lester S. *Medical Thinking: A Historical Preface.* 1982. Princeton, N.J., Princeton University Press, p. 173ff.

4. Cassell, Eric. J. Disease as an "It": Concepts of Disease Revealed by Patients' Presentation of Symptoms. *Social Science and Medicine* 1976; 10:143–46.

5. Feinstein, Alvan R. *Clinical Epidemiology.* 1985. Philadelphia, W. B. Saunders.

6. Feinstein, Alvan R. *Clinical Judgement.* 1974. Melbourne, Fla., Robert E. Krieger.

7. Wilcox, R. G., Roland, J. M. and Hampton, J. R. Prognosis of Patients with "Chest Pain ?Cause." *Br. Med. J.* [*Clin Res*]. Feb 7. 1981; 282(6262): pp. 431–33.

8. Cassell, Eric J. *Talking to Patients: Clinical Technique.* Vol. 2. 1985. Cambridge, Mass., MIT Press, Chap. 2.

9. The Heart Committee. Joseph H. Bainton and others, Harold E. B. Pardee, Chairman. *Criteria for the Classification and Diagnosis of Heart Disease.* 1928. New York, Paul B. Hoeber.

10. Engelhardt, H. Tristram, Jr. Doctoring the Disease, Treating the Complaint, Helping the Patient: Some of the Works of Hygeia and Panacea. *Knowing and Valuing: Vol. IV. The Foundations of Ethics and Its Relationship to Science.* Edited by H. Tristram Engelhardt, Jr. and Daniel Callahan. 1980. New York, The Hastings Center.

7

The Pursuit of Disease or the Care of the Sick?

The physician must be able to tell the antecedents, know the present, and foretell the future—must meditate these things and have two special objects in view with regard to diseases, namely to do good or to do no harm. The art consists in three things—the disease, the patient, and the physician. The physician is the servant of the art, and the patient must combat the disease along with the physician (1).

AS WE SAW IN Chapters 3 and 4, sick persons do not suffer solely because they have a disease but because they are persons in all their varied dimensions of personhood. On the other hand, to understand suffering, it will not do to simply dismiss the disease process as something mechanical or unimportant to truly human concerns. This chapter and the next, which together form one investigation, address the relationship between the sick person and the sickness, between the disease entity and its existence in a sick person.

Starting with the making of a diagnosis, it is helpful to examine the place of symptoms in medical care. Virtually all medical care starts with a symptom—a person notices that something is wrong. The experience of a symptom is the patient's first step toward illness. [For this discussion, illness is the affliction of the whole person, whereas disease is something an organ has (2).] When the symptom is taken to a doctor, it is the doctor's first acquaintance with the illness. As we will see, although patients and doctors speak of symptoms as though they are referring to the same thing, that is far from true.

"Doctor, What Is Wrong with Me?"

It is frequently troubling to patients to discover that most doctors are not primarily interested in finding out what is the matter with them but are concerned instead with discovering what disease is the source of their illness. To laypersons these two functions—finding the trouble and discovering the disease—appear to be the same, but a subtle but vital difference exists. They are the same task *if and only if* a disease is causing the illness. For example, if you have burning or hunger-type pain in the upper part of your abdomen that comes on about two hours after eating and is relieved by milk or some food, you may suspect you have an ulcer. The doctor agrees with you—his or her suspicions are sharpened by questioning you to discover that you have been awakening at about two in the morning with similar distress. Upper gastrointestinal X rays (a GI series) are taken which, in this instance, do not show an ulcer—or any other abnormality, for that matter. Perhaps the physician believes so strongly that an ulcer is present that gastroscopy (looking into the stomach through an instrument) is the next diagnostic step. Again, the endoscopist can find no disease. In all probability your doctor will reassure you that there is nothing the matter, and suggest that you try a drug such as Tagamet (an H_2 blocker that inhibits stomach-acid production) or some antacids. If the pain stops when you take the Tagamet, the explanation will likely be that the discomfort was related to stomach acid production. If the pain does not stop, your return to the doctor will occasion further tests—perhaps X rays of your gall bladder, then small or large intestines, and finally a CAT scan of the abdomen, as well as numerous blood tests. Ultimately, with no disease diagnosis having been made, you will probably be dismissed as a complainer, someone with a "nervous stomach" or perhaps even as having "imaginary pains." Of course there must have been *something* the matter, or you would not have pain. But the "something" does not seem to be a disease with a name or definable characteristics, or (so the doctor believes) the tests would have revealed it. Even if the pain is from "nerves" (not further defined), how does nervousness make pain? The pain is certainly not literally in your head, because truly imaginary pain—which would have to be like a hallucinated sight or sound—is probably unusual in the extreme. These are not issues of prime importance to most physicians—a patient appears with symptoms and a doctor endeavors to find the disease that is causing the symptoms, simple as that. Barring the uncovering of a disease, we clinicians being pragmatic folks, the next best thing is to find something that makes the patient feel better—and with the array of potent drugs and treatments presently available this is frequently possible. If that fails, we frequently act as if the whole thing must be the patient's fault. No disease, no relief, no problem! It is an unusual doctor who continues to pursue the problem until the reason for the pain becomes clear, whether the cause is an undiscovered disease—the previous hunt having stopped too soon—or some odd knot in a muscle that has pinched the nerve that goes to the place where the pain is experienced. Equally unusual, if the doctor believes that emotions play a part in the discomfort, the probing continues until he or she discovers what brings this pain to prominence in this person at this time.

To understand the frequent failure of physicians to continue searching for the origin of symptoms where no disease is found, one must understand how physicians make a diagnosis. On the first page of *MacBryde's Signs and Symptoms,* a well-known book about diagnosis, is written, "As broadly and generally employed, the word symptom is used to name any manifestation of disease. Strictly speaking, symptoms are subjective, apparent only to the affected person. Signs are detectable by another person and sometimes by the patient himself. Pain and itching are symptoms; jaundice, swollen joints, cardiac murmurs, and so forth, are physical signs. . . . In this [book] the word symptoms is often used to denote any evidence of disturbed physiology perceived by the patient or the physician" (3). The strange contradiction in which symptoms are both "apparent only to the affected person" and 'any evidence of disturbed physiology perceived by the patient or the physician" is a result of a change in meaning that has taken place in the twentieth century. Here is another example, taken from a text on the diagnostic examination: "But in diagnostication a symptom is usually considered to be an abnormal sensation *perceived by the patient,* as contrasted with a physical sign that can be seen, felt, or heard *by the examiner*" (emphasis in the original) (4). From antiquity until the nineteenth century, the word "symptom" (from the Greek for coincidence) meant *any* manifestation of disease, as in MacBryde's first sentence (5). Only in this era have symptoms come to be seen as purely subjective and signs as objective. Further, the word objective has come to have the connotation of real, in contrast to subjective things which are "only mental" and therefore unreal. This shift in meaning of the word symptom and the derogation of symptoms because of their subjective nature are results of the influence of scientific ideals on medicine.

Science is not only a way of uncovering nature's truths, it also promotes an ideal of knowledge. Acceptable knowledge, from a scientific point of view, is objective, reproducible, and predictable. Numerical data seem best to meet the ideal, but other artifacts such as X rays, electrocardiograms, spirometric tracings, and slides of tissue are also acceptable. In medicine, we call such information "hard" data. On the other hand, information that is subjective, value-laden, or cannot be measured is considered unscientific and believed to be of lesser value. It is often called "soft." Unfortunately, symptoms are *always* "soft," subjective (in that they have to do with a subject), value-laden, and nonmeasurable. Medical scientists believe that soft data should be replaced by hard data at all times. Most readers of this book will have been brought up on such beliefs. The Social Security Administration of the United States shares this notion, as one can see by the definition of symptoms employed in the determination of disability. In the book supplied to applicants for disability insurance under the Social Security system are found the following statements: "*Symptoms* are your own description of your physical or mental impairment. Your statements alone are not enough to establish that there is a physical or mental impairment. . . . We will never find that you are disabled based on your symptoms, including pain, unless medical signs or findings show that there is a medical condition that could reasonably be expected to produce those symptoms" (6).

Despite their problems, symptoms remain the source of the initial information guiding doctors toward a diagnosis. They point the way to the next diagnostic steps. In this role, symptoms have come to be considered the *direct manifestations of diseases.* The cough may come from the bronchial irritation that attends pneumonia, shortness of breath arises from the diminished pulmonary reserve of emphysema, and the pain arises from the pressure of the intervertebral disk on the nerve root. I believe it is fair to say that to conform to common medical practice, the above sentence should be changed to read: "*Real* cough may come from the bronchial irritation that attends pneumonia, *real* shortness of breath arises from the diminished pulmonary reserve of emphysema, and *real* pain arises from the pressure of the intervertebral disk on the nerve root." It follows from this understanding of symptoms as manifestations of disease, where nothing lies between the disease and the existence of the symptom, that if (in the case of pain) examination does not confirm pressure of the disk on the nerve root, the pain (in this example) *may not be considered real.* Currently, if symptoms suggest any disease of importance, there will be further diagnostic examinations. The net effect of current diagnostic technology is to allow *direct* access to the disease. By X ray, sonography, endoscopy, biopsy, or other methods, diseases have become accessible in a manner never before possible. In previous eras, even if diagnostic suspicion was considerable, actually visualizing the disease almost invariably meant surgery or some other intervention which was, in itself, risky. It is not surprising, therefore, that physicians would come to see symptoms as inherently unreliable (because they are subjective and "soft") sources of information in which the patient may, metaphorically, get between the symptom and the doctor and distort the symptom so that it no longer appears to be a lineal manifestation of disease.

When pain is a symptom, it is possible to demonstrate conclusively that a lack of direct correlation exists between the message in the nervous system that signals a painful stimulus (nociception) and the patient's report of pain. This unarguable finding should have ended any conception of symptoms as unmediated manifestations of disease. I would not be surprised to find the same conclusion drawn from the study of cough, nausea, diarrhea, or shortness of breath. Henry Beecher's observation that men wounded in combat frequently did not report pain even with terrible wounds was one of the first clues that the report of pain is influenced by factors other than the painful stimulus (7). Similarly, it is a common clinical observation that other severe symptoms may be obscured in certain situations such as delirium, great external danger, or the pursuit of some vital goal where illness would interfere. Medicine persists in its older view that symptoms result directly from the pathological process because of the history of the concern of disease theory and medical science with only the objective aspects of disease. Medicine's conception of symptoms also follows from the fact that medical science, like all science, is concerned with generalities. Patients, however, are not generalities; they are necessarily individual—but there is *no* science of individuals. Because science does not and cannot deal with particular instances, symptoms, from the point of view of medical science, must remain essentially generalities. A patient's report of pain or any other symptom, on the other hand, is irreducibly particular and individual.

Some symptoms have such dire meaning that physicians are instantly alerted to the possibility of danger. Certain kinds of headache speak of hemorrhage in the brain. A stiff neck as part of an infectious illness warns of meningitis. A kind of feeling of severe swelling in the back of the throat with tonsillitis is a sign of a very serious abscess. The fact that a person was bitten on the knuckles yesterday and today the hand is very swollen tells of a hand-threatening infection. Each of these, and others, represent *emergencies* that must be acted on immediately. We doctors train ourselves to keep our ears ever vigilant, waiting to hear these terrible symptoms in order to conform to a basic axiom of medicine: "Never miss life-, sight-, or limb-threatening disease." There are straightforward physiological and anatomical reasons why each of these symptoms occurs when it does. This virtually one-to-one concordance of disease and symptom again gives the impression that the disease is speaking directly through the mouth of the patient. In these circumstances the metaphor at first seems apt. But every physician knows that the same symptoms may be reported by patients who do *not* have serious disease. That a symptom may be a direct manifestation of disease does not mean that it is so *in this instance* or even in most instances.

The doctor's view of symptoms, arising from a consideration of their history in medicine and the perspective of medical science, diverges widely from the understanding of symptoms that result from an examination of their origin in a particular patient. Yet patients and physicians employ the same term—symptoms—and all believe they are the direct manifestations of disease. This is the reason why patients are often puzzled when discomforts from their bodies, things they know to be abnormal because of their difference from a lifetime of function, are dismissed by physicians as unreal. A forty-five-year-old woman, Caroline Preskauer, had congenital heart disease in which a portion of her blood was shunted away from her lungs, thus preventing her blood from being properly oxygenated. She had been expected to die in adolescence but instead lived a productive life, married, and worked regularly. Always somewhat bluish because of insufficient oxygen, she became sick with pneumonia and heart failure and required oxygen and other supportive treatment. At a certain point she complained that she was not getting enough oxygen. The staff argued with her, keeping the oxygen level where they had originally set it. She could not understand why they would not believe her. Ultimately, it had to be increased. Of course she knew. Her success in life depended on her ability to assess the degree of blood oxygen and keep her activities attuned to it. This is true, in fact, for all of us, but most of us are not aware of it because the way the whole world of humans is set up—for example, the height of stairs, the weight of packages, the duration of tasks—is guided by our level of blood oxygen.

The view of symptoms as the disease directly making itself known, inherited from antiquity in medicine and exaggerated by current scientific views of disease and evidence, has more profound effects than the disappointment experienced by patients who discover that physicians are not hunting for the source of their symptoms. It separates the patient from his or her own disease as though the patient were merely the wrapping in which the disease came—it could equally well have come wrapped around by another person. Since treatment is directed at disease, the treatment would be the same no matter which person carried the disease to the doctor. This formulation seems quite congenial to most people, but let us look further into the origin of symptoms to see what is wrong with it.

How Symptoms Get To Be Symptoms for the Patient

People frequently visit physicians because they feel ill, believe that they are ill or will become ill, or as a consequence of the fear of illness. They act in this manner because alterations in their customary manner of function have been perceived as events that can be explained as illness rather than, for example, overwork or fatigue. When people reflect about illness in order to understand doctoring, the example they usually bring to mind is something dramatic, like pneumonia, with striking symptoms such as fever or pain. In attempting to comprehend patients and doctors, however, this is misleading, because most sicknesses, even the dramatic ones, do not start with a bang. They begin, instead, with perhaps a little tiredness (possibly manifested as the common-enough desire not to get out of bed), or some difficulty concentrating ("The job is a bore"). Perhaps lunch does not taste as good as usual or is followed by a tiny sensation of queasiness, the kind that makes you wonder whether the fat the cook used might have been rancid. Your nose might be just a little stuffy or your throat dry—you blame it on cigarette smokers at the meeting or the office air-conditioning. Sleep is restless; perhaps you are worried about something. And so it goes. If it *is* pneumonia, the nice old-fashioned kind, by evening you will probably have a high fever, teeth-chattering chills, cough, and pain in your side. If these things happen, you will not have a doubt in your mind—you will *know* that you are sick and had better call the doctor. But usually sicknesses are not like that. Instead, the next day's symptoms are much like the first, indistinct and attributed to this and that, but not illness. If these vague discomforts continue, they will usually be credited to psychological sources (especially in the more "sophisticated" populations of large cities) or assigned to some nonthreatening illness—a "virus" or a cold. Gradually, the growing weight of slight disturbances in function forces itself into a consciousness that something is wrong and that what is wrong is *not* just a "virus." But when it becomes clear to someone that real illness is present, the person does not believe that some blurry blob of sickness has occurred; he or she wonders actively which specific disease has struck.

Thus, symptoms are perceived occurrences whose explanations come from the domain of illness. The key word is "perceived." There is no understanding of symptoms that does not start as an understanding of a special aspect of perception, the perception of self. But when the symptoms start, they are not yet symptoms—just happenings. And the happenings are even less organized than the examples given above for the beginnings of pneumonia. Symptoms are necessarily experienced against the background of function that is normal for a particular person. All of us know ourselves and our bodies to behave in certain ways in the multitude of circumstances that make up our daily life. Although we vary in the ease with which we can come to *awareness* of our bodies, our actions, or even the words that come from our mouths, attentive or not, we are always learning what is normal for ourselves. Our constant self-exposure provides the experience on which the learning is based—and against which change can be evaluated. To understand these phenomena, we must disregard the place of explicit awareness. It is also necessary to consider self-observation on a moment-by-moment basis. Thus, for example, a person compares this moment's operation of a thumb against its operation a moment ago and "expects" it to do as anticipated in the upcoming fraction of a second. The quotation marks around "expects" are necessary because the word has the connotation of conscious attention to something, while in this instance no conscious effort is involved. While consciousness plays no part in the process, the flow of experience is being monitored and captured in a manner that makes its recall into consciousness possible. This is similar to those instances when one does not quite hear the words, but many seconds after they have been spoken (and the sound has disappeared) the jumble of noise in immediate memory resolves itself into a meaningful utterance.

These moment-by-moment alterations in functions are still not, in themselves, symptoms, although they are the raw material from which symptoms are formed. A symptom is inevitably a symptom *of* something. There must be an addition to the experience of altered function—the "something" of which the experience is the symptom. In other words, symptoms are more than merely dysfunctions. We have only to focus on our own bodies for a few minutes to appreciate the barrage of information about dysfunction and discomfort that is constantly being received and disregarded. The sensation of discomfort or alteration in function rises to consciousness, in part, through experiment. My finger (or any other part) does not behave as envisioned or its use gives rise to unexpected discomfort. I repeat the action and perform "experiments" that test the dysfunction until the altered function is dismissed as irrelevant, circumvented, or perhaps is moved the next step toward awareness symptomhood.

Pulling any phenomenon out of this constant barrage of information is an act that immediately distorts the occurrence—removing it from the context of the ongoing function of the person. When we examine any aspect of function—moving, bending a finger, breathing—the phenomenon begins to have a life of its own. Putting it into words—essential for reporting the happening—further categorizes the matter, and thus even more definitively removes the phenomenon from its place in the process of which it was a part. It becomes part of other processes: first perception and then verbalization. Both perceiving and forming into words add feelings, values (in the sense of personal degrees of importance, goods and bads), and beliefs to the phenomena. These feelings, values, and beliefs then begin to influence how the phenomenon is perceived—what in the perception will be suppressed and what emphasized. What I have described is the flow of process, tiny drops of time (and space), if you will, that flow together to make our actions and selves unfold, creating the minutes, hours, days and years of our lives. Process—change—is constant, continuous, and extremely difficult to discuss—which explains Marcel Duchamp's painting, *Nude Descending a Staircase,* as an attempt to portray Henri Bergson's concept of process, *durée*—change through time. The person's perception pulls together aspects of the flow as an occurrence of a "something" and in that fashion removes it from the flow of process and changes it into (in some cases) a relatively static event of illness.

In the following two examples of women explaining why each came to the doctor we get a view of how they arrived at the conclusion that a recognizable thing—a disease—was present by forming a whole out of a series of smaller happenings with their associated feelings, values, and beliefs. Here is the first:

> Actually, for myself, first I thought it was a pulled muscle. But then when it took so long to go away. . . . Then I was beginning to watch for, like a shingles kind of thing. Ye know, an' I thought. It just seemed to go. . . . Because it was spreading . . . and goin' across my back. An' I thought, well maybe it's, like, following a nerve trunk. You know. I never saw any rash, or anything. Ye know, I mean it's, it's nothing that was serious. I just felt like you just shouldn' have a pain in your . . . ; You should be able to lay on your left side without its being, having to move. And . . . then I thought of neuralgia, and so on. . . . I kep' ruling out all these things. Then I began to think, Well, what if it's something really serious. An' I began te try and remember how you could diagnose Hodgkin's, and all these various malignancies. An' I thought, Is there something in my ribs an' in the bones 'n' so on an' so forth . . . And thats what made me pursue it (8).

Note that this woman (who is a nurse) did not go to a physician for her pain merely because it hurt but because she began to think of Hodgkin's disease. In other words, the visit to the doctor was prompted by the combination of pain plus meaning.

Here is a similar dialogue showing how a patient's knowledge endows bodily occurrences with meaning. In this instance, the doctor's questions bring out the chain of logic that led her to believe she had kidney disease. Usually the system of meaning remains below the surface.

> Ah, and then the other thing connected with it. I realize this in retrospect only. I've been doing this all the time. Strrettchingg. As if I had a pulled muscle or something. An' I go to exercise class once a week. An' I noticed

that when I bend to left I felt weak on that side. But I reeely didn' pay any attention to it. Because I could get a puuuled something. An' Suddenly it began to hurt HORRIBLY, an' I realized it was my Kidney! It wasn' my back at aaall. An' it hurt verrry badly.
What made you . . . wha' made you to realize that it was your kidney.
An acute pain here.
How do you connect them?
I connect it with Sansert [a drug used for a type of migraine-like headache]. Now I may be Absolutely wronng but its the only, eh. . . .
How long have you been on the Sansert?
About two years. A year an' ahalf, two years.
How, howdya connect these ankles an your kidneys?
Only that it has to do with water, somewhere. I mean its compleetly amateuur . . . commonsense analysis. Somepin', somepin' being retained somepla . . . I don't know why, I shouldn't even presuume to answer that, I don't know the answer. Only that [Dr.] Greenglass did tell me, I suddenly remembered, that, a', He read me the textbook thing. The contraindications an' all that, an' he said the only Real danger is . . . for even have urinalysis is there is potential damage to the kidney.
Right. Now . . .
An' that suddenly came back at me, an from then on. . . .
Right. Up until, an' not counting these three events, ankles-knees-kidneys, an' up until this week have you been feeling well?
Yes (9).

Notice that in both examples, particularly the second, once the perceptions have been assigned a name (and thus a belief or a concept), events of the past are reinterpreted—"I realize this in retrospect only"—in light of the new idea. This further pulls the happening out of the flow of everyday life because, while some happenings in the past achieve new significance, others that might not fit into the idea must be suppressed. This is what Danny German, a patient with AIDS, did with his symptoms in the beginning of his illness. The soreness in his mouth that turned out to be thrush (moniliasis) was attributed by him for weeks to his cigarette smoking. The discoloration on his face he thought was an odd bruise (although he could not recollect what it came from). Only when he began to have fever and some shortness of breath in addition to his cough (which previously he considered to be from cigarettes) did he know he was sick—and simultaneously he *knew* that it was AIDS. At that point he found a hundred little pieces of evidence from the recent past that supported the diagnosis—nailed the coffin shut, as it were.

Events and perceptions are initially assigned meanings that represent the least threat—for example, Danny's sore mouth and the cough were considered at first to be from cigarette smoking. Disturbances in bodily function, when they become severe enough, are assigned significance in disease terms. Disease nomenclature—pneumonia, cancer, viruses, kidney diseases, neurosis, AIDS, sinus trouble—is the culturally accepted language for illness. It is also a human characteristic that once a person believes there is really something wrong, they think the worst—Hodgkin's disease (as in the case above), brain tumor, multiple sclerosis, schizophrenia, or AIDS—nothing less will do! I may have given the impression that meaning is always assigned to alterations in function in terms of concepts for which there are words. Certain circumstances exist, however, where this seems not to be the case. Catastrophic symptoms, such as unendurable pain or inability to breathe, require no interpretation—they carry their meaning in the immediate threat to existence that they pose. Other symptoms, while not so instantaneously terrifying, may be interpreted in terms of dread or terror with no specific disease name attached. It is as though "dreadful" is a concept in itself. What is unendurable or dreadful implies the disintegration of the person.

When a patient has forged a symptom into independent being through the process described above, he or she views it in the same manner as do physicians—it is a disease talking directly through the patient's mouth. The process of perception, emphasis and deemphasis, and interpretation is no longer employed.

The Relationship of a Symptom to Suffering

Because pain is probably the most common cause of suffering, it would be helpful to trace how pain becomes what we mean when we say "my . . . hurts." Awareness of pain, like any other symptom, starts with perception. In the case of pain the sensations perceived are part of a specialized function of the nervous system known as nociception—the mechanism involved in receiving painful stimuli. Dedicated receptors—nociceptors—exist for painful stimuli whose neural impulses are conducted over specialized pathways in the peripheral nerves, spinal cord, and brain. It is an understandable and common error to confuse nociception with pain, but it is an error nonetheless. The mistake has led some to believe that pain is merely subjective and therefore perhaps unreal or culturally relative—some experiences are reported as pains in some cultures but not in others. Others have pointed out that some pains are reported as ecstasy and thus are not really pain at all. Most of this nonsense arises from the confusion between the experience of something and the meaning assigned to it. To dispel these confusion, it would be helpful to dissect the pain experience into its parts.

Certain kinds of stimuli elicit the sensory response of nociception in every culture, now and forever. The sensory response is perceived (above or below awareness). As a consequence, the sensory response is an event for the perceiver as with every other symptom we have been discussing. All events are assigned meaning—integrated into the perceiver's ongoing flow of experience. This percept, like all others, is a percept of something—every pain is a *something* pain. As I have pointed out previously, meaning includes both significance and importance. The significance of something is what the thing implies. A pain in the chest implies heart disease, a pain in the ear is an earache, or this pain in my thigh signifies something sticking me from my pocket. The importance of a thing is its value. The sticking pain from the pin in my pocket is of little importance, but the pain of a heart attack is very important. We know the significance of something from past experience, the experience of others, the experience with our bodies, general knowledge, and so on. The aspect of meaning that is importance—the value dimension—also arises from all facets of person.

Assigning meaning to the noxious sensation continues the pain process by influencing further perception and predicting the future. As the sensory responses to the stimuli continue to be perceived, within the nervous system they are intensified or suppressed, contrasted or blended (with other responses) to intensify and support the significance that the process has been assigned or (less commonly) to weaken and make uncertain the original interpretation. Other sensory impulses that put in doubt the assigned implication will tend to be surpressed. Awareness is focused by important meanings. The spotlight of awareness further influences perception and reinforces or changes meaning. These continued influences may occur at the level of sensation or in transmission of the nociceptive message from peripheral nerves through the spinal cord to the brain.

Meaning also predicts; it is a statement about the future. For example, "cancer pain is terrible," the pain of burns is . . . ," "coccygodynia goes on and on." The prediction further influences the perception. Given the choice of interpreting new events as trivial or threatening, as noted earlier, people usually assign the worst possible meaning. Because of this bias, patients frequently remember only those features that would support a fatal diagnosis, suppressing extenuating information.

A statement about the future may contain a threat exemplified by the belief that cancer pain is unendurable. When the threat is sufficient, the sick person will believe that his or her intactness *as a person* is in danger. Suffering ensues at that point. Suffering influences perception by changing the individual's total focus toward the source of suffering. The entire apparatus of perception, including the assignment of meaning, then contributes to the suffering. As this occurs, the person begins to adapt to the threat, and the nature of the person begins to change. The entire process must be seen as occurring in little droplets of complex experience strung along a thread of time that may occupy minutes or years (10).

Which Is Real, Symptoms or Diseases?

Let me restate where we are (in somewhat exaggerated terms). Doctors pursue symptoms because of the belief that they are the direct manifestations of disease. Diseases are the "real" things—the things that count. Symptoms are a second-best access to the disease entity, the best being "direct" views such as X rays, tissue examinations, electrocardiograms, and so on. From the same perspective, sick persons, as persons, are an agglomeration of "soft" data—feelings, emotions, values and beliefs—in these terms, not as real as their diseases.

On the contrary, diseases are not real things in the manner they are generally conceived to be. Diseases are real in the same sense that ideas are real, concepts are real, and categories are real. Consider this definition of disease (to go back a step) from a medical dictionary: "A specific entity which is the sum total of the numerous expressions of one or more pathological processes" (11). The specific entity ("which is the sum total, etc.") can *never* be directly observed by a physician. Diseases do not have *independent* existence; they are not things like lungs or livers. Cancer of the breast does not have free-standing concrete existence and neither does pneumococcal pneumonia. Diseases are abstractions, conceptual entities that serve a concrete purpose. They are generalizations, categories that contain the facts about the abstraction in the sum total of its numerous expressions. Only the individual expressions of the disturbance in structure and function have actual concrete out-in-the-natural-world existence (12). Only the sum total of the expressions of the disease in this instance has actual touch-them-with-your-hands existence. But even though they exist, the expressions of the disease can never be observed by themselves, because while they have existence, they do not have independent existence. If it is sum totals that are of interest, then we can observe the sum total of all the facts of this afflicted person plus the sum total of the facts of the affliction in this instance. Further, we make these observations only in this moment. (We can, however, add these observations to the previous observations.)

It seems reasonable to ask how this strange turnabout took place. The disease came to be regarded more real to the doctor, while the patient, in all his or her dimensions except the biological facts of the body, came to be regarded as less real. In Chapter 1 I showed how the intimate relation between medicine and science resulted in medicine's adopting the world view of science, and that this had come about because modern disease theory finally made possible the application of science to medicine. Medical science and disease theory have become amalgamated in the minds of physicians (and patients). The way of science is admirably suited to understanding the liver, well or diseased, but unsuited, by itself, to the care of particular sick persons. The purpose of science is the pursuit of knowledge about universals (e.g., diseases)—a goal that is the direct legacy of Aristotle. Science is unable to give an account of particulars—individuals such as this or that sick person. As Samuel Gorovitz and Alisdair MacIntyre point out, "The scientist looks for law like relationships between properties; particulars occur in this account only as the bearers of properties, and the implied concept of a particular is of a contingent collection of properties" (13). Particulars, they point out, are things that exist in space and occupy time. As examples, their list includes, "salt marshes, planetary systems, planets, dolphins, snowflakes, hurricanes, cities, crowds and people" (14).

Recollect the so-called two-cultures problem of C. P. Snow. In a number of books he wrote about the widely disparate worlds of science and the humanities—which he called the two cultures of Western civilization—and the apparently unbridgeable chasm between them. In medicine, we have the same two-cultures problem in miniature: the *science* of medicine, which is conceived of as dealing with the hard facts of sickness (i.e., disease); and those aspects of medicine (not accepted by science) having to do with what is conceived of as the "soft," the *human* and seemingly unreal microcosm of individual patients.

Who Puts Humpty Dumpty Back Together Again?

Doctors, not medical science, deal with the hard facts of sickness. The gap between the two cultures of medicine is bridged in the person of the physician. The doctor (this person who does doctoring) is an integrator—someone who can "put a spin on" medical science that makes it "work" for individual patients. This aspect of doctoring is tacit, not manifest, and virtually invisible—we all think (wrongly) that medical science is tuned to the needs of this particular or that particular person with (for example) a heart attack. The doctor believes this to be the case and so does the patient. Of course, everybody knows that the "human" aspects of doctoring—compassion, caring, empathy, and so on—need the doctor as a person. But there is more to it. The heart muscle (in this example) needs the person of the doctor; so does the blood pressure, support for renal blood flow, and all the other technical aspects of care medical science is directed toward. This is because medical science is only directed at heart muscles (or blood pressures or renal blood flows) in general, and this or that particular person's heart muscle will behave differently from heart muscles in general. The person of the doctor must relate the generalities of medical science about heart muscles to this individual heart muscle. If an individual heart muscle was not distinctly different from another one, we would not need statistical methods to arrive at general truths about the heart.

I may have set up a false distinction. One can say that the function of the doctor in making medical science work for particular patients is not tacit or invisible at all. Rather, it is judgment, and everybody knows that doctoring requires judgment. This is correct, but think how little is known about judgment aside from the fact that experience is necessary to acquire it, and that some people (including some doctors) never have it. One would think that if judgment is necessary to apply general truths about the heart muscle (or virtually anything else) to this particular person's heart muscle (or anything else), then we would have studied judgment at least as thoroughly as we have studied the heart muscle! Judgment is precisely the ability to deal with the particular—a science of particulars would inevitably be a science of judgment. No such science exists, although it is sorely needed, especially in medicine. Further, if it is so well known that general truths cannot be applied to individual instances without the intervention of judgment, why do medical scientists keep bloodying their heads fruitlessly trying to develop computers that will make diagnoses in this or that individual case? The person of the doctor is also necessary to add values to medical science so that it will work for particular patients. The classical view of medical science excludes values from the realm of science. Values are, however, an inherent aspect of persons (patients—the subject of medical science—or otherwise) in groups and singularly; consequently applying medical science to particular patients mandates thinking in terms of values as much as in terms of the objective facts of the body. Classical ideas of science not only exclude values, they also exclude qualities, both simple and complex, on which thinking about values depends—qualities such as warm, old, frail, blue, tall, brave, head-nursy (that almost undefinable mix of qualities that are implied in any usage of the term "head nurse"), bad- appendixy (the mix of qualities that are part of a colloquial usage such as, "He had a bad appendix"), good-patienty, and so on. Qualities are related to values because it is the qualities of a thing that help us decide whether we like it (value it) or not, and how much. The values each of us places on something—for example, the ability to run and jump or be free of discomfort—depend on the qualities of personhood that we associate with those activities. Thus, when doctors apply medical science to individual patients, they must not only consider how scientific facts about the heart apply but must also be able to think about values and qualities in terms of this particular patient. For these values and qualities, in addition to biological uniqueness, make each individual the particular person he or she is.

This aspect of science can be seen in medicine in the way diseases as entities are not considered to include their manifestations or symptoms. Pneumococcal pneumonia, as I described it, is a disease characterized by inflammation of the air sacs (alveoli) of the lung caused by the microorganism known as *Streptococcus pneumoniae.* Patients with pneumococcal pneumonia have fever, cough, chest pain, a certain appearance of the lungs on X ray, certain sounds in the lungs when listened to with a stethoscope, etc. These things (fever, cough, X-ray appearance, etc.) are considered manifestations of the disease. They are not, from the scientific perspective, part of the disease. The disease is only the thing in the lung. These manifestations are the qualities associated with pneumonia medical science does not deal with. In fact, no instance of pneumonia exists without manifestations. The confusion is not limited to medicine. Is the smell of Limburger cheese (or a rose) part of the cheese (or the rose)? If you believe (in defiance of common sense) that one can have the cheese without its smell or the disease without its manifestations, then you have excluded human beings from your considerations. To repeat, pneumococcal pneumonia, except as an abstract category used to contain knowledge for a concrete purpose, does not have independent existence. Doctors never treat pneumococcal pneumonia, they only treat this or that particular person with pneumococcal pneumonia. Consequently, they have never seen pneumococcal pneumonia apart from its qualities (manifestations). Being human, they have never considered these qualities—fever, cough, X-ray appearance, death-inducing ability—without notions about whether these qualities are good or bad, important or unimportant, for themselves, the patient, or someone else. Therefore, they have never dealt with pneumonia without thinking in terms of both qualities and values.

As the person of the physician bridges the gap between the knowledge contained in the abstract scientifically described disease category called pneumococcal pneumonia and the biological facts of this case of pneumonia, here again the doctor is the "Fixer"—the bridge—who applies that same value-free and quality (manifestation)-free abstract disease category to a person with the disease pneumonia who can never exist sick or well apart from values and qualities. Undoubtedly, appreciation of the patient's values and the role of qualities (fatigue, invalidism, the nursey quality of nurses, the sterile quality of hospital rooms, etc.) related to the illness in the patient's values and meanings is part of the skill known as judgment. Once again, see how much is required of the person of the physician to make up for the deficiencies in the care of patients when diseases as considered by medical science are the clinical entities—the primary focus of medicine. I believe that these functions of physicians are largely tacit, not manifest, and most often described in the word "judgment," whose use hides more than is revealed because we know so little about what constitutes the ability to judge. If these functions of physicians were not largely unnoticed and unheralded, were, on the contrary, manifest, open to view and written about, then they would be the subject of discussion in the literature of medical decision making. In recent years it has become clear that doctors are decision-makers who have never been properly trained to make decisions. In fact, a new field of special study has developed devoted to clinical decision making. However, up to now the specialty has concerned itself almost exclusively with the mathematics of probabilistic decision making (15). It has actively dismissed the problem of values and their meaning to individual sick persons or converted them to numbers, detracting from their importance. Alvan Feinstein, who is largely responsible for the development of the field known as clinical epidemiology, is aware of the necessity for coming to terms with the personal nature of clinical practice and has struggled with the problem, to date largely unsuccessfully, I believe (16).

We came to this point in the chapter by contrasting what symptoms are to doctors and how they actually arise. Raising the question about which view is "real" is most important to the care of the sick. Doctors tend to see symptoms as the unmediated expression of diseases. In fact, the bodily occurrences that lead to the process of perception and then verbal expression of symptoms are inevitably subjected to interpretation and distortion by the patient. The effect of the addition of the patients' personal meanings ineluctably individualizes and personalizes the altered physiology that is the disease process, so that what emerges and is presented to the physician is the unique illness unfolding over time that is the expression of the disease in a particular person. This raised some doubt about whether what the physician was seeking to do was possible—to pull the disease free, so to speak, from the obstructions and entanglements of the patient, much as one might deliver a baby. It turns out that the object of the physician's search, the disease entity, does not exist in concrete reality but is merely an abstraction without independent existence. The only thing the clinician can work on (a paradox for medical science) is *this* sick person.

"Have You Found the Cause of My . . . ?"

In Chapter 1, I discussed how ideas about cause were basic to classical disease theory. In 1911, Lewandosky wrote, "The principle of etiological specificity of disease implies that every disease entity is produced by a quite particular cause, that different diseases cannot arise from the same cause, nor can different causes produce the same disease" (17). And from Faber, "*Only when we have penetrated to the underlying causes and described the etiologic entities of disease will the goals of nosography* [the classification of disease] *have been reached*" (emphasis in the original) (18). I pointed out that this idea of cause was essentially artificial because it does not adequately explain the sick person's illness. For example, pneumococcal pneumonia is clearly caused (in these terms) by the specific bacterium, *Streptococcus pneumoniae* but many people harbor that germ without developing pneumococcal pneumonia. Thus, it obviously requires more than the pneumonia organism for someone to get pneumonia. As another example, tuberculosis may manifest itself by a kind of meningitis or widespread foci of tuberculosis bacilli (miliary tuberculosis) or by cavities in the lung. Clearly, other causes must operate that determine what kind of tuberculosis (or pneumonia or typhoid fever or HIV infection) a person has. To solve this problem, a language of causation was invented (19). The tubercle bacillus was considered a "necessary but not sufficient" cause. There were also "contributory causes" and "occasional causes." It turns out that the idea of determining the cause of most diseases in the sense of Lewandosky's quotation was somewhat naive. Few diseases show the inexorable relationship between cause and manifestation that is exemplified by, for example, smallpox (20).

That medicine should want to find *the* definitive cause for a disease or illness seems quite natural; we all share that desire. Once, while teaching a course, I used hidden speakers to broadcast the sound of an old-fashioned mechanical adding machine. The volume was gradually raised until the sound was distinct but not loud enough to interfere with my speaking voice. The students turned this way and that, looking for the origin of the strange noise, apparently unable to put the sound out of mind so that they could concentrate on the lecture. So it is with all of us. Whenever anything occurs, we are driven to know its origin or cause. Illness is such an occurrence. All patients want to know the cause of their illness. If questions about cause are not raised directly, they show up in some other manner. In seeking the cause of their illness, most people develop some interesting notions about why it occurred—something about themselves, their diet, motivations, or behavior.

But although the desire to find the unique cause is natural, it stems from an incomplete view of how illness occurs. An example may make the point (21). A man in his seventies was admitted to the hospital with pneumonia. He had been found on the floor of his fifth-floor walk-up apartment by police responding to a call from a neighbor who had not seen him for a few days. From an examination of the patient's sputum, the intern believed that the pneumonia was caused by the pneumococcus (a belief later confirmed by the laboratory), and the patient was accordingly treated with penicillin. By the next day his fever was down and within a few days he was much better—a good example of the utility of knowing the cause of a disease. At the time of the initial examination in the hospital, one of his knees was found to be very swollen. Initially his doctors thought it was an unusual kind of joint disease, but it turned out to be osteoarthritis—the kind of degenerative joint disease that is a common source of disability in the aged. In the ensuing days the whole story became clear. His wife had died about a year earlier, leaving him virtually alone in the city (his two children lived in different parts of the country, both far away). The knee had become increasingly swollen in the weeks before his illness, and walking was extremely painful. Because of this he restricted his activities markedly, going out to shop as infrequently as possible. In common with many elderly bereaved, he knew few people of his age (most of his friends had died or moved away) and had withdrawn from most social contact. Having little interest in food, he lost weight and became malnourished. It is common for pneumonia to occur in this setting.

What *did* cause his pneumonia? Obviously he could not have had pneumococcal pneumonia if the *Streptococcus pneumoniae* had not invaded his lungs. But if he had not had that pneumonia, then perhaps he would have had a different kind, a bladder infection. The severity of his malnutrition practically guaranteed that he would develop some kind of infection. Perhaps the malnutrition should be seen as the definitive cause of his illness. Would he have been malnourished, however, if he had not been grieving, or if he had been able to walk normally, or if he lived on the first, not the fifth, floor, or if he were wealthy? The factor considered the cause of his illness will differ according to the perspective of the person asking the question. From the intern's point of view it is the pneumococcus. The man's children might point to the fact that he lives alone, and others might attribute the whole thing to grief. Some public health physicians would focus on the malnutrition, because undernourishment is a common problem among the elderly. Still others would blame the social system that permits old people to be neglected. Trying to cut through this welter of causes, physicians might point out that aside from the pneumococcus, none of those other features of the case are specific to the pneumonia. At first glance, that seems to be correct. Given the pneumonia, the pneumococcus *is* specific, whereas the other factors are not. But given only the pneumococcus (which may have inhabited the old man's throat for years), no such specificity exits. After all, he might as well have gotten pneumococcal meningitis or an infection from an altogether different microbe. Each of these differing perspectives is correct but incomplete.

In this century, knowledge about sickness has grown in opposite directions. This is the era of molecular understandings of disease. It is also the period in which it has become clear that what happens to human beings can only be comprehended by seeing them (and their parts) as only aspects of a much larger living system. General systems theory suggests that the search for the definitive cause is fruitless (22). At every level of organization—molecular, cellular, organic, bodily, personal, interpersonal, familial, communal, national (and perhaps even international)—can be found elements which, had they been different, meant that this particular man would not have had pneumonia. The contribution of general systems theory has been important in the growing understanding that illness cannot be viewed from the perspective of disease alone. It is the basis from which George Engel's proposal arose a number of years ago that illness is a biopsychosocial rather than merely a biological phenomenon (23).

Wider understandings can be confusing, however. If everything is a cause, what good is the notion of cause in medicine? As Stephen Toulmin has pointed out, questions about causation lead directly to questions about such issues as responsibility, and different ideas about causation presuppose different modes of intervention (24). The beauty of the concept of cause in classical disease theory was that it narrowed the responsibility of physicians and determined what interventions could be considered specifically medical. The importance of looking for the specific cause of a disease was that it provided the basis for the hunt for a cure. We are forced now to reopen the exploration of cause because of the inadequacies of the medicine that followed from the ideas of classical disease theory. The care of the old man with pneumonia, for example, is simply incomplete if it stops at the treatment of his pneumonia with antibiotics. We hold physicians responsible for more than merely patients' bodies (although there is considerable confusion about what the limits of their responsibility should be). In addition, most patients believe that doctors should do more than simply mechanically intervene in the disease. Rather, they expect the doctor to help them find and remedy the factors that led to the illness, and assist them in returning to their best possible function whatever the outcome of the disease. They require care directed at the relief of suffering, whose causes, as we saw in Chapters 3 and 4, are as much within as external to the patient. It remains imminent good sense that ideas of causation in medicine should be in the service of the care of sick persons rather than primarily in the service of the philosophy of causality. So, given the weaknesses of medicine's view of the cause of disease, something must take its place that will better serve the care of the sick.

An Illness Is a Story

In the case of the old man with pneumonia, a change in each aspect of the situation would lead to a different scenario. Suppose, for example, that because of the pain in his knee he had started taking large quantities of aspirin. Ideally, this would have controlled the arthritis sufficiently for him to buy food; he would not have been malnourished and he might not have developed pneumonia. On the other hand, it is not improbable that he would have developed bleeding from his stomach, leading to a progressive anemia (aggravated by the malnutrition) and also ending in his collapse and hospitalization. In that instance the disease would be gastritis (or gastric ulcer) and the cause would be considered aspirin. Or, in sorrow, he might have started drinking one night, become intoxicated, vomited, aspirated the vomitus into his lungs, and developed a lung abcess or aspiration pneumonia. Increased alcohol consumption is a common event in the bereaved and may also lead to gastrointestinal bleeding or pancreatitis—both serious illnesses. It is of some interest that perhaps no one would mention the arthritic knee as the cause of the illness. But if the knee had not been troubling him there might have been no "case" at all. At the very least he would have been able to go out to buy food.

If the person in the story were different, so too would be the disease. Make him ruggedly independent, happy with only his own company. If he had been habitually gregarious, he would have sought out friends of all ages as he might have been doing all his life. Give him a lifetime of devotion to exercise and there might have been no knee problem. Change any of these features of the person and the story is changed. Everybody knows that the story changes when the protagonist is changed. Here it appears that if the story is changed, the disease in the story also changes.

The story of the man with pneumonia is just that—a story, a series of events that happens to characters, in some specific place and over time in a specific period in history. Medical stories are different from everyday stories in one crucial respect: They always have at least two characters: a person and that person's body. (There are no persons without bodies, but there can be bodies without persons, as we have discovered in this age of long-term artificial support of the almost dead. Indeed, most people make a distinction between themselves and their bodies.) The story of the man with pneumonia is the story it is because of what happened to his body. Classical medicine might hold that the story is *only* concerned with what happened to his body, but we know that stance to be insufficient because what happened to his body would have been different if some nonbody features of the narrative were changed—putting his apartment on the first rather than the fifth floor, for example. On the other hand, while novelists may be able to disregard what happens to his body, no one wants doctors to do that, so the medical story continues right *into* his body. This part of the story tells what happens when the pneumococcus invades his lungs, and how that invasion is promoted by the loss of immune functions (among other things) that follows from malnutrition. It goes on to show how the loss of functioning lung tissue deprives the man of an adequate respiratory surface to transfer oxygen from the air to the blood, and the effect that has on other functions, and so on, if you are interested, right down to the molecular level of his organism. As physiology is the story of function (how things work) in the healthy body, pathophysiology is the story of the altered function of the body in disease states. Pathophysiology shares that characteristic of all stories—change one feature of the story and the story itself is changed. An older body versus a younger one. The concurrent existence of another disease like diabetes. A history of cigarette smoking. Alcoholic intoxication at the time the pneumococcus invaded the lungs. All these things change the story that is the pathophysiology, and in so doing change the problem presented to the doctor.

Understanding illness as a story is useful in examining the idea of cause in illness (25). In a story, what causes this step in the narrative is what just preceded it. One step in the story "causes" the next step. Even if there seem to be some overriding causes, they are inherited in each moment of the story from the moment before. The fact that I am a male is certainly one of the determining facts in the story of my life, but it is more useful to see the effect of that fact being passed along at every step in my life's unfolding than to see it as being some big overriding cause of this or that. This view of illness—illness as a process rather than an event—diminishes older medical views of cause. It may be a useful shortcut to say, as one of his neighbors might, that the man got pneumonia because his wife died and he stopped eating. Or, as the hospital physician might say, his pneumonia was caused by the pneumococcus. But these comments about cause should be seen for what they really are: shortcuts that implicitly contain an understanding of the whole process—the story—that is the person's illness. To the extent that using the shortcut obscures seeing how illness is a process, a story unfolding, the shortcut does harm, just as seeing cause in the classical disease sense artificially narrows physicians' responsibilities and opportunities for intervention.

From the standpoint of the process that is an illness, it is artificial to stop at the boundaries of the body. The story of the old man includes the social facts of his solitude, the personal matter of his bereavement, his living conditions, his bad knee, his failure to maintain proper nutrition, the invasion of the pneumococcus, its progress in his lungs, his worsening infection, collapse, being discovered, being brought to the hospital, antibiotics, respirator support, and so on. Thus, the search for the cause of an illness is not helped by classical disease theory, which does not account for all the facts.

References

1. *The Genuine Works of Hippocrates.* Translated by Francis Adams. 1939. Baltimore, The Williams and Wilkens Company, Of the Epidemics, p. 104.

2. Cassell, Eric J. *The Healer's Art.* 1985. Cambridge, Mass., MIT Press, p. 48.

3. Robert S. Blacklow. *MacBryde's Signs and Symptoms.* 6th ed. 1983. Philadelphia, Lippincott, p. 1.

4. DeGowin, Elmer L. and DeGowen, Richard L. *Bedside Diagnostic Examination.* 4th ed. 1981. New York, Macmillan. p. 31.

5. King, Lester S. *The Philosophy of Medicine: The Early Eighteenth Century.* 1978. Cambridge, Mass., Harvard University Press, p. 89.

6. Social Security Regulations: Rules for Determining Disability and Blindness. U.S. Department of Health and Human Services. Social Security Administration. Office of Disability. 1986. SSA Pub. No. 64-014 Para 404.1528 and 404.1529.

7. Beecher, Henry K. Anxiety and Pain. *JAMA* Aug. 18, 1969; 209(7):1080.

8. Cassell, Eric J. *Talking with Patients: Vol. 2. Clinical Technique.* 1985. Cambridge, Mass., MIT Press, p. 124.

9. Cassell, Eric J. *Talking with Patients: Vol. 2,* op. cit., p. 125.

10. Cassell, Eric J. The Relationship Between Pain and Suffering. *Advances in*

Pain Research and Therapy, Vol. II. Edited by C. S. Hill, Jr. and W. S. Fields. 1989. New York, Raven Press, p. 61–70.

11. *Blakiston Gould Medical Dictionary* 1972.

12. Samuel Gorovitz and Alisdair MacIntyre. Towards a Theory of Medical Fallibility. *The Hastings Center Report* 1975; 5:13–23.

13. Gorovitz and MacIntyre, op. cit.

14. Gorovitz and MacIntyre, op. cit.

15. Pauker, Stephen G. and Kassirer, Jerome P. Decision Analysis. *NEJM* 1987; 316:250–58.

16. Feinstein, Alvan. *Clinimetrics.* 1987. New Haven, Conn., Yale University Press.

17. Lewandowsky 1912, quoted in Faber, Knud. *Nosography.* 2nd ed. Revised. New York, Haber. p. 183.

18. Faber, Knud. *Nosography.* 1923. New York, Paul B. Horber, p. 210.

19. King, Lester S. op. cit., pp. 209–32.

20. Englehardt, H. Tristram. Causal Accounts in Medicine. In *Changing Values in Medicine.* Edited by Cassell, Eric J. and Siegler, Mark. 1979. Washington, D.C., University Publications of America. p. 76.

21. Cassell, Eric J. Changing Ideas of Causality in Medicine. *Social Research* 1979; 46:728–42.

22. Miller, James G. *Living Systems.* 1978. New York, McGraw-Hill, Chap. One.

23. Engel, George. The Need for a New Medical Model: A Challenge for Biomedicine. *Science* 1977; 196:129–36.

24. Toulmin, Stephen. Causation and the Locus of Medical Intervention. In *Changing Values in Medicine. op. cit.*, p. 61.

25. Kleinman. Arthur. *The Illness Narrative.* 1988. New York, Basic Books.

8

Treating the Disease, the Body, or the Patient

IDEAS ABOUT CAUSE lead inevitably to considerations of intervention. Classically, doctors searched for the specific cause of each disease to find a cure, seeking something that would remove the cause and thereby remove the disease. Treatments have been developed that intervene at some point in the process of disease. Even when antibiotics are the treatment, things are rarely as direct as one might at first assume. Characteristics of the patient, social factors, or even the political or economic setting in which an illness occurs may modify treatment. For pneumococcal pneumonia, penicillin is the treatment of choice. But what if the patient is allergic to penicillin, or has severe diabetes, or refuses treatment? What if the pneumococcal pneumonia occurs as the last stage in the disease of someone dying of cancer? Each of these circumstances modifies "best treatment," but none is part of the disease. It is obvious that therapeutics are rarely as straightforward as textbook treatments of choice would indicate; otherwise all one would have to do is look up the disease, find out its treatment, and—Bingo—it's done.

Identifying the Best Treatment

The increasing recognition in the middle decades of this century that factors other than disease influence the outcome of treatment and the choice of therapeutic agent has led to the dominance of the randomized controlled clinical trial (1). It was quite common in even the recent past for drugs to be introduced as treatments for specific diseases because one, two, or even several patients with the disease had shown improvement when given the drug. These so-called "anecdotal" cases neglected the possibility that these patients might have gotten better even without the treatment. To counter this criticism, it became popular to compare groups of patients who received a new therapy with those who did not. These controlled trials, although an improvement over the anecdotal evidence of the past, still sometimes led to the adoption of treatments that subsequently proved worthless. Finally, in one of the major advances in medicine, the randomized controlled clinical trial came to be accepted as the only good way to test new therapies. In the best of these trials, patients who meet the rigorously defined criteria for a disease or condition are assigned truly at random to receive either the active treatment or a placebo in a manner that completely blinds both the patients and the investigators as to who is receiving what. The trial proceeds toward a predefined and recognizable therapeutically meaningful stopping point. Sufficient patients are enrolled to assure that a significant and clinically important result can be demonstrated that will stand up to appropriate statistical scrutiny. A moment's reflection will demonstrate how difficult it must be to meet the requirements in the preceding three sentences. Controlled trials are cumbersome, expensive, and time consuming—and they demand disciplined adherence to research protocol. They require investigators to subordinate their own theories and hard-won experiential knowledge to the power of the method.

Randomized controlled trials have won the respect they enjoy because the number and strength of "outside" factors that can influence the apparent success or failure of therapy have been repeatedly demonstrated. These other factors include biases introduced by the investigator; biases by the patient; the placebo effect; demographic characteristics such as age, sex, and social status; other therapies; the stage of the disease, and patient behaviors such as cigarette smoking, exercise, and compliance with the treatment. Controlled trials have even demonstrated that a current treatment cannot be compared with past treatments—so-called "historical" controls. While the disease may have remained the same (adenocarcinoma of the bowel is, by definition, the same in 1970 as in 1990), factors such as diet, antibiotic treatment of infectious complications, and surgical technique, all of which may have changed in the intervening years, may exert an effect on the survival of patients with the disease. The principal task of randomized controlled trials has been to eliminate the effect of these confounding biases and nondisease factors so as to assess the "pure" effect of the treatment on incontestable and rigidly defined instances of disease. During the same period in which investigators have come to subscribe to the uncompromising attitude toward research knowledge that is represented by randomized clinical trials, clinicians have had to learn to guide their therapeutic and diagnostic actions on the basis of objective evidence generated by such research.

Regarded from a different perspective, the rigor and success of modern clinical research illuminates the power of the biases that must be controlled in the randomized trial. It is predictable that in our effort to protect against the distortion of knowledge produced by such factors, we overlook their importance in the day-to-day practice of medicine. Remember that the object of the randomized clinical trial is to show what a drug has to offer to patients with disease in its ideal form—isolated from the confounding variables of the usual treatment situation. But sick persons are taken care of in "the usual treatment situation" where the variables that confound research cannot be eliminated. Let's look at some of the features of the therapeutic setting to see what part they play.

One of the most important sources of error in earlier clinical research was the physician's belief in the treatment or procedure being tested. The occasional instance of intentional dishonesty is much less frequent than the inherently more interesting unintentional distortion of research results that leads to confirmation by the clinical scientist of his or her original ideas. The history of medicine is filled with examples of enthusiastic endorsement by medical authorities of therapies that later proved to be worthless or, worse, detrimental. Such enthusiasm is based on the belief that the treatment really works and all kinds of theoretical justifications are usually provided. When I was a resident, gastric freezing was advocated for the treatment of bleeding ulcers. The surgeon who advocated that therapy was world famous, and doctors all over the United States were soon pumping freezing saline solution into the stomachs of patients with bleeding ulcers. Special machines were devised and sold to maintain the proper temperature of the solution. At Bellevue Hospital, we did not have such a device available, and so we did the best we could with bottles of saline nestled in buckets of ice. The treatment was a mess, and the patient was not too comfortable either, but the bleeding stopped in the majority of cases. Of course, the bleeding also stopped in the majority of cases if one did nothing, as a subsequent controlled trial proved. All the gastric freezing machines were rolled into backroom closets to take their place by the side of all the other equipment similarly converted into junk by the ultimate disparagement of treatment enthusiams by dispassionate randomized trials. On the other hand, would you want your doctor to offer you some treatment in which he or she had no belief and little or no enthusiasm? Scientists with the most impeccable credentials have fallen into the trap of searching for evidence that supports their beliefs rather than subjecting their beliefs to the test of impartial evidence. Linus Pauling's advocacy of Vitamin C in the treatment of cancer may be such an example.

How do enthusiasm and belief make some medical maneuver seem useful when it is, in fact, useless? There is no need to duplicate Alvan Feinstein's excellent discussion of these sources of distortion and bias, but some should be mentioned here (2). Doctors enthusiastic about a treatment tend unconsciously to seek out persons to treat for whom it will work best and avoid those for whom it will not be as useful. At first glance that seems reasonable enough, but some doctors act as if the best way to make sure a treatment works is to use it in people who do not need it at all. During the era when pneumonia was a killer, there used to be "pneumonia doctors" who specialized in the care of this often fatal condition. Their reputations depended on how many people with pneumonia they saved. It is obvious that if they made the diagnosis of pneumonia in patients with bad colds or even severe bronchitis in addition to those who really did have pneumonia, their success rates would be higher. In a similar manner, physicians who do a special procedure, or whose office is specially equipped in some way, tend to do that procedure or use that equipment not only in the most appropriate circumstances but also in situations where their use is marginally necessary. These practices may seem venal, but that is not usually the case; more often they are simply an expression of the uncritical enthusiasm people have for their work and their desire to look—and do—good.

Such so-called "selection biases" may also arise from patients themselves. When a doctor gains a reputation for treating a particular condition, this draws patients with similar illnesses. Often the diagnosis is self-made and not subjected to rigorous definition. This frequently occurs with the diagnosis of hypoglycemia but may just as well be true of the diagnosis of heart disease based mostly on symptoms. The manner in which diagnostic tests are done and interpreted may also lead to selection bias, and there are other sources as well. Physicians' and patients' enthusiasm also lead to bias in instances where patients are considered to have improved when, in fact, they have not. The doctor wants them to be better, the patients want to be better, and, as a result, only signs of improvement are heeded. In time, however, the condition is seen to be unchanged. The doctor may not like to concede failure—who does?—and the patient may be embarrassed or even feel guilty at having failed the doctor. In any case, a bias was introduced into the treatment situation that obscures what has really occurred.

What is important here to recognize that with the best of intentions, physicians—both investigators and practitioners—can come to see only what they wish when they wish and where they wish. The increasing understanding of the influence of these distortions on medical knowledge has not produced an equivalent understanding of the mechanisms that make these biases so powerful, only of their universality. But the treatment of an individual patient is *not* a randomized clinical trial. The same inherent sources of bias in the selection of therapies, in the manner in which they are given and the evaluation of the outcome of treatment, must operate in the care of individual patients. Which patients will be considered appropriate for which therapy is not simply a matter of making a disease diagnosis. The rigor and rigidity of definition of disease required for a good clinical trial *cannot* operate in the care of individual patients. The strictness with which treatment will be given to any individual patient, particularly if it is discomforting or has unpleasant side effects, rarely approximates the research setting. The circumstances that will be accepted as success or failure are only infrequently specified in advance for a particular patient. Each of these factors, and many more, determine the nature of treatment. They result from the beliefs and theories of the individual physician, as well as from his or her knowledge and personality. Thus, even in circumstances where a treatment has been shown by randomized controlled clinical trial to be appropriate (or inappropriate) to a specific disease, the treatment of a *particular* patient with that disease will not be determined by the disease alone. Inevitably, and necessarily, the doctor is part of the therapy. I do not mean simply that the doctor administers the treatment, but rather that the person who is the doctor is a central part of therapeutic medicine. This is an inherent part of doctoring, just as in making a diagnosis and fitting the generalities of medical science to *this* particular patient, the physician is a necessary bridge. Here also it would seem reasonable that doctors be taught the part they, as *individuals,* play in treatment so that they will master rather than be controlled by distortions and biases.

The Effects of Patients on Treatments

Patients also demonstrate the same sources of bias that distort physicians' judgment. After all, sick people want to get better—so much so that they will seek out treatments that are questionably effective simply because of their desire to *do something.* Sick people will follow diets that they would not feed their pets, swallow unbelievable numbers of vitamin pills, take coffee enemas, and do innumerable other things based on their own theories and beliefs about illness. Witness the faddish popularity of various diseases and treatments based on minimal or poor information. At this time food allergies are again having their fling, as is generalized fungus infection. Osteoporosis is being treated in many different ways, since an absence of good evidence about the best therapy is not accompanied by an absence of therapy. In the tragic circumstance of AIDS, where no effective cure for the underlying human immunodeficiency virus has yet appeared, many people flock to treatments that are untried, untested, and even potentially dangerous (3). Even when a fatal disease is present, a dangerous treatment can further shorten life, produce devastating side effects, or make treatment with more effective therapies impossible. People who are not feeling well will take potent treatments even when they know the therapy is inappropriate—"I had a bad cold, so I started myself on penicillin which I had left over from a gum infection and which I know doesn't help virus colds. But I hoped it would help me get better faster."

The Placebo

The factors thus far discussed that interfere with basing treatment choices on rigorous evidence of effectiveness are distinct from one of the most interesting, confounding, but constant features of therapeutic situations, the placebo effect (4). The word placebo was originally used in medicine to denote things given more to please than to benefit the patient. While still employed in that sense, it presently also denotes effects of treatments that cannot otherwise be explained and are assumed to be psychological in origin. Such usage may have started with the early research on the common cold where negative as well as positive placebo effects were described. In an attempt to find out what caused colds, volunteers were exposed to either the nasal secretions from persons with colds or, in a controlled and blinded fashion, saline solution. A percentage of persons who got the nasal secretions went on to develop a full-blown cold. To the investigators' surprise, the same thing happened to a definite although lesser fraction of those who got only saline solution; they too developed colds indistinguishable from the others. These effects, even though not related to treatment, have come to be included in the meaning of placebo effect. With the positive placebo effect, persons receiving the placebo derive benefit like those receiving the active drug.

My own exposure to the phenomenon is illustrative. As a medical student I regularly worked in an emergency room at night. Every evening patients would come in because of their asthma, and it was frequently necessary to give them intravenous theophylline (Aminophylline) to stop their attack. At that time I read an article that reported that the blood sugar fell considerably in patients with acute asthma. I decided to try giving a strong (50 percent) glucose solution intravenously to the next patients with asthma that I saw. It worked. Their asthma subsided and they went home. I was pleased, but some skepticism crept in, and so subsequently I tried the same amount of intravenous saline. That was just as effective as the glucose solution. It is important to note, however, that while the same degree of relief from asthma was afforded by glucose and then saline as by the active drug, theophylline, patients who received the placebos would much more commonly return to the emergency room later the same night with a resurgence of their asthma. There is a limit to the placebo effect.

A literature has grown up around placebos, criticizing their use (properly, I believe) as unethical because they involve subterfuge and a process basically similar to lying. However, one of the most interesting aspects of placebos is the demonstrated fact that a placebo effect can exist *even when the person knows the drug is a placebo.* The placebo effect is regularly invoked to explain the otherwise unexplainable effects of treatments, both positive and negative. Most often, the words placebo effect are used in a derogatory sense, as in, "That's just a placebo effect." However, I would happily give up the use of (say) digitalis preparations, as important as they have been in the treatment of heart disease, if I could be assured a similar mastery of the placebo effect—it would be useful in many more patients. One would think that something as potent as the placebo effect would have been subject to at least as much study as most pharmaceuticals, but that is unfortunately not the case.

The attitude of the individual physician toward a treatment affects the outcome of that treatment in a manner similar to the placebo effect. Doctors' enthusiasms give rise to patients' enthusiasms, just as their pessimisms lead to patients' doubts. In some patients, the exact opposite occurs. Although this fact (along with the placebo effect) leads to well-known biases in therapeutic research that must be controlled for by randomized clinical trials, little is known about how the doctor's attitude influences the patient. It is one of those things that seems so obvious as to need no further exploration. Like the biases that must be controlled for in clinical research, it is most often regarded as an incidental feature of the medical landscape. But that cannot be the case, since the effect of the doctor on the patient (and vice versa) is *always* present. In the care of sick persons, it cannot be otherwise. Rather than being seen as incidental, these influences, the placebo effect, and the other sources of bias noted above are so powerful as to make clear the fact that the model of a drug treating a disease is as artificial and removed from the care of actual persons as is the belief that diseases exist in and of themselves, separately from sick persons.

In the years since World War II therapeutics in medicine has moved further and further from the classical ideal of specific treatments directed at specific etiologies. In fact, some of the most successful and dramatic therapeutic actions in medicine are not directed toward the cause of the patient's sickness. Arnold Lauffer is a good example. Mr. Lauffer, who is seventy-two, has had angina pectoris for about ten years. Two weeks before entering the hospital, his angina worsened, and he began to have chest pain after eating. At about the same time he developed swelling in his right leg for which no cause could be found. (Specifically, he did not have thrombophlebitis, or clots, in the veins of the leg.) On the day of admission to the hospital he became short of breath and fainted. He was admitted to the coronary care unit when, in the emergency room, his electrocardiogram showed evidence of a heart attack.

For the first couple of days things seemed straightforward enough. Laboratory tests confirmed the heart attack. His breathing remained labored and his chest X ray had the appearance of pulmonary edema (fluid in the lungs following from heart failure). Despite what should have been adequate treatment for heart failure, however, day by day the chest X ray looked worse and the amount of oxygen in his blood dropped critically. He was put on a respirator and given high levels of inspired oxygen to support his lung function. By this time his doctors (there were now many—his attending physician, a lung specialist, a cardiologist, and an infectious disease specialist, in addition to the director of the CCU and the fellows, residents, and interns of the unit) believed that he must have pneumonia in addition to his heart disease, and he was given several intravenous antibiotics. No causative organism was grown from his blood or sputum. His condition worsened as his kidneys began to fail and then stopped making urine. Peritoneal dialysis was instituted and successfully substituted for the function of his kidneys. All the while his chest X ray failed to show any improvement and it was considered possible that he had pulmonary emboli (clots in the lung). Heparin was started to counteract that disease, if it was present. There was no improvement. He became progressively more anemic, to a degree for which no explanation could be found. He was given repeated transfusions to keep his blood count normal. His intestines stopped working and to maintain his nutrition he was started on total parenteral nutrition. At one point, because of remittent airway obstruction (wheezing) he was given high doses of corticosteroids. There was no improvement. The heparin was discontinued, the corticosteroids and then the antibiotics were stopped, and he neither improved nor worsened.

After three weeks, to the amazement of all the doctors, his kidneys began to make urine, his lungs improved, his blood count stabilized, and he became mentally clear (he had been delirious for two weeks). One month after admission to the hospital, he was breathing without the respirator and sitting up. He left the hospital alive and functioning. At the time of discharge from the hospital, the cause of his recent illness was unknown; a diagnosis was never made. His wife and family believed his recovery was a miracle. What led to Mr. Lauffer's remarkable recovery? Quite obviously, to the chagrin of his many physicians, it was not the discovery of a disease whose cause could be contravened or whose course could be predicted. To the contrary; Mr. Lauffer was kept alive by the successful intervention in and support of one failing body system after another without any knowledge of why they were failing. Because these support systems—respirators, methods of dialysis, blood pressure supporting drugs, cardiac drugs, and total parenteral nutrition—are so effective and can be utilized with relative ease, Arnold Lauffer was given time to "get better on his own."

Make no mistake, the treatments that Arnold Lauffer received do not simply represent technical feats. They exemplify some of the peak achievements of medicine of our era. This is all the more true since they are probably done in every intensive care unit all over the country and virtually every recently trained physician can administer them or be trained to do so. This kind of therapy epitomizes the success of treatment directed toward the mechanisms of disease. Unfortunately, *the problems of treatment based on pathophysiology come from the fact that it is blind to any larger goal.* Mr. Lauffer got better because his underlying disease (whatever it was) got better. If these catastrophic events had occurred (as is not uncommon) in a person with widespread unchecked malignancy, then his family might not have viewed their effectiveness as "a miracle," but rather as a curse that merely kept him alive when he would have been better off dead.

Treatment of This Patient

If each malfunctioning system of the body is treated and supported, then treatment becomes a matter of one interventional event after another, not necessarily related to what the sick person may want or to what would be best for the sick person by anyone's standard. In intensive-care units all over the world this is precisely what is happening. It is difficult for physicians to decide how to adjust the level of treatment to the needs of this particular patient. It is easy to start advanced support systems and difficult to stop them, a fact that has led to current moral problems related to the termination of life support. Angelo Costa had cancer of the kidney that had spread to his lungs and his liver. When he went home from the hospital he and his doctor decided that he would be best off in a hospice program where he could get care at home and where he could ultimately die. When the visiting nurse made her first visit, she found him acutely ill—he was short of breath and had a high fever. She thought that because he appeared mortally ill, he ought to go to the hospital. When he arrived in the emergency room he was very short of breath and in great distress. The physicians were confused about what to do. He was dying from his cancer, knew his diagnosis and its meaning, and had chosen to be a part of a hospice program and die at home. Should he be placed on a respirator, which would be the best action if he were not otherwise dying, or should he just be made as comfortable as possible? Mr. Costa chose the respirator and then lost consciousness. He had no family. What should have guided his treatment? Whatever answer you give, I believe you will see that it is not determined solely by his disease or the technical capacities that exist for doing things to him.

It would be an error, however, to think that medical interventions based primarily on the ability to perform them, whether directed primarily at causes as with antibiotics or at physiologic mechanisms as with, for example, dialysis, cause problems solely in the terminally ill. Treatment of diseases or therapy determined by pathophysiology has to be designed with the needs of the sick person in mind, otherwise difficulties ensue. What is good for the patient's lungs or kidneys is not necessarily good for the patient. Experienced clinicians usually establish treatment goals (beyond the vague desire to make the patient better) and base their therapeutic decisions on those goals. Therapeutic goals almost always have an aspect of timing. Thus, as Arnold Lauffer started to get better, it was necessary to get him out of bed and walking, with the anticipation that he would leave the hospital in ten to fourteen days. He had to have special nursing assistance and be disconnected from all but the most essential equipment. He did not want to stand or walk because he felt so weak. We had to bargain with him, promising relief from this or that onerous test or task, if he would stay in the chair for a length of time rather than returning to bed. The goal of ambulation was given precedence over other things that the doctors might have wanted to do.

Caroline Preskauer's heart is on the right rather than the left side of her body. In addition to dextrocardia, her congenital heart disease was marked by several complex defects so that her blood was always inadequately oxygenated. As a "blue baby" (to whom surgery offered no help) she had spent much of her childhood in the hospital and seen one after another of her similarly afflicted friends die of heart failure or infections of the heart valves. Despite its severity and the restrictions in activity that her heart disease imposed, she had gone through college, gotten a master's degree in school counseling, and worked regularly. In common with most people who had had considerable illness in childhood, she neither liked nor trusted physicians and hated and feared hospitals. She also had her own firmly entrenched ideas about what treatments were or were not in her best interest. In the beginning of February she developed a bad respiratory infection. Over the next three weeks her breathing became more labored, but she did not stop working or call her physician. Her ankles started to swell and her stomach was upset. After a few days, Rolaids did not help any more, so she took Brioschi (an antacid preparation that, she was unaware, is loaded with sodium). Two days later she was forced to go to her doctor because she could hardly breathe. When he examined her it was obvious that she was very sick; she had pneumonia and was in deep congestive heart failure. Despite his pleas she refused to go to the hospital. They negotiated a deal. She would try to get better at home by starting antibiotics, diuretics (water pills), and oxygen, and if she did not improve she would go to the hospital. In twenty-four hours she gave in and entered the hospital. Within hours she became much worse, lost consciousness, and was placed on a respirator. When she awoke to find herself on the respirator, she was terrified and could barely be kept calm by the combined efforts of her family, the nurses, and her doctors. To obtain her cooperation and reduce her panic, despite the danger, the respirator was discontinued before she had returned to her optimal lung function. She was sent home within a week of leaving the intensive-care unit and returned to work a month later. Each step in her care required a compromise between what was best for her heart and lungs and what seemed best for her, as distinct from her body. She was willing to take considerable risks to continue living independently and working because these goals were so important to her.

Most of medical care takes place not in hospitals but at home. And there it is even more imperative that treatment be designed with the particular patient in mind. Persons, sick or well, have lives to lead. They must work, continue their social obligations, live with their families, and play their parts in their interpersonal and intimate relationships. Medical care—treatments, medications, doctor's visits—should not be so intrusive that a person is involved full time in following the doctor's instructions, because when that happens, people simply stop following the medical regimen. They forget their medications or take more or less than requested, break their diets, are more (or less) active than instructed, overdo or do not do their exercises, and so on—not some people, *most* people, including doctors when they are sick. When patients become ill again because they stopped their medications or breached the medical regimen, physicians often blame them for being foolish. In fact, it is difficult to adhere to a routine of medicines or treatments. For example, in the treatment of some afflictions of the kidneys or bladder, a high water intake is frequently advised. Consistently increasing water intake would seem to be the easiest thing in the world, but even such a trivial change in habits can be difficult. I tried it, and found that on the days I made an effort to remember, I drank the extra water. It took many weeks before I began to drink more water as a matter of course. I even put a water carafe on my desk and asked my staff to keep it filled. Gradually, after more than six months of drinking at least three extra glasses of water daily, I lost interest in the project, and, despite my original intentions, my water intake returned to its initial level. The water pitcher remained on my desk, unused. I was chastened by the experience, and suggest it to others quick to criticize patients' failure to adhere to medical advice. I believe that people behave in this manner not only because of the enormous force of habit, but also because they have other, more important (to them) things on their minds, or because they have given meanings to the illness and treatment that are distinctly different from their doctors' meanings. Or, because after the acute phase of an illness passes and normalcy begins to supervene, the doctor and sickness become irrelevant, as they usually are to normal people. Normal persons do not consciously place the demands of their bodies in the central position.

Treatment in Chronic Illness

In chronic illness, the ideal of a drug or a treatment directed without the mediation of the ill person at a disease or pathophysiologic process is even further removed from reality. Doctors do not treat chronic illnesses. The chronically ill treat themselves with the help of their physicians; the physician is part of the treatment. Patients are *in charge of themselves.* They determine their food, activity, medications, visits to their doctors—most of the details of their own treatment. The chronically ill person's personality, character, intelligence, store of knowledge, previous experience, goals, relationships to the body, relationships to society and to others, socioeconomic status, living circumstances, quality of medical care, and relationship with the doctor(s) all influence the nature, content, and adequacy of treatment. Doctors who are oblivious to these factors or who believe that they are peripheral or removed from what is really important—the treatment of the disease—risk doing a bad job. And if their treatment *is* effective, it is because their patients rescue themselves from their doctor's detachment. Often the only effective treatment, or the element in treatment that makes the difference, is changing some aspect of the person's circumstance or behavior. May Prissel had extremely severe valvular heart disease with congestive heart failure. By religiously taking her medications and achieving maximal salt restriction, she was able to continue the work that was so important to her, but it was becoming increasingly more difficult to maintain the same pace or level of work. As the hours of the workday went by, she became more and more tired and would press harder to get her work done before she ran out of steam, thus aggravating her fatigue. She became depressed at the idea that she would soon be an invalid. Teaching her how to expend effort at a pace that was always within her body's work capacity (which, in this instance, was done with the aid of hypnosis) allowed her to continue her work and not feel herself becoming immobilized by the reduced capacity that was the natural effect of her disease.

Making such changes in aspects of the person's circumstances or behavior is quite difficult, and is rarely accomplished by simply telling a patient to do this or that. Instead, the physician is required to teach why it is important and how the changes are to be accomplished and then to reinforce the desired activity at every opportunity. People require their physicians' active help in the treatment of chronic disease, even when it would seem that nothing new is to be accomplished. Deterioration in the body's function—increasing breathlessness in emphysema, for example—may be interpreted not as arising from the disease, but rather as a personal failing. The person believes he or she is "just getting old," or is losing motivation, or just does not "have the stuff" anymore. The previous "will power" that was given credit for surmounting so many difficulties is seen as deserting the person. Making it clear that the diminished performance is due to the disease, and that a shift in medications (or something else) will restore ability, may return optimism and the ability to cope with the disease. Sometimes it is necessary to change the patient's expectations to conform to the diminished physical capacity. Constantly finding new ways to surmount this or that difficulty is the physician's job as part of treatment as surely as knowing the appropriate drugs. That is why the statement "There is nothing more that anyone can do" is so devastating. In addition, it is usually untrue—there is virtually always *something* that can be done to improve the patient's situation, no matter how small or seemingly inconsequential. Occasionally what is accomplished merely undoes some previous change. This is similar to the general illusion of progress, the illusion that humankind is always moving forward. I believe that for the patient as for populations at large, the idea of progress is necessary to forestall feelings of helplessness and hopelessness. With the dying, making it clear that the physical losses that accompany the inroads of disease *cannot* be combatted may be properly used to set in motion the patient's active intent to die—to withdraw the life force that has been the person's ally throughout life and in the preceding losing battle with disease. It should be clearly understood that although there is nothing more that can be done for the body, this does not mean that there is nothing more that can be done for the sick person (5).

In acute illness, chronic illness, or terminal illness, the active presence of the physician is a part of the treatment. I believe that it is accurate to put it even more strongly: *The physician is the treatment.* Antibiotics, other potent medications, modern technology, or even the ministrations of others in the medical setting (whatever they may be in their own right) are the physician's tools, but the physician is the treatment. In this era of egalitarianism, of "medical care teams," the nurse as an independent professional, the professionalization of social workers, physical therapists, and many others in medicine, to speak of the physician as the treatment may seem like fighting words. They are not meant to be; they are merely words that recognize a fact of the social nature of the biology of humankind. Other professionals may stand in the role of physician and also be the treatment, but it is inherent in the role of physician. It is not possible to understand the treatment of disease or patients without seeing that at every step the doctor, the sick person, and their relationship are woven into therapy. To understand what the next step must be, let us return to the old man with pneumonia, described in Chapter 7.

He has been treated with penicillin and supported with intravenous fluids and the respirator until the infection has subsided; malnutrition has responded to a standard hospital diet, the man will be well again. But for how long? If he returns home and nothing else changes, experience tells us that he will soon be sick again. Malnutrition will recur and pave the way for another infection, or he will fall and fracture his hip, or some other illness or accident will occur. In recognition of this, in most American hospitals the social worker will be called to deal with the "nonmedical" aspects of the case. But despite the best efforts of the social workers, the man will still be widowed and alone.

(Although it is possible that the attention paid to him in the hospital and afterwards by the visiting nurses and social agencies will serve to reconnect him to the social world. With his interest in others and in social interaction reawakened, he may overcome the other problems himself.) The usual pessimism of the hospital staff in cases like this is warranted; little can be changed in the basic social situations. His knee will always stand in the way of attempts to help him. Therefore, *the first key to the case is the knee.* It it true that osteoarthritis cannot be cured. However, with physical therapy and medication, most such joints can be made considerably more functional and less painful. All these activities can change the meaning of the arthritic knee. Changing meaning is itself a potent (but neglected) therapeutic force (6). The painful knee need not be a symbol of aging that diminishes physical activity through the inexorable passing of time. It can be a painful knee that needs treatment if this man is to get on with his life—nothing more, nothing less. Total knee replacement is available if simpler measures fail. The second key to the case is probably nutrition. Improving the knee will take time and, unless attention is paid to his diet, malnutrition will return and complicate everything. Seeing treatment in these terms is natural if the illness itself is understood as a story, only part of which occurs in the body; or if pathophysiology is understood to extend into the personal, interpersonal, familial, and even communal dimensions of the sick person.

The point of abandoning outmoded concepts of cause and seeing illness in terms of events unfolding over time is to realize that *proper treatment is what most simply and effectively changes the story.* Of course this man is subject to forces—social, psychological, and biological—over which neither he nor we have control. Grief is enormously potent, and so too are the changes in the social fabric caused by the modern geographic mobility available to his family. So too are the erosive effects of poverty and aging in a society unprepared for longevity or the negative biological effects of aging. But why should we feel helpless in the face of these things, regardless of how potent they are? Throughout most of its history, medicine has been a David facing Goliath, looking for a place where its weapons would be most effective. And throughout its history it has been helped by equally potent biological, psychological, and social forces that are also present in this man's story—the tendency of the body to heal itself, the inexplicable resurgence of hope (7), the drive in all of us to remain connected to the group, the sense of responsibility the larger society has for a sick person, and, ultimately, the magical bond that permits a sick person to be healed by a stranger.

Doctor, What Is Going To Happen to Me?

Hippocrates' *Book of Prognostics* opens with:

> It appears to me a most excellent thing for the physician to cultivate Prognosis; for by foreseeing and foretelling, in the presence of the sick, the present,

> the past, and the future and explaining the omissions which patients have been guilty of, he will be the more readily believed to be acquainted with the circumstances of the sick; so that men will have the confidence to entrust themselves to such a physician.
>
> . . . Thus a man will be the more esteemed to be a good physician . . . from having long anticipated everything; and by seeing and announcing beforehand those who will live and those who will die . . . (8).

While foretelling is vital to physicians, it is something all of us do all the time because we would be paralyzed if the future were not known to us. A goodly part of our life experience is given over to acquiring the information necessary to accurate foreknowledge. This may seem strange, because the usual meaning of predicting the future is knowing what will happen next month, next year or in ten years. While ten years from now is certainly in the future, so also is the next fraction of a second. The next minute, the next hour, day, and so on. It is a *necessity* to predict these futures with accuracy to live your life. Starting to cross the street, you require assurance that the street will still be there and will support your weight, that the moving car will not have gone beyond a certain spot, and that the pedestrians will move this way rather than that. The trains must be running an hour from now, the stores must be open tomorrow, Easter holidays will start next week. With a foresight that is remarkable (if the future is as opaque as it is usually thought to be) you are generally correct on all counts—but not precisely correct. Some uncertainty attends all these prognostications. Generally, however, your knowledge also permits a calculation of the accuracy of your prediction. The street will almost certainly bear your weight, although on the rarest of occasions a foot does go through a weakened surface. More often than that, automobiles lose control, difficulties with train schedules occur, stores sometimes close inexplicably, but Easter will most certainly be next Sunday if you have your dates right. If you live in the country, accurate predictions about the earth, trees, cows, barns, agricultural agents, and a myriad of other things make life possible.

All of this is true because part of knowing about almost everything includes the ability to make predictions about the thing, predictions in relationship to everything else of concern to you a moment, minute, hour, day, year, and so on in the future. In other words, all knowledge includes foreknowledge. As accurate predictions of the future are essential to getting along, uncertainty is the big problem of life. There cannot be one without the other. Every moment is filled with actions of one sort or another—smiling, opening the door, striking the next key on the keyboard, taking a sip of coffee. So too, of course, are choosing a physician, calling the doctor, starting chemotherapy, entering a hospital. Every action implies a choice, a decision of one sort or another. Every choice involves alternatives, and alternatives imply uncertainty about the right thing to do. Whether something was the right thing to do will not be known until that thing's future has arrived. Right or wrong, the choice and the action involve predictions about the future. It seems quite clear that the more knowledge of something one has, the more accurate one's predictions will be. An irreducible degree of uncertainty will always exist not merely because human knowledge is imperfect, but because knowledge is always gained about the present and the past and then applied to the future. The past of any thing, after all, is made up of instances each a little different from one another. So we take the previous examples and distill from them a somewhat abstract version that is our knowledge of them and which we can apply in predicting the future. But the future instances (the events we are trying to predict to reduce our uncertainty so that choices can be made on which actions are to based) will each be unique. To the degree that they *are* unique—different in some detail, however small, from the past similar events from which our knowledge came and on which we based our predictions—our forecast will be in error. This degree of uncertainty can never be removed.

That such irreducible uncertainty exists is also part of our knowledge. Usually we accept it, cast our predictions, make our choices, and act, aware that "you never know." A much better-known source of uncertainty arises from the deficiencies of each individual's knowledge. There is, after all, only a limited amount one can know of one's world. (Keep in mind that I am not discussing the kind of knowledge found in encyclopedias but rather the information we have concerning our everyday world.) Thus, while one has an enormous amount of information about one's bedroom, clothing, kitchen appliances, and other everyday appurtenances that permits quite accurate predictions about them, as the car, the children, or one's friends become the objects of thought and action, then the lack of sure knowledge and uncertainty loom larger. Conscious awareness of huge gaps in the knowledge on which decisions and actions are based is a source of discomfort or anxiety. The more important the decisions required, the less tolerable the uncertainty becomes. If a correct decision is absolutely crucial to one's well-being, then virtually no uncertainty is acceptable. Matters of health or life and death are areas where one simply cannot tolerate unsureness, yet it is always present. The necessity for trust, it seems to me, arises because we can't tolerate uncertainty in crucial matters. "I do now know the best thing to do, but my doctor does. I trust him (or her) implicitly." Of course, everybody knows that doctors are not infallible; it is simply that in certain circumstances that knowledge is not tolerable, so physicians are invested with infallibility.

While all knowledge about persons, objects, and relationships includes foreknowledge, the kind of information about these things that makes up our day-to-day knowledge and predictions includes what we believe about them to be important or unimportant, good or bad, right or wrong, fitting or not fitting. Naturally enough, we care about what is important to us and tend to exclude from consideration matters that we believe to have little significance. So, to pick a trivial example, when a person looks up at the sky and guesses whether it will soon rain, that prediction is more often in terms of what clothing to wear or how the day's activities should be modified than what is happening to the water supply. On the basis of these prognostications, behavior may be altered and important plans may be changed, actions that may modify the direction of the person's life—all the more so when questions about the future revolve around sickness, disability or death. In fact, when sickness does come, all of us want to know what it means in terms of our future. We know about the present; we are living the unpleasantness of the day-to-day illness. But what about tomorrow. And next week, month, or year? When I told Kay Michaels that the pathology report following her modified radical mastectomy indicated that there was cancer in her axillary lymph nodes and that she would require chemotherapy, she kept saying "Chemotherapy. Chemotherapy. Chemotherapy." I said, "What does that mean to you, Kay?" She said, "You know what it means—it means chemotherapy." We know that she was talking about her future—about sickness, about endless involvement with doctors, about hair loss, about her upcoming marriage, about ever having children. Whether chemotherapy meant Vincristine, Adriamycin versus methotrexate, 5-fluorouracil, prednisone, or some other regimen was not her interest at that moment. It is also true that her foreknowledge of chemotherapy, however limited at that moment, was intimately involved with Kay Michaels—*her* hair loss, *her* sickness, *her* inability to have children. As such, the precognition contained no pretense of objective predictive probabilities. At that moment she would not have been reassurred to hear the actual percentage of women who lost what percentage of their hair or the actual percentage of women who were able to have normal babies after their chemotherapy. At that moment she *knew* she would lose all her hair, never have children, and so forth. Thus Kay, like all of us, made her predictions not only about and in terms of things that were meaningful to her but also constructed her probabilities on the basis of her dreads and wishes rather than on their objective chances of occurring. In time, if she is like others, she will construct a wished-for future that is as positive as the feared future is negative, and the two will coexist in her thoughts. But both futures will be intimately related to *her*.

For all persons, predictions of the future are a necessary part of their thinking. The forecasts are based on knowledge of objects, events, persons and relationships because all such information includes precognition. Predictions arise not only from the objective details but from the *personal meaning* of the facts. These same forecasts begin to influence the future as people alter their behavior to fit their predictions. This aspect of forecasting the future is the fundamental reason that the nature of an illness is inextricably bound up with the nature of the person in whom it occurs rather than only with the disease on which it is based. Kay Michaels, out of her fear of chemotherapy's effect on her future may refuse it outright; delay starting; find a physician who promises a less threatening treatment; begin diets, coffee enemas, or other unconventional treatments said to mitigate the effects of the chemotherapy; or take some other action whose net effect will be to alter the future that would have occurred if she had received the chemotherapy as initially planned. Perhaps considering herself altered as a woman, and by extension transformed in the eyes of others, she begins to change the kinds of relationships she has, and as a result of these modified relationships may find herself more or less alone. The issue is not whether these alternative actions are for the better or worse, but only that her forecasts of the future change the experienced story of her illness and may alter its outcome profoundly.

One often hears how a particular patient "brought the cancer on by . . . " Such a thing may be as possible as common belief has it, but many dedicated researchers have failed to find hard evidence to support this popular conviction. While we may not be able to determine the largest influences on the pattern of our lives, we certainly have choice on a moment-by-moment basis. In illness, in all of life, each of these tiny decisions—in relationships, activity, projects, diet, exercise, sleep, reading—add up to matters of great consequence. Each choice, large or small, is based on knowledge that includes both a forecast and its personal meaning.

Science is also engaged in forecasting. Scientific knowledge, however, is meant to be entirely purged of the personal. The methods of science are designed to ensure that the specific environmental circumstances, life history, or personal characteristics of the individual owners of livers, for example, do not bias scientific knowledge of the liver and its functions. Scientific knowledge is therefore abstract knowledge which, as noted earlier, is meant to apply to universals—*all* livers—rather than only my or your particular liver. One of the tests of the adequacy of scientific knowledge is its predictive value. Given the same well-defined preconditions as in an initial scientific observation or experiment, the same outcome should follow. Whether a molecule of protein or an entire organ, to the degree that some object of medical science has been well characterized, any similar object met in the future should be the same. Similar predictive accuracy results from the knowledge of physiologic processes. If you understand how oxygen is carried by the blood and how its transport is altered under given conditions, you should be able to predict how *this* patient's blood will carry oxygen. Conversely, and of more importance to clinicians, given an abnormality in the amount of oxygen in someone's blood, a physician can generally tell what abnormality of structure or function exists. When Caroline Preskauer was in the emergency room with not only very little oxygen in her blood but too much carbon dioxide, it could not simply be that heart failure and fluid in her lungs were interfering with the transport of oxygen from air to blood; there also had to be some condition keeping carbon dioxide from being exhaled. She had to have something that was trapping air in the lungs, such as failure of her lungs as a bellows or emphysema, in addition to her heart disease. Unless the laboratory was in error, *it could not be otherwise.* The pursuit of the clue might lead to a solution that would provide her with relief even though her heart disease could not be reversed. The same information would allow the accurate forecast that, without successful action, Caroline Preskauer will soon be unconscious. That is one tiny example of the predictive power of medical science and its utility for clinical medicine.

Diseases, since the early 1800s, have also been objects of science. Thus, it should be as true of diseases as of other objects of science that, to the degree to which they have been well characterized, knowledge gained about them in the past should apply to instances of them met in the future. Characterization of a disease requires that it be isolated from the persons who have it—delineated as a thing separate from the sick person. Otherwise the knowledge will be biased by the personal qualities or idiosyncrasies of the afflicted patient. It will be knowledge about the sick person plus the disease rather than only about the disease. What is known about diseases with regard to abnormalities of cellular structure, body chemistry, physiology, or molecular biology is also abstracted from the persons who have the disease. These fundamental mechanisms become the disease's hallmark. When they are present, the disease is present. When they are absent, there is no disease. In the minds of physicians, they have largely supplanted the previous structural definitions of disease. It remains true that most tumors, malignant or otherwise, are still defined by their typical cellular structure as seen microscopically. But ideally we would like to understand the basic molecular abnormalities present in tumors and define them in those terms. We believe that when we know why they (or any diseases) are the way they are we will know how they act to produce their characteristic picture. We believe that such fundamental comprehension will give us the basis for predicting how a disease will behave. In other words, in the modern era, knowledge of the molecular biology of a disease is believed to provide an enhanced ability to predict what the disease will do.

My use of the word "believe" in the previous paragraph underlines the idea that knowledge of the molecular basis of disease allows *prediction* of the course or action of and instance of disease in a particular person is purely and simply a modern article of faith. It is perfectly true that information about the molecular basis of a particular disease can explain the manifestations of the disease. *But first you must know the disease and its manifestations.* Knowing *only* the molecular facts of a disease will not allow you to predict what the disease would look like—not only in a particular person but in general—in the same manner that merely knowing that one can hook together two hydrogen molecules and one oxygen molecule would not allow the prediction that water will be wet. Myasthenia gravis is a disease in which muscle weakness occurs. Its molecular basis has been worked out in great and accurate detail. Based on that knowledge, therapy is rational. However, the knowledge of its fundamental mechanisms may allow prediction of the behavior of an afflicted *muscle* but not its behavior in an *individual patient.* The disease generally afflicts persons after the age of thirty. It may affect the muscles of the eyelids or the eyes or cause weakness in jaw muscles or the muscles in the chest employed during breathing. Patients may awaken without having muscle weakness, but as the day goes on the weakness gets worse. With repetitive acts, like chewing, the weakness progresses, improving only with rest. In some patients (particularly those whose eye muscles are involved) the disease disappears spontaneously after a year. In others it is inexorably progressive. The stresses of physical effort, emotion, or other sickness aggravate the condition, even to the point of inducing life-threatening crises. But the disease behaves differently in different individuals. Good clinicians who have worked with myasthenia gravis patients for a long time can often prognosticate what will happen to individual patients after they have had experience with the pattern over time of that person's illness. Pathophysiology—knowledge about fundamental mechanisms of disease—is of little use to clinicians unless they have had experience with patients with the disease. Once again it is apparent that the individual doctor is the bridge, the tacit partner of abstract knowledge that makes it work for each individual patient. This function of doctors, included (or, more accurately, hidden) in the idea of judgment, is necessary for the care of the sick not because medical science has more to learn—its knowledge is imperfect—but because the *ideal* of scientific knowledge will not work for *this* sick person without the aid of *this* doctor. Science is sometimes described as knowledge of reality. To achieve such knowledge it is necessary to remove the distortions that human interests interpose in the same manner that the randomized controlled trial protects against the biases of patients and physicians. But when we are sick we do not need impersonal knowledge; we require *personalized* knowledge. As I have emphasized, the individual physician's judgment personalizes the impersonal knowledge provided by medical science.

It is necessary to go further to demonstrate the inaccuracy of the concept of impersonal, dispassionate medical science seeking truth wherever the trail may lead; the blind embrace of this ideal keeps us from the pursuit of knowledge essential to the care of the sick. Recently, a group of scientists described how they have been working for ten years to find the "discrete pathogenic mechanisms" for the long-term complications of diabetes. They found that elevations of the blood sugar cause decreases in a certain substance (*myo*-inositol) which through a biochemical chain of events has an effect on nerve conduction (9). Abnormalities of nerve conduction (diabetic neuropathy) is one of the long-term complications of diabetes. They believe that their research may lead to an effective treatment. Their hunt for the molecular basis of these complications, however, could not have taken place if they had not known about diabetes, been able to identify persons with diabetes in whom the complications have occurred, and been able to cause diabetes in laboratory animals. Last but by no means least, these researchers would never have started their investigations if they had not known the importance—in terms of frequency, severity, and effects on the lives of persons with diabetes—of these long-term complications of the disease. The disease category is necessary to organize the search for its molecular basis. Its importance to sick persons is the motor that drives the research. The disease category is equally necessary to bring the knowledge back into medical practice. Disease categories are human inventions, as I stated in the previous chapter they have no independent existence like oak trees or snowflakes.

If their investigations are successful, and if you have diabetic neuropathy, I will know why your nerves are not functioning well and perhaps I will be able to make them better again. Possibly their research will lead to a test that will allow earlier treatment for the disorder. But no knowledge of basic mechanisms will permit more than an informed guess as to whether you, as opposed to another diabetic, are going to develop diabetic neuropathy and how severe or disabling it will be. In fact, we know about diabetic neuropathy because we know about the natural history of diabetes. That knowledge comes only from watching and recording what has happened to countless persons with diabetes over many, many years.

It may appear that I am contradicting myself. Earlier I stated that when Caroline Preskauer was in the emergency room, knowledge of the levels of oxygen and carbon dioxide in her blood allowed a firm prediction that she would soon be unconscious. But in these last paragraphs I have suggested that, except for extremes, knowledge of the basic mechanisms of disease alone is virtually never sufficient to allow a predictive statement about the events that will befall an individual patient in a particular circumstance. No contradiction is involved; in clinical medicine such knowledge never exists apart from other knowledge on which the application of basic facts depends for its utility. Given only the abnormal levels of her arterial blood gases, certain statements could be made, but no one could tell us what was going to happen without more information. At the very least our hypothetical expert prognosticator would need to know whether the arterial blood gases were a step in the process of getting better or getting worse. In the emergency room where the blood tests were drawn, the doctor knew what Caroline Preskauer looked like and how she behaved. The briefest examination would have revealed not only that she had heart disease but that it was congenital. Her husband was there to tell the vitally important story of the preceding hours, days, and weeks which set the stage for the immediate events. In clinical medicine, medical science is *always* applied within a context and as part of an ongoing process. Both the context and the details of the process enter into the application of science and have effects on prediction, because, if it is true that the prognosis that counts is about *this* patient, it must be recognized that an individual person can *never* be found apart from some context or outside the unfolding of a particular story.

There are at least two other reasons why molecular-level information alone does not permit predictions in individual instances. Levels of arterial blood gases are facts that fit into a system of knowledge about cellular metabolism, and that system of knowledge, not merely the laboratory numbers, is employed in making predictions. As previously noted, that system of ideas, like all other scientific knowledge, is an abstraction that cannot be applied directly to a patient without adding a guesswork factor. In a manner similar to all our predictions, whether based in science or common knowledge, what we say of the future, based on the laboratory report and our knowledge of physiology, will only have a certain probability of being correct. The prediction will be true, we say, within certain confidence limits. On the basis of the physiology and the blood gas information alone, our confidence in the accuracy of the prediction will be low (the confidence limits will be wide). As the rest of the information pours in from all the sources available to the emergency room doctor, the probability of an accurate prediction will increase (the confidence limits will narrow). The predictions are part of a process, and as the process unfolds, the probabilities can be corrected. Although some decisions in medicine are made final on the basis of probabilities where no new information will be possible—decisions to operate, for example—in most instances there is a continuous flow of information that allows corrections of predictive possibilities. The "go, no go" aspect of surgery is one of the important differences between surgery and medicine and between surgeons and physicians.

There is a second reason why knowledge of the molecular basis of disease alone is not sufficient for the care of sick persons. General systems theory tells that what we know of one level of organization in living systems is not sufficient to predict reliably how the next higher level of organization will behave. In other words, the understandings of the molecular basis of, for example, the contractile proteins of heart muscle will not alone tell us how heart muscle cells will look or act. Knowing how the cells look and act does not make it possible to predict how a whole heart will look or act. It is the same all the way up the levels of organization. Because the knowledge works so well in the opposite direction—knowing how heart muscle contractile proteins work helps explain how heart muscle cells look and act—it is usually forgotten that knowing about the parts of something is not sufficient to predict the behavior of the whole.

What doctors who treat sick persons know about how to apply medical science comes from their having taken care of person after person with a particular disease. What medicine as a profession knows about the life history of any disease is similarly abstracted from the profession's cumulative experience with the disease. In this regard, clinicians' knowledge of diseases is like the information all of us have about our world and the things that are of interest to us. Singing teachers have knowledge of singing and singers. They get the former by abstracting from the latter, there being no way to hear singing without hearing singers.

The tools of medical science—from exacting criteria for the diagnosis of a disease to molecular explanations for the abnormalities of disease—have added immeasurably to the ability of physicians to meet the Hippocratic ideal of prognostication, but it is physicians' knowledge of sick persons and of themselves, no less than their knowledge of medical science, that makes accurate prognosis possible.

What transpired in Arnold Lauffer's illness makes the interdependence of these kinds of knowledge clearer. Taking care of Mr. Lauffer in the intensive-care unit was difficult because no one was sure what the basic disease was, despite the plethora of information that had accumulated about the function of his various organ systems. After he left the intensive-care unit for a regular hospital room, more active and more himself, the amount of function that he had lost in the course of his illness became evident. Despite all the medications, almost any activity caused fatigue and shortness of breath. He finally went home because nothing more of benefit could be expected of further hospitalization. Within a few days he developed obvious heart failure and shortly thereafter died following a cardiac arrest. After an autopsy demonstrated how numerous recent heart attacks had left him with remarkably little functioning heart muscle, understanding his illness became possible. He was a tough-minded, strong-willed man—a survivor, as one of the consultants put it. Put that weakened, devastated heart into someone less tough and death would surely have occurred earlier. With the same heart, his initial recovery seemed miraculous. But, ultimately, his prognosis was determined by his underlying disease. Even Arnold Lauffer could not exist with a heart that pumped so little blood.

And so it was with Caroline Preskauer. Enormous force of will, intelligent and sophisticated manipulation of physicians, more avoidance of medical care than one would have thought possible, an uncanny ability to know precisely how much the oxygen level of her blood would permit her to do, and a loving and supportive family had combined to allow her to survive decades longer than any of the other children with congenital heart disease who were her friends in the clinic. Ultimately, two factors combined to bring about her death. One was the ineluctable progression of her heart and lung disease and the other was her inability to stop trying to be "just like everybody else." No single part of her could explain her remarkable life.

But other factors of importance in prognosis clarify where the physician fits into the process. A number of specific types of knowledge, which become part of judgment, are learned by experience in caring for sick persons. One of these is the rate of progression of events and diseases. If the diagnosis of pneumococcal pneumonia is correct, then the fever should fall to normal within twelve to twenty-four hours after the penicillin is started. The fever takes longer to return to normal when someone is treated for streptococcal tonsillitis (about thirty-six to forty-eight hours). If these predictions are wrong, the probability is that the diagnosis is wrong.

When I was a resident I took care of a man with severe chronic obstructive pulmonary disease (we called it chronic bronchitis in those days) who I was sure was soon to die. When I returned from the army two years later he was still alive and not much worse. I was too inexperienced to know how slowly the disease progresses. Physicians in training frequently behave as if catastrophe will follow in minutes if they do not act *now,* leading them into the error of precipitate therapy. Doctors whose entire experience is in hospitals often have exaggerated ideas of the speed of disease. Learning that each disease has a characteristic pace that is modified (within limits) in individual patients is one of the results of experience.

Learning to think in terms of probabilities and within their confidence limits is another kind of knowledge that comes with experience. Recent research in decision-making techniques, with their emphasis on probabilities, has emphasized how much a systematic approach to aspects of judgment has to offer. Students of this field are able to repeatedly demonstrate how counter-intuitive some of the statistics are on which these kinds of judgments must be made.

Good prognostication also requires learning how medical science must be modified in certain contexts: in the light of who *this* sick person is, with awareness of the limits of disease categories, and, finally, with a full awareness by the physician of his or her limitations of knowledge, experience, nerve, involvement, and physical factors (such as fatigue) which also influence a prediction. When they have acquired the skills that result from these kinds of learning, physicians become clinicians. It is a pity that every clinician has to take thirty years to rediscover the knowledge.

As Faber said so many years ago, clinicians cannot live or breathe without knowledge of the disease. To understand the fundamental biology of disease is necessary to rational medicine, but, in itself, such knowledge is inadequate to clinical medicine. Doctors must see instance after instance of the disease to understand its behavior in sick persons. They cannot help seeing instance after instance of sick persons who are ill because of that disease. In addition, they cannot help being molded and changed by their experiences. We have seen how the four tasks of the clinician—diagnosing, seeking cause, treating, and prognosticating—cannot be accomplished in the absence of knowledge about both the disease and the sick person. Physicians' manifest knowledge of disease has been the focus of medicine for these last 150 years while knowledge of sick persons and doctors has languished—left to intuition and unfocused experience.

References

1. Feinstein, Alvan R. *Clinical Epidemiology.* 1985. Philadelphia, W. B. Saunders, Chap. 29.

2. Feinstein, Alvan R., op. cit., Chap. 21.

3. Bishop, Katherine. Frustrated AIDS Patients Devise Their Own Therapies. *The New York Times.* Tuesday, March 17, 1987, p. C3.

4. Spiro, Howard M. *Doctors, Patients and Placebos.* New Haven, Conn., Yale University Press.

5. Cassell, Eric J. *The Healer's Art.* 1985. Cambridge, Mass., MIT Press, p. 10.

6. Cassell, Eric J. *Talking with Patients: Vol. 2. Clinical Technique.* 1985. Cambridge, Mass., MIT Press, p. 187ff.

7. MacIntyre, Alisdair. Seven Traits for the Future: Designing Our Descendants. *The Hastings Center Report* 1979; 9:5–7.

8. *The Genuine Works of Hippocrates.* Translated by Francis Adams. 1939. Baltimore, The Williams and Wilkens Company, *The Book of Prognostics,* p. 42.

9. Greene, Douglas A., Lattimer, Sarah A., and Sima, Anders A. F.. Sorbitol, Phosphoinositides, and Sodium-Potassium-ATPase in the Pathogenesis of Diabetic Complications. *NEJM* 1987; 316:599–606.

9

The Doctor and the Patient

IN THE PRECEDING chapters I have emphasized the difficulties that arise in the care of sick persons when medicine's exclusive focus is on diseases. Many have said that the solution is to train doctors to have more concern for the sick person. Two generations of attempts from within the profession of medicine to accomplish this goal have had remarkably little effect. One reason for this failure—surprising in view of the amount of time, effort, and thought expended—is that sick persons, is another way of stating that in the intellectual basis of modern medicine, patients and their diseases are not *logically* a part of disease-oriented medicine. Logical relationships are those in which one thing follows from, is an obligatory consequence of, or is necessarily related to another. Logically related subjects are connected in the mind—to think of one leads to thinking of the other. Disease theory has no logical relation to person—in disease theory it does not matter what person has the disease—therefore, the common complaint that patients are overlooked in the treatment of their diseases is another way of stating that in the intellectual basis of modern medicine patients and their diseases are not logically related. Emphasis during the training of doctors on something (person) not logically related to what is central in their education (science of disease) will not solve the basic intellectual problem that arises from trying to concentrate on two logically unrelated subjects.

If the patient as a unique and particular entity is not inherently and logically a part of disease-oriented medicine, then neither is the relationship between patient and doctor. Nor is there a place for the doctor *as a person,* although surely if the personhood of the patient is seen to be important, then the person of the doctor must also be a factor. (Only people—not questionnaires, computers, or diagnostic machines—can deal with other people as the complex entities they are. With the exception of scientific knowledge of disease, the doctor's most important skills do not derive from disease theory.)

The importance of the doctor's skills, apart from scientific knowledge of disease, is also not derivative from disease theory. The usual view of the art of medicine continues to see it as just that—an art that is not to be considered as seriously as science in the treatment of sick persons, although no treatment can take place in its absence. Because moral problems raised by modern medicine follow from the effects of biomedicine on persons, their consideration is also logically unrelated to disease-centered medicine.

When the patient as a person, ethical considerations, the doctor-patient relationship, and the art of medicine are logically outside the mainstream of medicine from the point of view of its dominant theory, surely a better theory must be sought. It may be argued that I have constructed a straw horse, that all good physicians always keep the patient in mind. Consider this excerpt from a medical encyclopedia, the *Oxford Companion to Medicine:*

> HOLISTIC MEDICINE is a doctrine of preventive and therapeutic medicine which emphasizes the importance of regarding the individual as a whole being integral with his social, cultural, and environmental context rather than as a patient with isolated malfunction of a particular system or organ. Though the term has recently become fashionable, the underlying philosophy is *nothing new and has always been inseparable from good medical practice* (emphasis added) (1).

I suggest that the author is incorrect for several reasons. First, a careful distinction must be drawn between an "underlying philosophy" and the degree to which it has an effect on practice. The evidence suggests that the influence of that philosophy has lessened. Second, although good physicians have always understood that they were "taking care" of persons, with all that the term implies, knowledge of the social, cultural, and environmental has never prevailed to the same degree as knowledge about the body and its diseases. Third, modern scientific medicine and, particularly, technology have become so compelling as to disturb the priorities that have ruled medicine for centuries. In this chapter I look more closely at areas of medicine such as ethics to see how they would fare if medicine's primary focus was on other than the disease itself, and I will begin to examine the problems that would arise if the sick person became the central concern of medicine and physicians.

The medicine of our era is marked, in part, by a concern for ethical and moral issues. Patients believe they have a *right* to take part in their own care—they expect their wishes to be a determining factor in doctors' decisions. The right of patients to refuse or discontinue treatment is now an acknowledged aspect of American medicine. The appropriate allocation of scarce resources—deciding who will get treatments or organs when there are not enough to meet prevailing needs—is a current issue in the face of budgetary restraints. Abortion on request, surrogate motherhood, involuntary sterilization, abortion of defective fetuses, and *in vitro* fertilization (test-tube babies) are all examples of morally problematic issues in human reproduction. If not the parents, who should decide whether a newborn infant should be treated for defects that will irreparably impair its personhood or longevity?

The field of bioethics has grown up in the past twenty years to deal with the moral problems posed by modern medical science and technology, and there are now many bioethicists whose expertise lies in the analysis of issues such as those mentioned above. In the light of the present intense and growing interest in medical ethics, it may be surprising that there is no logical reason why a medicine directed primarily at diseases should also encompass ethical problems. To be concerned with moral problems is to be concerned with persons. Where medicine is focused on diseases, the sick person *as person* is not central, and consequently neither are decisions that arise from the moral nature of the person. Indeed, clashes between technological and moral imperatives are currently a commonplace in medical practice. Few guidelines exist for resolving the conflict between the demands of the disease and the other needs of a sick person, which suggests the possibility that something might be considered appropriate treatment if it were, at the same time, unreasonable or inappropriate in terms of the patient. Moral philosophers have most often based their approaches to the moral problems of medicine on theories of ethics that have developed over the twenty-five hundred years since Classical Greece. Not surprisingly, there is often disagreement among ethicists about the best approach to many of the thorny difficulties that have come about as a result of medical advances. Recently, some physicians and philosophers, particularly Richard Zaner in his book, *Ethics and the Clinical Encounter* (2), have proposed that discussions of everyday moral problems of medicine are obscured by the emphasis on ethical theory. They believe that an understanding of the moral issues inherent in a particular clinical problem can be explored by a thorough discussion of the case as long as all the pertinent features—the disease, the sick person, the family and community, the institution (e.g., hospital), and legal concerns—are included in the analysis (3). What this approach makes absolutely clear is that in the case of a particular sick person the nature of the moral problem depends on the details of the case. Change the details and the moral problem is changed. I can illustrate this approach and its relevance by presenting the cases I used when teaching a second-year medical school course in clinical ethics, and by showing how the students viewed the problems.

> When Anthony Spatz, a 78-year-old retired attorney whose wife had died a year earlier, went for his annual physical examination, he felt fine. However, his physician of many years discovered that his stool was positive for occult blood. Six more tests for occult blood were also positive, although rectal examination and sigmoidoscopy were normal. When Mr. Spatz asked Dr. David Anderson what he expected to find, Dr. Anderson said that the most common reasons for occult blood in the stool were benign—things such as diverticulitis. On the other hand, Dr. Anderson pointed out, the tests were important because they made possible early diagnosis of cancer.
>
> Mr. Spatz was adamant. He said, "Dave, I must tell you ahead of time, even if you do find cancer, I'm not going to be operated on." "Tony," Dr. Anderson said, "if you are going to refuse permission for surgery, why

bother going ahead with further diagnostic tests?" "Because I like to know what the problem is—who my enemies are, so to speak."

The barium enema was negative, and Dr. Anderson was ready to quit. He told Mr. Spatz that colonoscopy was expensive and inconvenient and that it was foolish to waste his time and money. Mr. Spatz said, "It's my money, my time, and my decision. Arrange for the colonoscopy." Colonoscopy revealed an early annular carcinoma of the bowel in the splenic flexure. The biopsy diagnosis was adenocarcinoma. Despite the cancer and true to his word, Mr. Spatz refused to be operated on.

In August, when Dr. Anderson was on vacation, Mr. Spatz fainted on the street and was brought to the New York Hospital emergency room. Because Dr. Anderson was a Lenox Hill Hospital physician, there were no records on Mr. Spatz at New York Hospital. He was extremely pale. Examination of the abdomen was normal—specifically, it was not distended and the bowel sounds were normal—no emergency surgical condition was present. He was profoundly anemic from blood loss (his hematocrit was 15 percent). There was blood in his stool. There were no other abnormalities.

The doctors in the emergency room explained everything to Mr. Spatz and *very* strongly urged him to have blood transfusions, but Mr. Spatz was adamant about being returned to his home without treatment.

The students wanted to know whether an operation for the cancer when it was first found might have saved him and what would happen to Mr. Spatz now, if he did or did not have the transfusions. The class had two physicians (beside myself) to act as consultants. They agreed that an early operation might have cured him and would have certainly delayed or avoided the present problem. The consultants believed that Mr. Spatz would continue to bleed and surely die from the anemia within weeks to months. The students (and the consultants, who also voiced their opinions) were unhappy that the patient had initially refused surgery and wondered whether Dr. Anderson had worked hard enough at convincing him. Given the present situation, however, they were unanimous that Mr. Spatz should not be given blood transfusions over his objections. In addition, they were aware that the law protected Mr. Spatz's right to refuse treatment.

Later, in the same class, further developments in the case of Anthony Spatz were presented.

When they heard what had happened to their father, Anthony Spatz's two children, Clarice Arnheim, who lives in Minneapolis, and Edgar Spatz, who lives in Atlanta, came to New York to be with him. They argued with him constantly about his refusal to accept treatment, but to no avail. Dr. Anderson, whom they called, was sympathetic, but he pointed out that Anthony Spatz was an adult who "knew his own mind." When, one month later, Mr. Spatz slipped into a coma, the children had him brought to New York Hospital (to avoid Dr. Anderson). Although his refusal of treatment on the previous visit to the emergency room was recorded, they insisted that he be transfused.

The previous unanimity of the class and the consulting physicians disappeared. Some of the students believed that the fact of his being unconscious and his children's desire that he be transfused were sufficient reasons to give him blood. They had been uncomfortable with the death of someone who would be so easy to save, and now they had their chance. Others believed the children had the legal right to insist on transfusion. (In this case, that would not have been so. While in some jurisdictions they do, in New York State children do not automatically become legal surrogates for a parent in these circumstances.) Most students held to the belief that Mr. Spatz should not be given transfusions because he had previously expressed his desire not to be treated and had formed that opinion aware of the consequences, and he had not changed his mind over a long period of time. One of the consultant physicians and several students remained uncomfortable with the decision to allow him to die untreated. To stand by helplessly and watch him die with the possibility that he might have changed his mind was difficult for them.

The bare-bones doctrine of patient autonomy was not sufficient in itself to determine doctors' actions, the class and the consulting doctors believed. Patients, they reasoned, were not being treated by machines that could be turned on or off at will. Doctors were involved as persons, and that involvement was desirable for patients and necessary to good medical care. The conflict between empathy and objectivity of which Freud spoke was present here also. How could a physician be both empathetic and at the same time indifferent to the fate of the patient or to the patient's decision? To empathize with a patient's desire not be treated surely must mean coming to understand and being sympathetic with the patient's reasons for refusing treatment.

The way the class and consulting physicians dealt with the next case makes their attitude clear.

> Helen Case came into the emergency room two hours ago because of severe headache and fever. She is 24 years old and a second-year medical student. She says that she has been sick for several days, but she thought it was the "flu" so she did not do anything for it. But today, when the headache became so painful, she got frightened and came over. The resident knew in a moment that she was really sick. Her temperature is 104 F. and examination reveals a stiff neck and other signs of meningitis. She consented to the spinal tap, with which there was some difficulty. However, when it was finally done, the fluid confirmed the diagnosis of meningitis. Gram stain suggests that it is pneumococcal meningitis.
>
> There is no evidence of neurological impairment as yet. Despite the headache, she appears mentally clear, a fact that has been confirmed by many physicians, including a psychiatrist. This has become a crucial point because an hour ago she refused consent for any further treatment except analgesics.
>
> The treatment for Helen Case is intravenous antibiotics. Without antibiotics she will almost certainly die. Every minute of delay increases the chance that she will be left brain damaged even if she is treated. On the other hand, if she gets antibiotics promptly, the probability is that she will be home in ten days without any aftereffects of her meningitis.

In the beginning the class was ambivalent. The patient is mentally clear and has a right to refuse treatment. The fact that they do not understand the basis for her refusal is the central problem. On the other hand, they do not really understand why a Jehovah's Witness should refuse blood transfusion, yet they honor such a patient's rights. But the beliefs of Jehovah's Witnesses have stood the test of time and are shared by a whole religious group. Helen Case's refusal to allow treatment seems to have no logical or cultural underpinning—particularly since she is a medical student who should know the consequences. Ultimately the students decided (and the consultants and I agreed) that she should be treated against her will and forcibly restrained if necessary. To watch her die in these circumstances, they argued, would be like participating in her death. After she recovered she could go home and commit suicide if that is what she wanted to do. They were willing to take their chances on being sued by her for battery.

This case seemed to indicate that the students felt obligated to save lives in the absence of an understandable refusal of consent for treatment. Early in the course, in case after case the discussion showed that the students believed that doctors had an obligation, independent of their patients' desires, to utilize their knowledge and technology to save lives and do what could be done for individual diseases. Occasionally, as they saw it, this "medical" obligation came into conflict with "patient autonomy," and then the patient's right to refuse treatment overrode the independent medical goals. As the course progressed, they began to change their views. Two cases were important in this transition. The first was straightforward.

> Jen Liang Yee is a famous 72-year-old artist with advanced Alzheimer's disease. He has been cared for faithfully by his wife, Stella, herself suffering from severe rheumatoid arthritis. Mr. Yee fell at home and fractured his hip. The accident happened about a week before Mrs. Yee called an ambulance to bring him to the hospital. It had taken all her strength, over several hours, to get him back into bed. At first she thought he was all right—she certainly did not realize that his hip was broken—but yesterday he became obviously very sick with a high fever.
>
> Mr. Yee, who is clearly demented, is malnourished, has an intertrochanteric fracture of the right hip, and bilateral lower lobe pneumonia. Gram positive diplococci are seen on the gram stain of the sputum.
>
> While all the diagnostic procedures were going on, Stella Yee sat in the corner, tearful but quiet. But when she was told about his condition, she asked that he not be treated for the pneumonia. The doctor explained that he would surely die without antibiotics.

Here was a case in which antibiotics would save the patient's life, the patient had not refused consent for treatment (he was, in fact, legally incompetent), there were no advanced directives, and his wife was not legally his surrogate. According to the students' previous opinions, Mr. Yee should get antibiotics because the treatment was both available and life-saving. But they were reluctant in this instance. If they gave him antibiotics, he would just get another infection, and then another and another, until something finally killed him. If he recovered, where would he go? Back home to his wife who seemed to have done more than her best, but from whom not much more would be possible? A nursing home was a more probable—but clearly undesirable—destination. If they did not treat him and he died, what reason should they give? That he was old and had Alzheimer's disease and his treatment would waste societal resources was discussed, but it made them uncomfortable to make a decision about Mr. Yee on the basis of economics. That he was merely too old or infirm to save also bothered them, because they felt such criteria might be based on mere prejudice. They argued the matter for a long time because the alternative they ultimately accepted seemed so (to use their term) "soft." They should withhold treatment because Mrs. Yee, who knew him best, said to do so because for many years he had not been the husband she had known all her adult life, and no matter what they did he would not get better. Although to many readers their decision may seem obvious, it meant disregarding the goals of medicine with which they were most comfortable and which had been emphasized to them for their first two years of medical school.

The next case was even more troubling.

> Giorgio Frascatti has been brought by ambulance into a Jersey City emergency room because of severe chest pain. He was in early shock when he came in but was soon stabilized. He is an 86-year-old violinist who has survived many serious illnesses—always returning to performing and teaching. Twenty years ago he had a pulmonary embolus (clot in the lung) from thrombophlebitis of a leg following an injury. An abscess of the bowel had required surgery and a long hospitalization some ten years previous to this episode. Four years ago he developed a strangulated right inguinal hernia, which was repaired.
>
> At the time of hospitalization for the hernia, a large aneurysm of the thoracic and abdominal aorta was discovered. The potential seriousness of the aneurysm was explained to him (that he might die suddenly), and he was advised to have surgery. He refused, explaining that he had to die of something pretty soon and a ruptured aneurysm did not sound as bad as some other ways of dying.
>
> He had had two routine physicals since the hernia surgery, and on each occasion he had refused further investigations related to the aneurysm. On the most recent visit, in 1983, he had asked, "How's the hand grenade in my chest getting along?"
>
> In the emergency room Mr. Frascatti was conscious, although in considerable pain. The X rays and other studies strongly suggested that his current desperate situation was a result of a tear in the aneurysm. His wife, who had come with him and his son, who arrived later, were told that without an operation Mr. Frascatti had no chance of living. A vascular surgeon was called in who confirmed that opinion and talked for a long time with the wife and son to convince them of the importance of the surgery just on the "long shot" that his life might be saved. The wife and son finally consented and talked to Mr. Frascatti, who signed operative consent.

Mr. Frascatti died in the surgical intensive-care unit about five hours postoperatively.

After he died, Mrs. Frascatti wrote a letter to his internist expressing her sadness that she had consented to surgery—that she had not followed her husband's frequently stated wishes.

The class saw a slide showing the letter (with the real names removed). They were distressed about the surgeon's obligation. They already knew that the Hippocratic Oath (to which patients frequently refer when they say that "I know you took an oath to save life") did not require saving life. It actually says: "I will follow that system of regimen which, according to my ability and judgment, I consider for the benefit of my patients, and abstain from whatever is deleterious and mischievous" (4). (The concept that physicians are required to save life at all costs was introduced in the nineteenth century.) They thought that because the surgeon did not know the family and could not know how resolutely and for how long Mr. Frascatti had refused surgery, he was correct in strongly recommending the operation. Other students believed that the surgeon might have discovered this if he had questioned the wife and son with that end in mind. Everybody agreed that just because a patient says no does not mean that you should not do your best to convince the patient or family of the correctness of your views. The problem was, as they saw it, that a patient has a right to decide what treatment to accept because only the patient knows what is important to him or her. Only the doctor, they said, *really* knows what the options are and what they mean. In a case like that of Mr. Frascatti, the stakes are so high—life and death—that the students could not quite accept that the wife and son should have the last word. On the other hand, Mrs. Frascatti's letter was moving because she believed that he had been *injured* by the surgery—not only because of the physical discomfort, but by the failure to honor him as expressed in his frequently stated choice.

There were two other troublesome issues in the case. Despite the high probability of failure, the operation *might* have succeeded. If it had, Mr. Frascatti would have returned to his life and work. The question raised by the students puzzled the consultants as well. It is generally believed that to maintain hope and optimism in their patients, doctors should be optimistic about the future even when it looks bleak. Thus it seemed reasonable to them that the surgeon would stress the possibility of success (without being untruthful) despite the odds. On the other hand, since failure was much more probable, the family should have made their decision based on the high probability of failure—and thus of unnecessary pain, possible long and arduous hospitalization, and ultimately death—rather than the small possibility of success. To do that the surgeon would have had to stress the negative probabilities and their consequences in his discussion with the wife and son. As they explored what the surgeon might have said, it did not feel natural. It seemed clear to the students after the discussion that just as Mr. Frascatti brought complexity beyond his difficult aneurysm to the hospital, the surgeon had to bring more to his encounter with the patient then simply his surgical expertise. Was it right, they wondered, to expect such skills from a surgeon? But if the surgeon did not pursue all the details that would allow a decision based on Mr. Frascatti's wishes, who would? To believe in the patient's right to self-determination is pointless unless there is somebody present to find out what the patient *really* desires.

The second issue arose because Mr. Frascatti *had consented* to the operation. His wife was distressed because he had given consent to please her and his son. Who were doctors expected to listen to, the patient at the time of obtaining consent or the patient's opinions over several years prior to the emergency? The problem appeared to them to be the same as the question raised earlier as to whether Mr. Spatz, when in a coma, should be given blood transfusions because he might have changed his mind about refusing treatment. The students believed that most of their own such opinions came from durable parts of themselves—for example, personality, character, and cultural background—rather than dictated by a specific moment. The doctor should try to consider the long-standing opinion of the patient. Sometimes, however, opinions formed at the time of the sickness were more what the person actually believed because new information and understanding were contributed by the illness. In addition, the students believed, people should be able to change their minds. How were they to know whether Mr. Frascatti had truly changed his mind or was merely consenting because his wife asked him to? Was it proper to expect the surgeon or other physicians to help resolve the family problem?

No matter what formula they applied, the quandary remained. Doctors try to base their actions on their superior knowledge of results and chances for success or failure for a patient whose wishes and beliefs the doctors must somehow discover not only with regard to this moment of decision, but in terms of the patient's longstanding ideas. Since mistakes are always possible, doctors must err on the side of life without using this as an excuse to reduce the burden of discovering what the patient *really* wants. This seemed to the students almost impossibly difficult in light of the fact that their training provided only for mastery of the technical knowledge of medicine. What the students discovered from debating these cases is true not only in these difficult circumstances but in noncontroversial cases as well. Faced with a medical problem, the doctor decides on a course of action that is presented to the patient almost invariably accompanied by supporting reasons for the decision. The patient then consents or rejects the action. The proposed act and its grounds may be as simple as "You have an infection and I am going to prescribe antibiotics," or "I want to get a GI series because of the possibility of an ulcer." Subsequently the patient either takes or does not take the antibiotic or has or does not have the X rays. For more complex problems, the grounds and warrants may be more complete, as give-and-take between patient and doctor require the physician to further justify the decision. It is inherent in even the simple statement that the action is meant to benefit the patient. "You have an infection [which I can tell by the redness and swelling around the wound on your hand] and I am going to prescribe antibiotics [because untreated infections may lead to serious illness or death and antibiotics kill the infecting bacteria so that the wound will heal]." Whether the patient believes that the benefits outweigh the harms can be inferred from whether the patient follows the advice. Phrases such as "patient compliance" and "following doctor's orders" suggest both that one might naturally *not* want to comply or follow orders and that the physician tries to exercise the authority to make people do what is unpleasant. However, judging from studies which have shown that the majority of prescriptions written by physicians are never filled, most patients do not blindly follow doctors' orders. Research on compliance (a word to which many object) has demonstrated that patients more often cooperate if the doctor spends time explaining the reasons and answers the patient's questions—the more the patient understands, the more likely he or she is to cooperate.

Getting patients to collaborate in their own care requires persuasiveness on the part of physicians—an unpersuasive clinician would almost be a contradiction in terms. The facts of a case and its proper treatment *never* speak for themselves except through the mouths of physicians skilled in rhetoric. Rhetoric, the art of speaking persuasively, must be added to the other skills clinicians must have to make medical science and technology work for their patients (5). It has had a bad name for a long time—as in "empty rhetoric" or "political rhetoric"—because of its use in the service of questionable causes and the inflated language associated with the term. The cardiovascular surgeon who persuaded Mrs. Frascatti—over her objections and those of the patient—that her husband should be operated on did so on the basis of his successful argument for surgery. But, as the students concluded, there is good reason to question whether he was correct in trying to sway them. In other words, was his rhetoric properly responsible? Distracting symptoms, fear, denial, unsupported hopes, misconceptions, impairments in thinking, the stresses of the moment, impatience, or conflicting advice make sick persons and their families an especially vulnerable audience for a persuasive physician. The irresponsible deployment of rhetoric, which gave it its bad name, is all the more to be guarded against by physicians. We should have no doubt that the surgeon's argument in favor of the operation he was proposing for Mr. Frascatti was supported by the conviction that it was the best thing for Mr. Frascatti's aneurysm. That, as the students discovered, is not a sufficient reason unless it is also the best thing for the *patient.* Clinical rhetoric is only responsible if it is supported by *both* knowledge of medical science *and* the best interests of the patient *as defined by the patient.*

In the introduction to this chapter I pointed out that the response of the profession of medicine to the criticism of medical practice that I have described in previous paragraphs has been to enlarge the educational focus of the medical curriculum. This has been a continuing, intensive, and largely unsuccessful endeavor. A number of years back there was an attempt to deal with the personal concerns of the patient through programs in behavioral science. Although these were introduced into the curricula of many schools, almost none are still in existence, having met resistance from both faculty and students. Currently, there are very few medical schools that do not offer courses in medical ethics. These vary from a course or two in most schools to flourishing programs in some institutions. Students have generally been enthusiastic. Despite the widespread acceptance of the importance of ethical problems in medicine, the faculty involved in this teaching often do not find their efforts wholeheartedly embraced by their colleagues. Part of the difficulty arises from the Byzantine nature of the politics of curriculum time in medical schools, but a more important factor is the general faculty belief that teaching ethics takes time away from teaching medical science, the real business of medical schools.

Although in clinical medicine there is a need to move from the perspective of simple treatment of disease, it is equally clear that mere addition of the concept of person—with all that it implies—is not the solution.

The Search for a New Basis for Clinical Medicine

Pathophysiological thinking is a natural candidate for a new basis of clinical medicine that seeks to blend person and disease. It would solve certain problems inherent in the consideration of disease alone as a clinical entity and I will show you why it is so enticing, but ultimately fails.

Pathophysiology is the study of disturbances of function in sick persons, as physiology is the study of biological function. Focusing on function, disturbed or otherwise, requires paying attention to the process involved. One of the major problems that people—doctors or laypersons—have with thinking about diseases is the tendency to regard them as though they were either things or events. The old man got pneumonia; "it" (the thing called pneumonia) got into him and almost killed him. Arnold Lauffer was well and then this event befell him—he had a heart attack. President Eisenhower experienced a similar event when he had a heart attack. The viewpoint of pathophysiology, however, is much more like the story of the old man with pneumonia as it unravels the process—the series of moment-by-moment events through time—that is involved in the old man's illness. Similarly, the dramatic events that lead us to know that President Eisenhower had a heart attack are just steps (albeit visible and dangerous) in the process of the underlying disease of atherosclerosis.

The reason pathophysiology is such an attractive focus for clinical medicine is that there is *no* way of understanding what happened to Caroline Preskauer's body except as a process: the gradual thickening and stiffening of the usually diaphanous membranes of the lung's tiny blood vessels subjected to the pounding of blood in abnormally high volumes because of the congenital disease of the heart, reduces blood flow to parts of the lung. Because this happens unevenly, some of the blood in the lungs flows easily and is well oxygenated but mixes with other blood that is poorly oxygenated, producing an overall fall in blood oxygen. This exaggerated the problem resulting from the fact that from birth some of her blood was shunted so that it never went through her lungs (she was a blue baby). Little by little those thickened blood vessels not only failed to allow blood through with normal ease, but began to require ever higher pressures of the blood to force its passage through the blood vessels of her lung. The heightened pressure required for perfusion of the lung increased the strain on the heart. Her heart grew larger as its muscle thickened and took up even more room in her chest, diminishing the effectiveness of the chest as a bellows. To simply call what happened to her "pulmonary failure [or] congestive heart failure secondary to congenital heart disease" (the disease terms by which her illness was designated on the document that was sent to the insurance company to justify payment for hospitalization) is not only to fail to understand it, but leads to inappropriate treatment. It is a lot simpler to say "congestive heart failure" or "pulmonary failure." Not only are these terms written more quickly, but they are more easily thought about. Most people have difficulty in thinking in terms of processes unfolding over time. I had the symbol Δt (standing for change in time) put on all my T shirts to keep me constantly thinking in process terms; nonetheless I find it almost impossible to routinely see things in a constant state of change rather than as static. Yet, although complex, pathophysiologic thinking so much better approximates what actually occurs that I believe the simplicity of disease terms will eventually be discarded in favor of the greater understanding of process afforded by pathophysiology. Illnesses are poorly understood in any other terms.

While disease categories, as the abstractions that they are, can never be viewed, the moment-by-moment process of the disease in the body is frequently subject to observation. Whether the pathophysiology can be directly known, of course, depends on the availability of methods for observation. On the whole-person level, the eyes and ears of both doctor and patient may be sufficient, but as the process is pursued to ever deeper levels, the sophisticated diagnostic and research technologies of modern medicine become necessary. Even here, however, we rarely see the disordered processes of disease in "real time." We extrapolate from serial observations of the patient, repeated blood tests, X rays, or other tests in an attempt to make a composite picture of events in motion take shape in our minds. In this manner, and despite the fact that the process of the disease can never be known in its entirety, ideas that are formed about what is happening approximate the real-life nature of illness better than the static views of disease do.

Prognosticating, at least in the short term, is enhanced by pathophysiologic thinking. As one sees the process of the illness unfold, a trajectory is described that can be imagined as projecting into the future. We expected that Caroline Preskauer would come to the point of having to decide about heart-lung transplantation within a year or so because of our expectation that she would have increasing difficulty both in terms of the severity of her symptoms and the rapidity with which her heart and lungs were getting worse. (We did not forecast the sudden development of the abnormality of her heart rhythm that led to her death although, in retrospect, it was not a surprise, because life-threatening abnormalities of the heart's rhythm are more common in individuals who chronically carry lower than normal amounts of oxygen and higher amounts of carbon dioxide in their blood.)

It remains true, however, that no matter how knowledgeable physicians are about pathophysiology, they must also have knowledge about the disease. The *processes* set in motion by lack of oxygen are the same whether there is inadequate oxygenation because of smoke inhalation, pulmonary edema following a heart attack, or extensive pneumonia, yet the long-term consequences of each are vastly different. That is because the totality of each of the disease states is different even though they share one aspect—lack of oxygen.

The fact that doctors must have knowledge of the disease as well as the pathophysiology illuminates a problem in thinking about sick persons like Caroline Preskauer. Because pathophysiology reveals so much about what is happening in the course of a disease, we appear to have an edge in predicting her future if we are knowledgeable in both. But as we look harder, the illusion that we are better able to predict *her* future based on what we know about the dynamics of blood flow and oxygenation in the lungs melts away.

Pathophysiology is a way of looking at the process of disease by isolating and examining each step in the disease process. Medical science has contributed its brilliant best to pathophysiology by investigating each of these disease steps down to the molecular level. Each step in the scientific explanation of, for example, oxygen transport from room air through the lungs, into the bloodstream, and finally to the metabolic processes in the tissues is like a step of reasoning. From what is already known, each step implies the next. And, conversely, if something goes awry at any point, from the state of things at that point we can infer what has gone wrong. For example, on one occasion the amount of oxygen in Caroline Preskauer's blood was even lower than usual—probably her heart failure had worsened, we reasoned, and was exacerbating the mismatch between parts of the lung where oxygen was being transferred easily but bloodflow was insufficient and where the opposite was the case, an inference that could be acted on. The basis for the success of this reasoning—the ability to infer what will happen next or what has gone wrong—is that it duplicates the scientific method by which the physiology was discovered in the first place. What we know as the scientific method consists of breaking down bodily processes into steps and then subjecting each step to repeated experiments. The experiments are set up so as to completely isolate (to the degree possible) the physiologic step of interest from outside influences in order to elucidate it in a pure form. Repeated experiments are necessary to control for individual variation. The research procedures are chosen by reasoning from what is already known and from an underlying theory to what ought to be the case and designing experiments to test the inference. In scientific terminology the inference is called a hypothesis.

The test of the correctness of a clinical reasoning process is its ability to predict what will happen next—the same test applies to science. A prediction is like an inference. Given a theory about how the body or one of its systems works and this set of facts, we infer what should follow. If our facts are correct and our reasoning is good, our prediction (inference) should be right. Here pathophysiology (even with knowledge of disease added) fails us. As we have seen, pathophysiology is extremely successful in explaining what has already happened—why Caroline Preskauer's blood tests reveal so little oxygen in her blood. It is equally successful in telling us our explanation of her case is wrong. We predicted that she would not have too much carbon dioxide in her blood, but she had a large excess. Therefore (pathophysiology tells us), our explanation of what is wrong with her is incomplete. Then, after rethinking her case (reviewing the X rays and other tests) we came up with another explanation of her situation that matched the facts.

Why, in relation to Caroline Preskauer's CO_2 level, were we wrong in our prediction? Because our theory was wrong. We were considering her to be someone with congenital heart disease in whom the blood carried insufficient oxygen (our theory)—nothing about her congenital heart disease would make us expect too much CO_2. What we did not realize was that after all these years of overwork, her heart filled up so much of her tiny chest that her lungs were not working properly—like someone whose chest was too rigid, she could not blow off CO_2 adequately. One might argue that it is not fair to blame pathophysiology as a predictive tool because we got our beliefs about her disease wrong. Fair or not, pathophysiology is at fault because it gets us into a kind of circular thinking. As long as the sick person's clinical situation approximates the scientific and research methods that produced the knowledge of pathophysiology, then that knowledge will allow accurate predictions. But knowing whether the sick person is like the laboratory experiment requires knowledge that is wider and more extensive than pathophysiology. So pathophysiology *alone* works well as something on which to base predictions only in very restricted clinical circumstances. Another way of saying this is that pathophysiology, like all of medical science, is about generalizations—ideal cases. But Caroline Preskauer, like all patients, is a particular individual. To apply pathophysiology to Caroline Preskauer as a predictive tool you must know how closely she approximates the ideal case. To know that you must know a lot more about her than pathophysiology will tell you—at the very least you must know about her overall disease *as it has behaved in her.* Thus, if you believe her situation to be one thing, then certain predictions about the pathophysiology follow. If those predictions are not borne out—the test results are unexpected or she does not get better as expected—you know you are wrong in your ideas about what is wrong with her. Thus, *by itself,* pathophysiology is a poor predictive tool. Doctors, whether they are aware of it or not, prognosticate by constructing a whole picture of the sick person out of every bit of knowledge they have about that person and then base their predictions on the whole picture. To the extent that their picture-in-the-round accurately represents the sick person (including the process of the disease), their predictions have a chance of accuracy. Pathophysiology can tell them whether they are right or wrong, but in itself it does not prognosticate. In this regard it is like all reasoning. Each step in a chain of reasoning (clinical or otherwise) if carefully thought out, seems to bring you closer to the truth, or at least to give you greater confidence in the hypothesis. But that is an illusion. The success of the reasoning depends on your overall knowledge of the particular situation you are reasoning about. The more you know about your world, the better you can reason about any part of it. Sometimes, in medicine as elsewhere, when we are concerned about a part of something abstracted from the rest—like an aspect of a sick person (e.g., blood oxygen levels)—it appears that our thinking can isolate itself from the whole patient and still be successful. This is only true if successful thinking in clinical medicine is defined as being able to think about the pathophysiology of blood oxygen levels. Clinical medicine, as I have shown in previous chapters, takes place on a much broader landscape.

The way the word is generally employed, pathophysiology applies only to disease processes in the body itself, but such a restriction of scope is not necessary. Unlike disease concepts alone, the kind of thinking about processes and mechanisms used in pathophysiology can be logically extended to include aspects of the process outside the body and outside the person. In this fashion the whole story of the illness can be traced as far up or down in the system as one wishes. The story of Danny German's AIDS can be understood as an exciting tale of virology or immunology, the tragic human drama of one sick person, a problem of international politics, or the relationship between social behaviors and disease. The basic manner of thought—of thinking in terms of changing events over time—will serve in each instance. Further, each of these perspectives will reinforce the others. Factoring in psychological features as aspects of the total picture will require no shift in basic understanding. The idea of cause itself becomes realistic because thinking in terms of process allows one always to pick any point in the chain of events and know it to be the cause of succeeding events. Therapy is rational when the treatment is chosen because it interrupts the chain of events; it is arbitrary when the treatment simply fits into some artificial concept of diseases and their causes. Similarly, preventive strategies assume their place as merely another aspect of treatment, not a course of action that requires a whole new understanding. Finally, thinking in terms of process brings medicine to a concern with a knowledge of health as well as illness. Function, sick or well, is function. Methods and ideas developed to comprehend function apply equally well to understanding, improving, or maintaining the function of the well as they do to understanding or improving the dysfunction of the sick.

But Pathophysiology Just Does Not Work

For all its attractiveness, pathophysiology alone or even strongly combined with disease theory, as I have shown, shares certain disadvantages of thinking of diseases as the central focus of medicine. Some entity that is more inclusive than each aspect of disturbed body function is needed to organize thinking and direct the physician's actions. This becomes clear in the care of Arnold Lauffer. In the intensive care unit, his lungs, heart, kidneys, and blood system could each be (and were) successfully supported on the basis of modern understanding of pathophysiology. Making plans for Arnold Lauffer's future care, on the other hand, or deciding what to tell his family about the future, or even thinking about him beyond each day was impossible because we did not know what disease he had.

The pathophysiology of diseases is influenced by other processes within and outside of the sick person. To know the pathophysiology, at least in current terms, is not necessarily to know the whole story. However, as noted above, the basic kind of thought employed in pathophysiology is applicable to the process of the illness, no matter how inclusive the story. Here, as in disease, the doctor-patient relationship, physicians' doctoring skills, and the moral dimensions of illness have no logical relationship to current notions of pathophysiology. The problem of logical disjunction would not be solved by returning to a consideration of disease constructs. Although this century's major scientific contribution to medicine—understanding the process of disease to the molecular level—has been a vast step beyond classic disease concepts, the basic problems for medical pracitice of diseases as the focus of medicine would not be solved.

Could the Sick Person Be "the Clinical Entity?"

Based on the knowledge that suffering cannot be understood apart from the suffering *person,* the overall thrust of this book has been toward a medicine in which the sick person rather than the disease is the focus of medical practice. Yet such a change in orientation raises many problems, not the least of which is how to define a sick person. The operational definition of a person is not troublesome, but what *is* a sick person? Are sick persons simply these who define themselves as sick and because of that self-definition deserve to be treated by physicians? Most physicians would find such a suggestion upsetting, as though they were merely at the beck and call of anyone who wished to consider himself or herself sick whether as self-indulgence or because of true illness. Doctors and many laypersons would argue that there must be objective standards; otherwise people would be inclined to lapse into self-defined illness anytime life became difficult. On the face of it, such self-definition seems not to meet the test of practicality. Others would point out that medicine became effective only when objective definitions of diseases provided the basis for the beginnings of scientific medicine. To go back to patients' self-definitions of illness, these others say, would be returning to the chaos that existed before the nineteenth century. This is because definitions that are too all-encompassing are as defective as those that are too narrow. H. Tristram Engelhardt, Jr., discusses the issue well:

> I will thus be in disagreement with the notion that the world of illness, the world of the clinician can be deduced from or reduced to the world of the pathoanatomist. I [will contend] that the reverse is the case—the world of the pathoanatomist, the pathophysiologist, and the pathopsychologist is al-

> ways dependent upon that of the clinician for its sense and direction. Further, the world of the clinician is defined by people—by their complaints and vexations. One must, in fact, somewhat circularly say that the world of medicine is defined by the medical complaints of people and medical complaints are what medicine could, in principle, address.
>
> This definition loses its circularity when one notes that in the definition there is a difference in accent between the two meanings of medicine. From the side of physicians, nurses, and so on, the focus is on the abilities of the art. From the point of view of the patients, the accent is on complaints, upon what the art is there for. Physicians look to the capabilities of their technologies including the possibilities of their art, and patients to what is vexing (of course the distinction of patient vis-à-vis physician perspectives is artificial, and is made to illustrate two poles of medicine) (6).

For Engelhardt, vexations and complaints are medical when they come from processes, physiological or psychological, not directly under the voluntary control of the patient and recognized as dysfunctions, pains, or disfigurements. This last clause, "recognized as dysfunctions, pains or disfigurements" (7), enters another factor into the definition of the sick person as the clinical entity. People cannot be considered sick persons, entitled to be cared for by medicine, solely on the basis of their own definition. One might add that persons are (by definition) sick persons who qualify for the attention of medicine if they recognize themselves to have a complaint, condition, process, or disease that doctors, medical science, and their culture also accept as requiring the attention of medicine. The definition requires all these terms because it must permit determination by the patient, determination by doctors, and recognition that medical care is indelibly embedded in society. By definition, a person could not become a clinical entity except by agreement.

What about someone who is found unconscious? Despite lack of agreement with physicians, is that person a clinical entity? As in issues of consent to treatment in emergency circumstances, it is presumed that the person would make the same choice to be treated if he or she had the capacity to choose. When volition returns, the care can be accepted or rejected. Except in such emergency circumstances, a person can never unilaterally be made a clinical entity. This term may be disturbing because it seems to turn the sick person into an object. Because of the element of choice and self-determination, the sick person as clinical entity can never be an object of care, but rather the subject of care. Sick persons become the subject of medicine in both senses of the term.

The value-laden aspect of these definitions may trouble those who want only objective standards of sickness and health. I believe the inescapable conclusion is that medicine is a normative pursuit—it is guided by ideals and values. Definitions of health and illness *always* include value judgments by a society and its individuals about what constitute acceptable dysfunctions, pains, or disfigurements. While that element of norms is inescapable, it is also the case that there will always be objective, non-normative elements in definitions of illness. For example, although emotional illnesses may seem to have only subjective aspects, that is not the case. There must always be some manifestation of every illness, whether primarily physical or primarily psychological, in every dimension of the person. *Nothing can happen to any part of a person without having effects in all other parts. Therefore, every illness will have objectively observable consequences in the world of shared reality—all that is required is that they be looked for.*

Solutions

Certain difficulties of classical disease-oriented medicine are clearly solved when the focus of medicine is the sick person. The doctor-patient relationship, the person of the physician, and moral dimension become logically related to medical practice and a central concern of medicine because these features are aspects of persons and personhood—of both patients and caregivers. It remains to be seen whether changing the focus of medicine will solve problems in diagnosis, treatment, and prognosis. A person is not an abstract generalization, as a disease is, but is instead a particular individual sick person. It would be a mistake to believe, however, that because we have moved from the abstraction of disease to the concreteness of an individual sick person, all the problems of generalizations are solved. No person, sick or well, can be known in his or her entirety. The real is constantly and inevitably larger than our ideas about it. But the individual sick person is both our concern and under our direct observation. We do not have to abstract aspects of the sick person to make up the disease. What is there before us is also our central interest. Everything the doctor sees of that person is directly relevant to his or her care of that person—and there is much to be seen that can only be seen by those who care. What Francis Peabody said so many years ago as a moral precept for physicians finally becomes a fundamental necessity of medicine: "The secret of the care of the patient is caring for the patient." It remains true, however, that we can only know the past of the sick person by questioning rather than by direct observation, and the future remains a matter of probabilities.

When the sick person is the doctor's primary focus, the diagnosis will still frequently contain the name of a disease. (It should be understood that to move forward to a focus on the sick person does not mean losing all the understandings in medicine that came from the earlier focus on disease.) However, that is not the end of the matter, but only one step toward a complete diagnosis. The general form of the diagnostic question now asks what threatens this person's functioning at this time, so the answer will be incomplete if it stops at the *what*—the disease. The goal is to find out what is happening in the body (pathophysiology) as well as who the patient is; to uncover what (about the pathophysiology, the patient, or the context) threatens the patient, and why it does so at this time. To do this, it is necessary to pursue different kinds of information and then integrate the results into the more general formulation—what threatens this patient's functioning at this time? Only then can an appropriate therapeutic plan be generated. Finally, there is the definitional problem—the clinician must discover how the patient defines the problem and what has to be corrected before that patient will consider the problem solved. When all this has been accomplished, the physician will understand what is the matter, why it threatens the patient, and why it happened when it did. With this approach, doctors have defined the problem both in their own (medical science) terms as well as in the patient's and they are in a position to plan treatment for the disease that is suited to the individual and, almost as important, comprehensible by the patient.

Remember the old man with pneumonia who was widowed, had a bad knee, and lived in a fifth-floor walk-up apartment? With every patient there are questions that must be answered. What is there about this person that contributes to his being ill? (Why is this a sick person?) Aspects of this person must be part of the illness even if not part of the disease process. Another person might not have the sickness in the first place (not have the disease process)—someone who does not smoke, takes medications as directed, visits doctors, has different occupational exposure, different genes, more money, more education, etc. Another person with the same disease process might not have an identical illness. The usual meaning of the word "diagnosis" ("The determination of the nature of the diseased condition; identification of the disease by careful investigation . . . ; also the opinion [formally stated] resulting from such investigation." *OED*), which has only been in common use since the beginning of the nineteenth century, is inadequate to the modern task. The diagnosis must include individual factors that affect the "penetrance" (the degree to which it shows itself or can be known about) of the disease process. Factors concerning the person's physical, psychological, or social response to the disease process must be considered. Interpersonal relationships that bear on the illness must also enter the diagnosis. No person becomes ill in absolute isolation; except for trivial illness, relationships have a bearing on illness. For example: What is the person's family status? If the person is a dependent child, what is the relationship to the parents? Is the person single—living alone or with others, far from or close to family (in both senses)? Are there social supports? Is the person married? Is the family intact or disrupted? Are there children? Is the spouse alive? Is he or she divorced? Are there other stable partnerships or relationships? What is the relationship with the physician or other caregiver? What is the setting of the illness? What is the physical environment? Is it urban or rural? What are the occupational circumstances? In what era (year, month, etc.) has the sickness taken place? In summary, diagnosis, treatment, prognosis, and search for cause require knowledge about the person.

To be successful, doctors have to know more about the sick person and the illness then just the name of the disease and its pathophysiology. Focusing on the sick person seems to solve these problems—what can be known about them will supply what clinicians need to make them better. Stating that requirement and satisfying it are a world apart. The next chapter deals with the way in which we come to know about sick persons.

References

1. *The Oxford Companion to Medicine.* Edited by Walton, John, Beeson, Paul, Bodley Scott, Ronald. 1986. Oxford, Oxford University Press, Vol. I, p. 548.

2. Zaner, Richard. *Ethics and the Clinical Encounter.* 1988. Englewood Cliffs, N.J., Prentice-Hall.

3. Jonson, Albert R., Siegler, Mark, and Winslade, W. J. *Clinical Ethics.* 2nd ed. 1987. New York, Macmillan.

4. The Oath. In *The Genuine Works of Hippocrates.* Trans. Francis Adams, 1886. New York, William Wood, Vol. II, p. 279.

5. Pellegrino, Edmund. The Clinical Arts and the Arts of the Word. *Pharos* 1981; Vol. 44, No. 4: 2–8.

6. Engelhardt, H. Tristram Jr. Doctoring the Disease, Treating the Complaint, Helping the Patient: Some of the Works of Hygeia and Panacea. In *Knowing and Valuing.* Edited by Engelhardt, H. Tristram, Jr. and Callahan, Daniel. 1980. New York, The Hastings Center, pp. 226–27.

7. Engelhardt, H. Tristram, Jr., op. cit., p. 228.

10

Who Is This Person?

IT IS GENERALLY believed, with good cause, that individuals are unknowable in their entirety. This *must* be true for at least two reasons. First, people change constantly. The person we confront at this instant was different a moment ago and will be different a moment hence. The second, related reason is that we can only see one aspect of an individual at any moment. When I look at the front of you I cannot simultaneously see the back of you. If I shift my perspective, I lose my original line of sight. This is true of any viewpoint—emotional, social, physical, or conceptual—from which a person is considered. It certainly seems harder to know a person than a disease, which appears more easily knowable because it can be conceived as a static object in the here and now.

Despite the difficulties, we know the other people in our lives sufficiently to interact with them on a daily basis. We want to know whether the person in the marketplace is honest and worthy of our trust. Even there, trustworthiness is judged in relation to the risk of loss. More knowledge is needed about teachers because we expose our weaknesses to them to a greater degree. We want to know even more about the people we work with or our intimates because we may conceive ourselves to be in greater danger of injury from those close to us than from strangers. Knowledge of others is not gained in an instant, but grows over time as we interact with them and observe their behavior in relation to other persons or events. To know persons to the degree required by a medicine that focuses on sick persons demands of the doctor an accuracy of judgment greater than that called for in everyday life. Let us examine how this knowledge comes about.

We'll start with an actual case.

Amos Unger, a fifty-nine-year-old sales manager for a garment manufacturer, tells the following story. He had an argument with his wife one morning that made him both angry and late to work. As he was running to catch his bus he felt a tight feeling in his chest that stayed with him for a few minutes even after he sat down. It crossed his mind briefly that it might be his heart. The same sensation occurred later that morning as he was sitting at his desk trying to straighten out a feud between two of his salesmen. The sensation lasted about ten minutes and focused his awareness on the discomfort. After some silent dialogue, he was half convinced that it was his heart—that he had heart trouble. His father had died of a heart attack at seventy-nine, and he knew several men who had had bypass surgery. However, the thoughts, the feeling, and the little tinge of fear passed, to return only occasionally during his active day. He expected it to occur on the way home; walking to his house (briskly, as a test) the feeling seemed to be present, although less intense than in the morning.

The feeling recurred several times the next day, so he called a cardiac fitness center and scheduled a treadmill exercise stress test. He did not call his doctor, whom he rarely saw, because he thought his doctor would order the test anyway. He decided that if the test were positive, he could tell the internist and, if negative, he would forget the whole thing. While on the treadmill he did not get the sensation in his chest, but the cardiologist at the fitness center said that the test was "borderline positive" and that he probably should have a coronary arteriogram "to make sure one way or the other."

Mr. Unger was reluctant to have the arteriogram because he knew that the result might suggest the need for an operation. The cardiologist at the fitness center, who was affiliated with a well-known hospital, assured him that surgery was probably not in the offing. Currently, the cardiologist said, something called balloon angioplasty was frequently all that was required and was really safe. In this procedure, the cardiologist told him, a thin catheter with a balloon on the tip is introduced into an artery in the thigh and advanced to the heart. Then it is threaded into the coronary artery and positioned at the site of abnormal narrowing. The balloon is expanded, which compresses the material obstructing the artery and opens it up again so that blood can flow normally. The cardiologist's detailed explanation and the good reputation of the hospital reassured him, and he made plans to enter the hospital. By this time he was convinced that he had coronary heart disease and that the coronary arteriogram and the angioplasty (that he was sure would follow) were necessary. His family and friends shared his anxieties, but the consensus, after much discussion, was in accord with his diagnosis and his decision. Some thought he should call his internist, but others argued that this would be pointless since the internist was not a cardiologist; at any rate, the patient and his family were eager to have the procedure done, and they didn't want the internist's possible objection to stand in their way. Much to everyone's surprise, the arteriogram was normal. Mr. Unger was puzzled but relieved. The disturbing chest sensation recurred from time to time for a while, but it finally disappeared.

There are two problems facing a doctor who is consulted by Amos Unger. The first is whether Mr. Unger has heart disease (and the consequent question of what treatment, if any, is required), and the second is the kind of a person he is. Some doctors may consider only the first question important, but in previous chapters we have seen that the nature of Amos Unger as a person is intertwined with the nature of his disease. His personal influence on events is clear: his sense of urgency; his determination, indicated by the way he went about the matter; his knowledge of coronary heart disease; his familiarity with stress tests and how to get one done; his lack of attachment to his internist; and the place of his family in the decision. These factors influence the outcome because it is *Amos Unger's* chest discomfort. It is also the illness it is and not another because of the era in which it took place, the geographic setting, and all other visible and invisible details of its context and those of its participants.

There are physicians who believe that consideration of patients' personalities complicates clinical medicine and prevents it from achieving the precision of medical science. As I've already pointed out, I do not believe that the patient can ever be totally separated from his or her disease, but even if it were possible, how could this particular case ever be removed from its context? It is the need to know about the patient that distinguishes the practice of medicine—clinical medicine—from medical science. However, as you will see in the following chapters, clinical medicine not only has a different subject—the patient rather than the disease—but employs a kind of thinking distinctly different from scientific thinking. In fact, when clinicians look at facts, such as the results of Amos Unger's stress test, as if they were scientists rather than practicing physicians, they make a fundamental error.

But in understanding how doctors are to know who *this* sick person is, we must look more closely at precisely what *persons* are. In the pages that follow there is implicit a belief that persons do not exist except as imbedded in the matrix of their society, and that thinking about or trying to understand a person as separate from his or her society is like thinking about or trying to understand the word person apart from language in general and the fact that language is a human capacity that presupposes that humans live in groups. In Chapter 3 I offered a simplified topology of a person to provide a basis for understanding the nature of suffering. I said that persons have personality and character, a lived past, a family, a family's lived past, culture and society, roles, associations with others, a political dimension, activities, day-to-day behaviors, an existence below awareness, a body, a secret life, a believed-in future, and a transcendent dimension. The importance of these features for understanding suffering is that each can be affected by illness and become a source of suffering if the integrity of the person is thereby disrupted. For example, the person's past, though it seems no longer to exist, can become a locus for suffering if, for example, the events of the present illness put the truth of the past (as the person knows it) in question; or, more radically, if the recent or remote past is totally in doubt, as in the case of the amnesic patients described by Oliver Sacks(1). In Chapter 4 I extended this understanding of person by showing that the rules of society and the definitions of culture, although seemingly external, are inside each of us, contained in our beliefs, concepts, and definitions of words like mother, doctor, hard-working, weak, crippled. This leads to the knowledge that suffering in chronic illness may come from internal conflict—one part of a person trying to comply with the demands of society while another part resists such strictures because they place painful demands on the body or inner resources. It follows that persons are not necessarily unitary in their perspectives, desires, concerns, fears, or even their abilities or capacities (2)(3).

The beliefs, concepts, and definitions of words that arise from the world external to the person are not of a single origin. Each of us exists in multiple contexts simultaneously—familial, ethnic, cultural, religious, political, and geographical. The difficulties that American children born of immigrant parents have in trying to be true members of the American culture of their peers and at the same time part of the ethnic culture of their parents attests to the conflicts that may be generated when simultaneous contexts differ significantly. It is of interest that individuals transplanted from one society to another have disease patterns that show the influence of both the original culture and the host culture. Japanese who live in Hawaii have higher rates of heart disease than homeland Japanese, but lower than native-born Hawaiians.

The power of context is difficult to comprehend because, like water for fish or air for animals, it is just there. Having dinner one evening in 1981 in a restaurant on the Upper East Side of Manhattan I saw a woman in her early thirties who I thought could only exist in that milieu in 1981. Her hair color and style, makeup, clothing, tone of voice, gestures, manner of sitting—even the expression on her face—were typical of Manhattan's Upper East Side in the 1980s. Her absolute exemplification of a context, that complex set of features too many and diverse to enumerate that characterize a time and place, began to make me aware of the extent to which they become part of us. In this instance, the degree to which the context had formed the presentation of the woman to the world was remarkably apparent in her appearance. But before you dismiss the effect of the context as a surface phenomenon in the East Side woman, remember that context does not express itself merely as a set of appearances, clothing styles, slang, idioms, metaphors, gestures, values, attitudes, opinions, beliefs, and so on, all appended to a person as a costume or mask is worn in a play to signify a period. These things become incorporated into the person; if they are removed, there would not be a complete person left. They can only be changed—indeed, within limits, they *will* be changed as times and places change. As these features enter into the marrow of the person they provide the potential for suffering in acute and chronic illness. Consider what might happen to the East Side woman if the skin of her face had a permanent rash or became coarsened, or she had a prominent scar on her neck, she lost her hair, her abdomen became distended, her legs and feet were constantly swollen, and she had prominent varicose veins.

I was intrigued by the idea that the East Side woman's facial appearance was also typical of the time and place. In the ensuing months I compared photographs from different periods in the yearbooks of the Cornell University Colleges of Nursing and Medicine, photographs from magazines from different countries in the same year, and photographs of persons past and present. I became convinced that persons in distinct eras and dissimilar settings were of differing appearance. The distinctions were not due merely to variations in photographic techniques, hairdo, or makeup, as I and others had assumed; their faces were *literally different.* Slides of people's faces from various eras and places and slides and videos that showed the influence of society on body posture and gait were included in my lectures on the social determinants of disease. Although the students agreed that facial appearance was consistent only within the same era, they strongly resisted the idea that the actual appearance of each of *their* own faces could be socially determined. They pointed out that the bony structure of the face and the size and shape of the ears and nose were not plastic. They reluctantly conceded—the evidence before their eyes was convincing—that facial expression might to some degree be a product of social forces.

The hesitation is understandable. The face is prized for its individuality, its symbol of uniqueness—"I would recognize her face anywhere." If your face is not your possession, what is? The unhappy opposite of this idea is illustrated by the expression "He's just a face in the crowd." That our faces are not entirely our own is clear from the thanks that usually follow when someone says, "You're looking more like your father every day." The statement is complimentary because of the notion that characteristics of a favored person have been acquired, and it acknowledges that the face is the repository of those characteristics.

In the face (as elsewhere in the person) a tension exists between the desire for uniqueness and the recognition that its appearance comes to reflect external and internal influences (the basis for Oscar Wilde's novel, *The Picture of Dorian Gray*). Everyone wants to believe that his or her presentation to the world is self-determined—that others will see what the individual wants them to see. In the nineteenth century it was commonly believed that much of the interior world of persons—emotions, character, and personality, for example—could be read from their outward appearance. Charles Darwin's book, *The Expression of Emotion in Man and Animals,* represented an attempt to systematize the notion. The field of phrenology, popular during that period, was based on the theory that much about persons was to be read from the shape of their skulls, and was another expression of the belief. As the discoveries of Freud and subsequent dynamic psychologists have led to an appreciation of the complexity of the mental life and the forces that determine behavior, the simpler ideas about character and emotion that led to Darwin's book have been discarded. It remains true, however, that the moment-by-moment play of facial expressions, augmented by body motions and gestures, mirrors an individual's feelings and thoughts. This plethora of signals by which our inmost beings are revealed are apparent to any close observer. That so much of ourselves is there for anyone else to see underlines Stephen Toulmin's telling observation of the great extent to which inner life is as much outward as inward. In fact, aspects of our lives, which we believe to be private, are better known to others than to ourselves(4).

The medical students were helped to overcome their skepticism about the influence of society on the face by listening to the lyrics for "Seen and Unseen," from the Talking Heads album, *Remain in Light,* by David Byrne and

Brian Eno. The protagonist of the song decides that if he keeps "an ideal facial structure fixed in his mind or somewhere in the back of his mind," by force of will his face will very slowly change over the years. "A more hooked nose . . . wider, thinner lips . . . beady eyes . . . a larger forehead." The protagonist imagines that he shares this ability with other people who had also "molded their faces according to some ideal"(5). The song is not only persuasive, it is correct.

The historical time and place in which an illness takes place shape not only the person but the illness. Chest discomfort in New York City in 1990 had different consequences from those it had in 1960. People now have more knowledge; they are less passive in relation to their symptoms, to doctors, and to the process of medical care; doctors are also more active—angioplasty, surgery, exercise programs, and superior medications have changed treatment. Doctors know this, and so do patients. As a result, the attitudes of both are different and, in consequence, the illness is different. It is widely believed that New Yorkers differ from Californians, Alabamians, and Midwesterners, and, further, that urban and rural dwellers in the same state differ in some respects from each other. Places of residence also have an influence on people's medical care and perceptions of disease. This is what it means in medical terms to say that persons exist in multiple contexts.

It is obvious that while many—perhaps most—people in New York City today hold certain views or have certain attitudes about specific symptoms and diseases, this does not mean that a specific person holds the same views. (While this is correct, if the matter is at issue, the doctor has only to ask the patient.) If this person does not obtain his or her views at least in part from the context, where do they come from? My behavior differs because I am a New Yorker rather than a Virginian, of Russian-Jewish origins rather than English. So it is with all aspects of the context of illness. Birth and lifelong residence in New York is not merely a source of my attitudes, it is an inseparable part of me. As it has formed my accent, my word choice, and my fearless manuevers amid charging taxicabs it has played its part in the *construction* of me. To know New York is in part to know me. To know me is to have a view of New York in a certain era.

The general nature of the relationship between patient and physician (indeed, of all interpersonal relationships) varies from era to era, as do the participants. Patients have different expectations of physicians and medicine currently than they did in 1970, 1950, or 1930. Knowing my patient's expectations helps me to know something of my patient, a knowledge I need to understand our conversations.

When I entered practice in 1961, patients did not behave like Amos Unger. If (allowing the impossibility) the details of the case remained the same while all else returned to 1961, he and the physicians he encountered would have formed opinions of each other quite different from those they now hold. The 1961 appraisals would not be flattering. Doctors would think him intolerably arrogant and uppity. (In fact, in those days no cardiologist would have seen him without the personal referral of his own internist.) Mr. Unger would think that the doctors had no sense of responsibility or authority and that they probably did not know much medicine. (Otherwise, why would they keep deferring to his decisions as though he knew medicine, when that knowledge is rightfully theirs alone?) While words, sentences, conversations, and even whole interactions acquire meaning because of context, these entities do not exist in a vacuum. The meanings and intentions of persons become interpretable because the context is known. If we keep everything else in the story of Amos Unger the same but change the protagonist into a 68-year-old widowed, indigent woman who lives alone, the course of the narrative as it was related is unthinkable.

Persons also work. To know someone's occupation is to learn something about his or her social status, education, specialized knowledge, responsibilities, hours worked, income, muscular development, skills, perspective on life, politics, housing—and much more. The danger of bias and stereotyping is as acute as in issues of race, ethnicity, and gender, but it remains true that much can be discerned about persons by knowing their occupation. Their day-to-day behavior and even their personalities can be shaped by their work to a degree they are often unaware of. Reporting a stolen car, I waited a long time in a police station while the complaint was filed. Again and again the phone was either taken off the hook or went unanswered, and other tasks were set aside as the police and the clerks chatted with each other. A police aide who was perhaps 24 years old interacted at best brusquely and more often sharply with a number of inquirers as I waited for her much older colleague to finish my report. At one point, when we were alone in the room, the young woman looked up at me pleasantly and volunteered, "You know, I'm not like this outside here." She had been in the job about a year. Judging from the behavior and pinched appearance of her older colleague, I wondered how long her external attractiveness would last. When and if the transformation occurred, she would probably be unaware of the change in herself, cognizant only that, to her, the world had become a mean place.

Occupation has such a profound effect on illness that doctors routinely inquire about their patients' work. Imagine how different the story of Mr. Unger would be if he were a steelworker. From the presentation of symptoms to the impact on career, coronary heart disease behaves like a different disease in heavy laborers and New York businessmen. This is also true of many other diseases. Physicians come to know a great deal about each job, what it entails, the demands it makes on workers, the special stresses involved, and the attitudes toward illness of both employees and employers. Physicians who work in areas with a high concentration of specific industries become expert on the nuances of their patient's work-related requirements and skills and problems. For them this knowledge is essential.

Knowledge of persons is also derived from observation of their habits—for example, whether they smoke or drink—and their capabilities, skills, and talents. Many human capacities, such as digestion or urination, are taken for granted and assumed to be the same in all healthy humans, while others, such as muscular ability, intelligence, problem-solving ability, or musicality are distinguished as abilities or talents because they are known to be unevenly distributed and open to expansion through training. In fact, however, virtually every human faculty, including digestion and urination, can be altered through training or habituation. Differences in physical or mental powers have an impact on the expression of illness. This is one reason why age, intelligence, occupational history, educational attainment, parental training, special knowledge and abilities (such as self-hypnosis, Yoga, spirituality, outdoorsmanship), in addition to the effects of cultural background and social context discussed earlier, may alter the experience of illness in crucial ways. Many of these things are readily observable or can be uncovered with a few questions.

Let us go back a step. What I have written implies that many aspects of a person are both societal and individual, and that some of the most explicit details of another's personhood exist within the observer; that is, they are seen from the perspective of the observer's knowledge and experience. We do not really stand before each other as relative strangers, unknown to one another; we start each interaction with an enormous amount of information about each other, much of it stemming from the fact that to know what people are is also to know what they are not, will not, and could not be. What kind of knowledge is this, and where does it reside? When I say that the fact that Amos Unger is a New York businessman in the 1990s modifies the effect of the disease or that it would be different if he were a steelworker, clearly there are external factors—of technology, medical care, and lifestyle, for example—with which I am familiar. But I am suggesting more than that. Just as the meaning of his chest discomfort moves Mr. Unger to action, it is the meaning of the cardiologist's words, the meanings associated with heart disease in general, the hospital, the arteriogram, work in the steel mills, New York, the businessman's life, steel towns, and all the myriad details of context that contribute to making us the persons we are and determine the nature and course of our illnesses—and it is the observers' knowledge of these meanings that fuels their knowledge of others. Shared meanings provide the basis for knowing one another. In the modern era, because of education, geographic mobility, common interests, print media, television, and communication, individuals hold vastly more meanings in common than they did even thirty years ago. In other words, to know another one must delve into one's own store of meanings.

Rarely is this knowledge explicit. There is a long tradition that identifies self-knowledge with self-awareness, and I do not suggest otherwise. Rather we should call the knowledge we have of our own meanings part of our personal knowledge, as the meanings themselves are personal meanings.* Thus, our knowledge of the external world and our personal meanings together allow us to know others.

These unavoidable truths about persons—that we know so much about each other, that we are each inextricably part of society, and that just as we live in our social world, the world lives in us—may seem to contradict three

*This usage borrows from the meaning of the term personal knowledge as it was employed by Michael Polyani.

hundred years of increasing Western belief in individuality, perhaps especially now when individuality has become almost a religion. However, instead of being contradictory, these are complementary aspects of persons. We have many things in common, and we are also completely individual and particular.

Here is an example to prove the point. I worked on this chapter during a cross-country flight, and I did not wish to be distracted by the in-flight movie, in this case *Crossing Delancey.* Although I had not ordered earphones, I found myself watching the film. The setting was familiar to me—the cultural context was part of my personal knowledge, and I could easily follow the story and interpret the relationships among the characters—and the characters themselves—without hearing the words. On the other hand, the movie was the unique film it was because of the individuality of these particular actors. Other actors, same script, different movie.

We *are* all different from one another. How from so much sameness is difference wrought, and does this effect the task of knowing who the person is? To begin with, we are all subject to a capricious fate, regardless of our attempts to repudiate that uncomfortable fact. However, although we are flung into a torrent not of our choosing, once in it we determine our own ways of swimming through it—we individualize our route. In every moment of time all of us make choices and act on them. Think of choice here not only in the large sense of choosing a mate or a career, but in the smallest moment-by-moment sense—turning this way rather than that, reading this book instead of another, eating this now rather than that later, smiling instead of frowning, saying yes instead of no, taking the second as well as the first dose of medication instead of discarding it, choosing this physician rather than that, calling him or her now rather than an hour later, resting, running or calling home. Even what we see, hear or feel are choices by which we individualize each moment of our existence; moreover, the same object may be perceived in a significantly different way by different people. Our perceptions personalize our surroundings, and thus it can be said that the context makes the person and the person makes the context.

Although the verbs "to choose" and "to decide" imply conscious intention, it is incorrect to assume that all of our decisions and choices are consciously made. It is one of the errors of our time to give too much weight to consciousness instead of realizing it for what Whitehead called it, "a vague flickering on the surface." We do not give much thought to most of our daily actions, but they are nevertheless our own.

Knowing Persons Through Their Narratives

Our innumerable actions, small and large, write the narrative of our lives, which in turn describes us. The narrative is not only an assemblage of empirical facts; it is an aesthetic whole—a tapestry woven from individual threads to form a coherent pattern that is complete in itself but that also tells of the weaver. To choose is to value, to rank in importance, and thus in the pattern of a person's actions can be read what that person considers important. We express ourselves as moral beings in the same fashion. Honesty, courage, forthrightness, patience, and all other virtues are expressed not only in momentous events, but in the tests posed by daily life as well. To illustrate this point, obtain a minute-by-minute account of yesterday from someone. Leave nothing out, consider no detail too small. It will take an hour or two, and when you are finished I believe you will be amazed at how well you have come to know the person.

Perception, choice, decision—life as it is lived—occur in the stream of time. It is natural that the increasing concern of philosophy with time in this century should lead to an interest in narrative. The idea that narrative, or story, is necessary to an understanding of the human condition has grown in recent decades.* Those who emphasize narrative views of human experience do so because, whether an event is important or insignificant in the life of an individual, the event itself cannot be understood apart from its history. Each of us gets to our illness our own way, it becomes part of our story, and we individualize it by its place in the narrative of our lives. To know that illness one must know something of the person. To know the person, one must know something of the narrative.

The idea of the centrality of the personal narrative in understanding the person and diagnosing the illness may seem to complicate the physician's task of knowing the disease, but I think not. Whenever two people sit opposite each other they tell stories.† Doctors may try, in the usual fashion of history taking, to restrict their patients to simple yes-or-no answers to questions designed to reveal some diagnostic pattern, but patients almost always respond by telling stories. As the tape-recordings made for my study of doctor-patient communication, *Talking with Patients,* demonstrated, doctors also frequently tell stories to their patients. When people attempt to answer doctors' innumerable questions—about their habits, education, jobs, marriage, family, illnesses past and present, and the rest of the information obtained in a

*I was extremely fortunate to be a member of a project of the Hastings Center entitled "The Foundations of Ethics and Its Relationship to Science," which was supported by the National Endowment for the Humanities and lasted for several years in the mid-1970s. My early and unsophisticated ideas about process in medicine were given enormous impetus by discussions of the narrative and story in those meetings. Of the many members of the group whose thinking on narrative influenced me, I am particularly grateful to David Burrell, Stanley Hauerwas, Alisdair MacIntyre, and Stephen Toulmin for their papers and subsequent work. A narrative understanding of life as lived is central to the thesis of MacIntyre's rich and important work, *After Virtue.* More recently Howard Brody has discussed the place of narrative in the philosophy of medicine, Richard Zaner has dealt with its importance to medical ethics, and Arthur Kleinman sees no comprehension of the importance of illness to the sick person apart from the narrative of the illness.

†The anecdotal has come to stand, in medicine, for the epitome of unscientific information. This is because anecdotes are viewed as individual stories about singular events. In fact, as Katherine Hunter has pointed out, stories play a very important role in medicine because they are most often used, as were the parables, to demonstrate a general point; the cautionary tale is an old-fashioned useful device for training. Charles Bosk, in *Forgive and Remember,* has shown its importance in the training of surgeons.

standard medical history—it is impossible for them not to tell stories about themselves, what they did, do, and expect to do, how they behaved in relation to illness and doctors (and many other things) present and past, what attitudes they have about doctors and illness (and many other things). The static facts of the person's life are the framework on which is hung the narrative revealing them as the particular persons they are.

The physician must understand that the patient's story is not an intrusion but a legitimate requirement for the clinician's effectiveness. With that understanding, the multiplicity of tools for extracting the information from the narrative is likely to be employed effectively by the doctor. The single most important tool that reveals persons through their stories is their use of language. In one of the earlier considerations of persons in this century, George Herbert Mead stated his belief that the self (his word) is a social phenomenon constructed by language. As a person speaks or a patient answers questions, more language is inevitably displayed that in its verbal style, choice of words, and logic adds to the characterization of the speaker.

It is one of the interesting facts of the spoken language that each word employed by patients to describe their symptoms tells the attentive listener not only what the symptoms are but how the patients feel about them. Put another way, the choice of words to describe something tells not only about the thing but about the speaker as well(6). Even the nonword portions of utterances—pause, pitch, speech rate, and intensity—contribute to our knowledge of the speaker's beliefs and attitudes. As Collingwood has made abundantly clear, all spoken language expresses a speaker's emotion(7). It follows that it is virtually impossible for a patient to report a symptom as an "objective fact" in a computerlike manner. The patients' adjectives for describing pain, nausea, shortness of breath, or any other symptom not only describe the symptom's emotional meaning for the patient and the person's attitude toward the symptom, they place it on a scale of relative values. Since physicians are concerned with severity of symptoms, they must disengage this information from the patient's scale of values and give it a rating on a "medical scale." How is this to be accomplished? The language used to describe other events allows the attentive listener to learn whether, for example, the speaker's palette contains vivid emotional colorings or whether taciturnity is more usual. If a patient states that the chest pain is "not so bad" but also uses moderate language for everything else, it should be suspected that by medical standards the pain may be worse than reported. On the other hand, if a pain is described as "excruciating," but everything else is "horrible," "terrible," "simply awful," "magnificent," or "sensational," a doctor may be justified in probing further before calling an ambulance.

Personal Logic

Popular belief has it that people are often illogical in their speech and actions. But if that were the case, if we were all, or even some of us, illogical, how could there be meaningful communication? All normal conversation is logical, by which I mean that it consists of premises, ideas that follow one from another and lead to conclusions supported by the premises. It *is* true, however, that the logic in some conversations is so convoluted that it would take Aristotle himself to follow it. This is not because people are illogical but rather because they are often of more than one mind. As a consequence, two or more concurrent ideas may be expressed in the same series of statements, as illustrated by the following:

> I know myself, and that pain in the stomach is nothing but nerves, considering the work I do and working with my family. So I was wondering whether I shouldn't get an X ray or something of the esophagus and stomach as I've lost a little weight.

Notice that there are two logically separate clauses in this utterance. In the first is a warrant that the conclusion is correct ("I know myself") then the conclusion ("that pain . . . nothing but nerves") followed by the two premises on which it is based ("the work I do" and "working with my family"). If he really believes that his stomach pain is the result of "nerves," why is he requesting the X ray of his stomach which would, he knows, be normal in that instance? The second clause contains an implied contradictory conclusion, that there is an organic lesion such as a tumor. That conclusion leads him to request an X ray, which (he and I believe) is of use in demonstrating such things. The pain and loss of weight suggest the possibility of cancer. In this brief utterance, which may appear illogical—if it is nerves, why request an X ray?—two separate reasonings exist. One presents the argument for the pain being "nerves" and the other for its being an organic lesion, perhaps cancer. Seen in this manner, the overall utterance is logical. The frequently stated idea that people in actions and speech are not logical stems from the fact that on the surface we are not a consistent breed—we say one thing but do another. We *are* logical, but we are frequently of more than one mind and our words and actions permit an attentive physician, or any listener, to know what it is that we believe as well as the conflict we have over the conclusions to which our beliefs lead us. Since such conflicts may be a source of suffering in illness, knowledge of their presence may be essential to its relief.

We know a lot about the man with stomach pain from this snatch of conversation. His premises (about the effect of nerves and the meaning of weight loss) reflect his beliefs, which include the following: (1) A doctor is a proper person to tell this to; (2) one can know oneself; (3) he knows himself; (4) things are caused by other things; (5) "nerves" are a possible cause of illness; (6) "nerves" come from some kinds of work; (7) working with his family (we can assume from his comments) is aggravating; (8) many beliefs about X-ray examinations; (9) weight loss is not a symptom of "nerves" (at least for him); (10) weight loss is a symptom of things that show up on X rays; (11) it is important to find out whether such things are present.

Physicians clearly have the opportunity to learn an enormous amount about an individual patient in a short time. I believe, however, that *most doctors do not know nearly enough about their patients.*

Disinterest in the Nature of Person

Of all the information, formal and informal, that interactions with patients offer, doctors characteristically take but a small bit and discard the rest. The patient's disease interests them but the *person* of the patient seems at best intrusive. Physicians and others accrue only the knowledge they think they need (although as more knowledge is required, more is often sought).

Lack of Perceptual Focus

Another reason for doctors' lack of knowledge about their patients arises from the fact that anything in which there is no specific interest is not likely to be perceived, even when present and obvious. To demonstrate this, ask someone to look at his or her watch to see the time. After the person has glanced away, ask what the second hand looks like, or whether the numbers are Arabic or Roman. You may be surprised that the person does not immediately know, considering that he or she has just seen them—now and probably a thousand times before. Long training and the development of strong perceptual habits are required for physicians to register the details of a physical examination when they are not completely focused on what they see, feel, or hear. Physicians rarely train themselves to perceive who their patients are, although they do learn to perceive their patients' bodies.

Knowledge of Persons Seems To Infringe on Their Personal Freedom

It would seem that some aspect of freedom is compromised when someone is too well known by others. It is a tenet of prevailing Western—and especially American—political and social philosophy that individuals have virtually unlimited freedom of potential. Anything, so the belief goes, is open to us. Of course, we know that is not true, but that idea is the heart of the dream of autonomy and freedom. However, what prevents us from being anything that we want to be is not geography, economics, or other limitations of opportunity (although each may affect us), but the fact of who, precisely, we are. Any description of me must include factors—age, gender, place of birth, physical type, education, talents and lacks thereof, personality features such as competitiveness and ambition, even my ideas and beliefs—which preclude some futures while allowing others. I cannot be whatever I like, even if I set my mind to it.

Bias and Reluctance to Criticize

There is hardly anyone whose complete description will not involve terms or phrases that carry the specter of bias. We are so sensitive about prejudice that it is difficult to use words like black, Jewish, gay, Southern, old, adolescent, rich, poor, housewife, doctor, and lawyer without the listener's taking offense at what he or she hears as a stereotypical comment. To demonstrate the effect of culture on the body and its functions, I showed my students a videotape of people walking. The tape, made by my staff in Greenwich Village, demonstrates the contrasting walking patterns of black, Hispanic, and white young men, among others. Gaits, like speech patterns, hand gestures, and posture, are influenced by culture. The medical students did not seem troubled, but several faculty members in two different medical schools were upset by what they considered my portrayal of stereotypical behaviors.

Walter Lippman first used the term stereotype in a 1922 book called *Public Opinion* to highlight the danger of forming opinions about people from sources other than first-hand experience. Lippman further pointed out that stereotypes influence perception, thereby affecting direct experience. Since the publication of Lippman's book, so strong a fear of stereotypical thinking has developed among many that it prevents people (including many physicians) from seeing what literally is in front of their eyes. Denying differences among people for fear of arousing bias, as in reaction to the videotape, precludes the skills of observation necessary in good clinicians. The same fear blocks the ability to know, from the medical history and other sources, who the patient is.

A somewhat similar obstacle to knowing who a person is comes from the social convention that discourages critical remarks about others. This may not seem to be the case since criticism of others is the stock and trade of gossip—a most popular pastime—but gossip is a special kind of conversation. Generally, if you say, "Harry is a short-tempered man these days," a listener will reply, "That's because he's sick," or something similar. An excuse or rationalization tends to follow anything perceived as critical. Hardly any characterization of a person is possible without saying something that someone may consider derogatory; consequently, full knowledge of others is prevented by the social requirement to be polite.

Walter Lippman was justified in his concern that stereotypes influence perception. Our beliefs about people determine to a large degree how we interpret their words, facial expressions, gestures, conversational behavior, actions, and the way they position their bodies. In addition to interpretations based on preconceived expectations, listeners tend to understand a speaker in terms of what they themselves would have meant had they made the same utterance. It requires a truly attentive listener to be able to hear what a person says apart from an interpretation of what that person means. In most instances listeners do not separate their observation of the speaker's language from their assignment of meaning to the conversation.* Knowing what kind of a person another is similarly requires separating judgments about a person from the information on which the judgments are based. To do this one must attentively observe, listen, and be receptive to the person before making a judgment. Further, the information on which the conclusions are based must remain available for recall (at least while one is learning this skill) to avoid incorrect characterization and allow modification as further information becomes available. Just as a listener gives meaning to the speaker's words on the basis of the listener's understanding of the words, the doctor's personal knowledge of people—their language, behaviors, emotions, and values—provides the foundation for knowing about the individual person. For this reason, physicians' knowledge of persons is often called *subjective* (with the implication that it is idiosyncratic) to distinguish it from the *objective* knowledge available from tests and measurements.

Converting the Patient into an Object

Once a doctor has described someone, that person has, in some important sense, become an object of medical interest like a specimen in a bottle. The act of description can convert the person from a dynamic and changeable subject into a fixed and unchanging object, especially if the doctor sees people as being of one or another type and thus comes to know them only well enough to fit them into categories: this one is a type-A personality, that one an obsessive, she's self-destructive and he's noncompliant. All people—not only doctors—cherish their categories, as is clear from everyday conversation.

Thinking in terms of categories is the enemy of thinking in terms of process, and the habit is difficult to break. Although the richer and more complete the description, the less danger there is in the objectivization, it remains true that as soon as people are described they are, in some sense, made into objects.

Concern for Privacy

Another social reason, probably more fundamental than all the others cited, prevents us from bringing to consciousness all the knowledge about a person we acquire through conversation and from within ourselves. The fact that doctors can know so much from taking a history is discomforting for some who do not like the idea that they are so easily revealed; it seems to them an invasion of their privacy. These same people will allow physicians access to the

*The subject of how listeners know what a speaker means is discussed in depth in my *Talking with Patients: Vol. I—The Theory of Doctor-Patient Communication.* Also discussed are the distinction between observation and interpretation of the speaker's utterances, and how listeners can learn to overcome the problem of prejudging a speaker.

secrets of their bodies, but they are uneasy about invasion of their person. They are accustomed to (but not usually happy about) the idea of undressing in a physician's office, an act they believe to be voluntary, while there seems something involuntary about the exposure of their persons that occurs during the history-taking interview. It is one thing to open your body to view but quite another to open your person.

Alisdair MacIntyre discusses the importance of this aspect of social existence:

> Each of us, individually and as a member of particular social groups, seeks to embody his own plans and projects in the natural and social world. A condition of achieving this is to render as much of our natural and social environment as possible predictable, and the importance of both natural and social science in our lives derives at least in part—although only in part—from their contribution to this project. At the same time each of us, individually and as a member of particular social groups, aspires to preserve his independence, his freedom, his creativity and that inner reflection which plays so great a part in freedom and creativity, from invasion by others. We wish to disclose of ourselves no more than we think right and nobody wishes to disclose all of himself—except perhaps under the influence of some psycho-analytic illusion. We need to remain to some degree *opaque and unpredictable,* particularly when threatened by the predictive practices of others. The satisfaction of this need to at least some degree supplies another necessary condition for human life being meaningful in the ways that it is and can be. It is necessary, if life is to be meaningful, for us to be able to engage in long-term projects, and this requires predictability; it is necessary, if life is to be meaningful, for us to be in possession of ourselves and not merely to be the creation of other people's projects, intentions and desires, and this requires unpredictability. We are thus involved in a world in which we are simultaneously trying to render the rest of society predictable and ourselves unpredictable, to devise generalizations which will capture the behavior of others and to cast our own behavior into forms which will elude the generalizations which others frame [italics in the original](8).

This universal need and concern for privacy are acknowledged in virtually all physician's oaths, which throughout history have emphasized protecting the privacy of patients. (The Hippocratic Oath enjoins the physicians to promise "and whatsoever I shall hear in the course of my profession, as well as outside my profession in my intercourse with men, if it be what should not be published abroad, I will never divulge, holding such things to be holy secrets.") The necessity of maintaining the confidential nature of information obtained in the history-taking interview (and all other patient-doctor interactions) is the same with knowledge of the person as with knowledge of the body. It is the threat of sickness and death that *forces* patients to allow physicians to breach their privacy.

Understanding the importance of privacy is central to understanding the curious dichotomy of the human condition. We are at once particular me-myself-and-I individuals, each different from other individuals in the very nature of our biological existence, while at the same time members of a group which can only survive through the bond of our similarities. Privacy threatens the group and the group threatens privacy, creating a constant tension. In one era identity is stressed, in other times differences become more important. But the privacy of individuals is essential to their survival within the group. As a group and individually this fact is known so that we protect the privacy of others so that our own will be protected. The constitutional right of privacy has been recently stressed in many court decisions including *Roe* v. *Wade* which supported womens' right to abortion. Conversely, in *Discipline and Punish,* Foucault shows that part of the power of prisons and even of schools lies in their ability to invade the privacy of their subjects(9). The inescapable conclusion is that we do not allow ourselves to know about others what is plainly revealed in conversation and in the everyday presentation of self because it would reveal to us *how fragile our privacy is.* Here, as in matters of the body, people are especially uneasy about what doctors know.

Social Constraints

Physicians are subject to the same social constraints as others, but must learn from their training and experience to overcome them in the service of the sick. A number of years ago I discovered that I never looked as closely at a patient's face—the details of skin and features—as I did at other parts of the body. To see these aspects one must peer intently at the face, an act that is usually precluded by social rules. (Try staring at someone's face and see what happens!) When I became aware of this, I would ask the patient to close his or her eyes for the few moments that were required to examine the face. After a while I became proficient enough so that virtually no time was required to see the minute particulars of a face. I had learned discretion in my examination. Discretion preserves the social conventions and privacy.

In *The Birth of the Clinic,* Michel Foucault equates the ability of doctors to see the disease below the surface, where laypersons cannot gaze, with the power of medicine(10). The great advances of nineteenth-century medicine involved the invasion of the body—gazing, to use Foucault's term, into its depths. Opening the body not only revealed it but demonstrated the body's powers—the miraculous complexities of human biology. Opening the body permitted the entrance of science into medicine, and there has followed not only effective knowledge and treatment of disease but amplification of the body's powers. Telecommunication, computers, aerospace exploration, automobiles and airplanes, television, hearing aids—an endless list of modern achievements—depend not only on engineering and the physical sciences for their development but also on human biology for making them of use to humans. A central task for the twenty-first century is the discovery of the person—finding the sources of illness within the person, generating methods for the relief of illness from that knowledge and revealing the power within the person as the nineteenth and twentieth centuries have revealed the power of the body.

References

1. Sacks, Oliver. *The Man Who Mistook His Wife for a Hat.* 1985. New York, Summit Books, p. 22ff and 103ff.

2. Cassell, Eric J. Self-Conflict in Ethical Decisions. *The Foundations of Ethics and Its Relation to the Life Sciences. Vol. III Morals, Science and Society.* 1978. New York, The Hastings Center.

3. Cassell, Eric J. *Talking With Patients. Vol. I: The Theory of Doctor-Patient Communication,* 1985. Cambridge, Mass., MIT Press, p. 101.

4. Toulmin, Stephen. The Inwardness of the Mental Life 1979. Nora and Edward Ryerson Lecture The University of Chicago, Center for Policy Research.

5. Byrne, David and Eno, Brian. "Seen and Not Seen." From the album, *Remain in Light.* Talking Heads. 1980. New York, Site Records Company.

6. Cassell, Eric J. *Talking With Patients. Vol. 1: The Theory of Doctor-Patient Communication.* 1985. Cambridge, Mass., MIT Press, Chap. 2.

7. Collingwood, R.G. *The Principles of Art.* 1938. New York, Oxford University Press, p. 264.

8. MacIntyre, Alisdair. *After Virtue.* 2nd ed. 1981. South Bend, Ind., University of Notre Dame Press, p. 104.

9. Michel Foucault. *Discipline and Punish: The Birth of the Prison.* 1975. New York, Vintage Books.

10. Michel Foucault. *The Birth of the Clinic: An Archaeology of Medical Perception.* 1975. New York, Vintage Books.

11

The Measure of the Person

IN OUR ERA of medicine the only *real* knowledge is thought to be scientific knowledge: that which is gleaned from natural science and is objective, or measurable. Other kinds of knowing are considered of lesser value. Scientists believe that science must deal only with facts about the objective world because only facts can be valid. Facts can be verified—empirically demonstrated; everything that is not a fact is unavoidably doubtful and uncertain. However, it is not doubtful and uncertain things in themselves that are therefore suspect, but rather things that can *never* be other than doubtful and uncertain. For example, the manner by which certain genes express themselves to cause Tay-Sachs disease is at present doubtful and uncertain, but how these genes do their work is open to eventual discovery and subsequent verification.

From the scientific perspective, on the other hand, whether the man with a broken leg is in pain or the woman who has lost her hair from chemotherapy is suffering are questions which, not being open to empirical verification, can *never* be answered with certainty. If the question of whether someone is suffering is not open to scientific knowledge, then the relief of suffering—medicine's fundamental purpose—cannot be achieved by purely scientific medicine. Because this conclusion is unacceptable if medicine is to achieve its enduring goals, we must clarify what kind of knowledge is represented by knowing who a person is, and mediate any conflict that exists in medicine between the two kinds of knowledge which we can call the *scientific* and the *personal.*

Perhaps the best way to attack these problems is to examine some literary descriptions of persons. Where better to begin than with Shakespeare?

Caesar: Let me have men about me that are fat;
Sleek-headed men and such as sleep o'nights.

Yon Cassius has a lean and hungry look;
He thinks too much; such men are dangerous.

Anthony: Fear him not, Caesar, he's not dangerous;
He's a noble Roman, and well given.

Caesar: Would he were fatter! but I fear him not:
Yet if my name were liable to fear,
I do not know a man I should avoid
So soon as spare Cassius. He reads much;
He is a great observer, and he looks
Quite through the deeds of men; he loves no plays,
As thou dost, Anthony; he hears no music;
Seldom he smiles, and smiles in such a sort
As if he mock'd himself, and scorn'd his spirit
That could be mov'd to smile at anything.
Such men as he be never at heart's ease
Whiles they behold a greater than themselves,
and therefore they are very dangerous.
I rather tell thee what it is to be fear'd
than what I fear, for always I am Caesar(1).

Here is Herman Melville's description of Captain Graveling, master of the *Rights of Man,* in his novel, *Billy Budd.*

The shipmaster was one of those worthy mortals found in every vocation, even the humbler ones, the sort of person whom everyone agrees in calling "a respectable man." And nor so strange to report as it may be—though a ploughman of the troubled waters, lifelong contending with the intractable elements, there was nothing this honest soul at heart loved better than simple peace and quiet. For the rest, he was fifty or thereabouts, a little inclined to corpulence, a prepossessing face, unwhiskered and of agreeable color—rather a full face, humanely intelligent of expression. On a fair day with a fair wind and all going well, a certain musical chime in his voice seemed to be the veritable unobstructed outcome of the innermost man. He had much prudence, much conscientiousness, and there were occasions when these virtues were the cause of overmuch disquietude in him. On a passage, so long as his craft was in any proximity to land, no sleep for Captain Graveling. He took to heart those serious responsibilities not so heavily borne by some shipmasters.(2).

Let me conclude with one more. Can you identify him?

[He] was certainly not a difficult man to live with. He was quiet in his ways and his habits were regular. It was rare for him to be up after ten at night, and he had invariably breakfasted and gone out before I rose in the morning. . . . Nothing could exceed his energy when the working fit was upon him; but now and again a reaction would seize him, and for days on end he would lie upon the sofa in the sitting-room, hardly uttering a word or moving a muscle from morning to night. On these occasions I noticed a dreamy, vacant expression in his eyes. . . .

> In height he was rather over six feet, and so excessively lean that he seemed to be considerably taller. His eyes were sharp and piercing, save during those intervals of torpor to which I have alluded; and his thin hawk-like nose gave his whole expression an air of alertness and decision. His chin, too, had the prominence and squareness that mark the man of determination. His hands were invariably blotted with ink and stained with chemicals, yet he was possessed of extraordinary delicacy of touch(3).

He is, of course, Sherlock Holmes.

In each description three kinds of information are given. First, and most obvious, there are empirical facts. Cassius is a Roman noble who is thin. He is a penetrating observer, he does not like plays, or listening to music, and he does not smile. Captain Graveling is a ship's captain who had been at sea all his life. He is fifty years old, somewhat heavy, and does not have a beard. Holmes is tall and thin, sharp-featured, and sometimes energetic. (The actor who played Holmes in the movies, Basil Rathbone, will forever epitomize him.)

Another kind of information is prominently featured in each description. Cassius' lean and hungry look results from his uneasiness in the presence of others more powerful than he—he is a thinking man who is ambitious, envious, and untrustworthy. Captain Graveling, on the other hand, is respectable, honest, prudent, and conscientious, while Sherlock Holmes is quietly determined, energetic, alert, and decisive. These are value-laden terms in the vocabulary of morals. They have to do with goodness versus badness, rightness versus wrongness and correctness or appropriateness versus their opposites as they describe categories of human activity. They are all matters of degree according to some criteria held by the authors of these passages.

The final type of information involved in the characterization of persons is aesthetic. It is the intention of the authors that each of these descriptions, although composed of separate facts, should become a whole for the playgoer or the reader. We, the observers, are being prepared for the further appearance of each of these individuals, and when that happens we must—if the author has been successful—believe the next materialization of the character and his actions to be fitting in light of what we already know. It is as necessary, if this is to come about in our minds, that the persona created with those few sentences be a recognizable, cohesive totality as it is that the character fit the action that will take place. The domain of the proper "hanging together" of the parts of a whole—whether as a portrait of the character alone or the character as he or she appears in an unfolding work of literature—is aesthetics.

This chapter will show that each of these three kinds of information about sick persons—brute facts, moral, and aesthetic—are necessary to the work of clinicians. Here, as in everything else that is important in human existence, the classical categories of truth, goodness, and beauty apply.

I must make it clear that I do not suggest here—nor in anything I have written—that medicine can progress by emphasizing anything in opposition to its scientific aspects. There are no advantages in returning to prescientific medicine; the task is to go forward—to add, to enhance. This cannot be emphasized too much, because for the past several generations of physicians it has been an article of faith that medicine is scientific—lives up to the model of any scientific study of natural phenomena—when the information on which physicians base their actions in behalf of patients meets the criteria of objective scientific facts, and it stops being scientific and becomes "subjective"—or even sloppy—when it bases its actions on any "lesser"kinds of knowledge. However, I believe that the objective facts which are the basis of medical science, as necessary as they are, are in themselves insufficient to the clinician's task.

The simplest way to put the problem that we are attempting to solve is to restate the well-known fact that clinicians treat particular patients in particular circumstances at a particular moment in time, and thus they require information that particularizes the individual and the moment. Science, on the other hand, deals with generalities in which particular circumstances and particular moments in time have been systematically excluded. We have to ask what it is that makes a particular individual this explicit individual rather than an abstraction. Then we must ask how a physician applies knowledge about generalities or universals to specific individuals? How does knowledge about congestive heart failure in general pertain to this particular patient who has congestive heart failure today? The answer must lie, in part, in the way the physician finds out about the particular person. There are ways of apprehending knowledge of a person that are more or less true to the person and the person's circumstance. If I am to apply general knowledge about pneumonia to you as the particular patient I am treating, then it seems sensible that the more I really know you as the particular-person-*with-pneumonia,* the more successful I will be. If being a particular-individual-with-pneumonia in some way modifies pneumonia—makes it *this person's* pneumonia (and thus different from another person's pneumonia)—then the task of the clinician, as opposed to the scientist, is to consider the pneumonia-in-the-person rather than as an entity in itself, which is the scientific mind's natural tendency and the very goal of science. The solution to the problem of applying the general to the particular is to particularize the general.

This may sound circular, but it is not. It is a movement from the immediacy and relatively elementary idea of the sick patient to discrimination, differentiation, and analysis producing separate ideas of the disease and the person then again to a particular unity—*this sick person*—about whom these ideas are systematically integrated(4). Medical science comes to its knowledge of pneumonia by analyzing a multitude of cases and finding out what characterizes pneumonia *in general,* stripping away, in the process, those features that are idiosyncratic. By abstracting in such a fashion, pneumonia can be so characterized that it can be studied scientifically *as pneumonia,* apart from the patients who have it. By seeing its particular exemplification in *this* patient, on the other hand, we see what it is about this particular patient that modifies the abstract category of pneumonia but still allows us to employ the knowledge that has been accumulated about pneumonia. The great majority of patients have temperatures between 37.5° and 39° Celsius; only rarely is the temperature normal or higher than 39° Celsius. Pneumonia is individualized when the clinician is prepared for unusual levels of fever without their occurrence in any way invalidating the clinician's general knowledge of pneumonia. Atypical body temperatures in pneumonia is a trivial example; the point can also be made by using values for cardiac output in congestive heart failure, degrees of narrowing in coronary artery disease, or blood gas determinations in chronic obstructive pulmonary disease. What is there about *this* patient that allows him or her to function, go to work, be free of pain, have no difficulty breathing (or their opposites) in a manner not predicted by the diagnostic category? The general categories of medicine—its diagnostic and scientific concepts—are individualized when the clinician understands how this particular patient modifies the disease and the clinician can thus accept things that don't fit into the picture or see things that would otherwise be disregarded during the detailed search for evidence of disease.

The same concepts of diseases, however, can blind the clinician who substitutes the concept for what actually exists in the sick person. If an older person has pain in the back that makes motion difficult and the doctor categorically attributes it to arthritis as a prelude to saying there is nothing that can be done about it, then the general idea has been employed to hide what is actually to be found in the sick person. An equivalent danger exists in the characterization of the patient where generalizations, stereotypes, and biases are substituted for a true understanding of the person as discussed in the previous chapter. General or universal categories, therefore, can either promote or hinder individualization; the choice lies with the person utilizing them. The problem of applying the general to the particular does not lie in the general category—the universal *qua* universal—it lies in an inadequate knowledge of what makes this individual a particular—an inadequate characterization of the individual. And also in the difficulties faced in integrating the knowledge of the universal with a rich characterization of the individual.

Particularizing the general notions of medical science is also difficult because the process of making a diagnosis leads the clinician in the opposite direction. The problem for the diagnostician is to select some general category, diagnosis *X* (pneumonia, for example), that will best make sense of the cluster of phenomena displayed by the sick person. Pneumonia and the other medical *X*'s of this world do not proclaim themselves but, like oak trees, purple finches, salt marshes, and hurricanes, they are identified according to their adherence to criteria. The better they are known, the more exact the criteria and the sharper the distinction between an *X* and a non-*X*. Of course, the more exacting a set of specific criteria for a diagnosis, the more universal it will be, with all the atypical or inexact characteristics having been discarded as confusing the diagnosis or overlapping other diagnoses. It is a characteristic of particulars that they do not fit completely into any generality; that they have fuzzy edges and fall between distinctions. We see a strange bird on the lawn and rush to the bird book to identify it. The beak is more similar to this one, the tail feathers more like that one, the coloring and the size together make it seem more like this one after all. But the bird on the lawn is not similar in every single characteristic to the drawing in the book, and finally we decide it is a purple finch after all. Once we have used our powers of generalization to characterize it as a purple finch, we will tend to look at the bird and see what the book says about purple finches rather than seeing and knowing *this particular* purple finch.

Thus we can appreciate the difficulty for the clinician. He or she is confronted by a patient presenting a mass of evidence, some that is pertinent to particular disease categories and much that is not. The process of deciding on a particular diagnosis is an abstractive one—discarding the evidence that does not support the diagnosis and searching for information that does. Once a diagnosis is made, however, the process should proceed in the opposite direction, searching for what it is about the patient that modifies the disease. Let me reiterate. The process is dialectical—from the confusion arising out of the jumble of information that naturally exists in and around the sick person, a disease category (the diagnosis) is chosen. Then the abstract knowledge about the diagnosis is brought back and integrated with what has, at the same time, become known of *this* sick person to produce a more rounded, individualized, and whole interpretation of the disease that applies to the care of the particular sick person. This is not a step of addition—integration is not addition. Too often what is lacking is this last step of integration. As soon as doctors say that the patient has pneumonia, they will tend to discover in that patient what they already know about pneumonia rather than being open to discovery about this particular patient with pneumonia. The problem is exacerbated by the tendency to believe that the only legitimate knowledge is scientific. Therefore, we will better understand the problem of applying the universal to the particular and move toward its solution by examining the nature of scientific facts.

Science sets the standard against which empirical facts in medicine are measured. In this view, a fact is a "good" fact if it is scientific. A scientific fact can be relied upon, it is not dependent or contingent on other facts, it will not lead the doctor astray, and it will be consistent. What makes a fact a scientific fact? First and foremost, a scientific fact is objective. In physicians' terms this means it can be known independently of the doctor who knows it. If the doctor—or you or I or Aunt Tillie—come across the fact, in this idealized concept of scientific facts, it will be the same for each of us. The question of whether a patient has a fever can be decided by what seems to be a scientific fact; no matter who looks at it, the thermometer reads something greater than 37° Celsius (or 98.6° Fahrenheit). The degree of anemia as measured by hemoglobin or hematocrit determinations seems to qualify as a fact. These ideas about facts are extensions of the earlier scientific belief that facts are derived from sensory information: if you can see it, hear it, touch it or smell it, it is a fact, as in, "I'll believe it when I see it." Ultimately, scientific facts are *believed* to have existence that is independent of human observers, and they became knowledge or information when they are observed in one fashion or another. Finding methods to produce objective facts about disease is one of the goals of research. Patients also like tests because they *seem* to produce reliable, real facts unsullied by biased human observers. From the perspective of twentieth-century scientific medicine, a fact is like a pebble on the beach; whether or not you see it or pick it up, it will always be the same free-standing ultimate, logically simple atomic fact.

You may wonder where such strange ideas about facts came from. It is certainly impossible that anyone ever discovered such a fact, because there are no facts that can *ever* stand alone and independent, for at least two reasons: first, for something to be a fact in medicine it must be observed by someone; second, a fact is always part of some larger whole. The process of observation, whether simple as with the unaided eye, or complex as with a diagnostic test, is inevitably guided by the observer's ideas. No observation is free of interpretation; rather than facts being independent atomic entities, they are the facts they are by virtue of the observation. If this were not so, I would see the forest merely as a blur of unnamed color and indistinct shape. Instead I see trees, grass, weeds, stones, and earth in various shades of green, yellow, and brown. My concepts and ideas about colors and these objects of nature allow me to see them for what they are, just as these colors and objects of nature form my ideas and concepts. The two processes take place in continuous interplay.

It is the same when physicians examine an X ray or look at the cells of a tumor under the microscope. Even the fact of how much cholesterol is in the blood as it appears on the numerical printout of an automated blood chemistry machine is not independent of the observer. The test reveals the amount in the blood of a substance that interacts with the chemicals of the test and that is presumed to represent cholesterol. No biochemist believes that the test result represents all the cholesterol and nothing but the cholesterol. In this instance the concepts of the observer that allow the cholesterol to be known are the ideals about the biochemistry of the test and its relationship to "actual" blood cholesterol. The numerical result of the cholesterol test is adequate for clinical purposes, but it is not—nor is anything like it—an independent fact of nature.

In the examples of facts given above, the degree of fever expressed by the thermometer is an idea that allows the interpretation of a number on a instrument that registers the temperature inside a mouth or a rectum that is believed to represent the temperature of the body. The degree of anemia expressed by a hemoglobin or hematocrit determination is likewise a human interpretation of the numerical reading on an instrument. Both the thermometer and the hematocrit produce useful information, but not independent facts. This is not to say that the facts of clinical medicine exist only in the eyes or minds of the observers; these are the basic facts of the body, the given world of nature. But it is only when they are registered by an observer in medicine that they become facts of medicine with this rather than that significance.

Facts do not stand alone; they derive their meaning from their relationship to the other facts with which they form a whole, and also from that very whole of which they are a part. What this thing is it is partly because of what it is not. A fact that is distinguished from the background of other facts implies the background. We never consider things in isolation—a single fact of kidney function at this moment is not independent of other things happening in the kidney (or even the liver) at this moment or moments past. This is of great importance to us as physicians. We elicit medical facts because of our need to understand, and what we want to understand are not isolated facts but wholes—whole kidneys, whole bodies, whole persons, and even whole communities.

As we move forward in our attempt to understand the information required for the care of sick patients (about both person and disease), we must remind ourselves that we constantly think in terms of wholes, even when this is not our intention. Practicing physicians, because of the nature of their perception and reasoning, cannot completely isolate their knowledge of facts about patients' parts from whole patients living in a real world. If that is the case, a skeptic might ask, why do they so often seem to pay no attention to the whole sick person, much less the world in which the patient lives? It is because their theories of disease and the science on which modern medicine is based pull them away from their natural inclination. Thus, physicians who work from within that understanding abstract themselves from their own natural inclination *not* to abstract, not to isolate their knowledge from the experiences of whole persons in the real world.

Objective and Subjective

These words have special connotations in medicine, as distinct from their meanings in philosophy, for example. It is essential, therefore, that we understand what these highly charged terms mean to the physician. As noted above, the reading on the clinical thermometer is an objective measure of an elevation of body temperature. The feeling of feverishness is subjective because a feeling can only be experienced by the subject. The patient who has the fever has ideas about its meanings that are also considered subjective. But subjective in this instance has the connotation of idiosyncratic—unique to this subject. Subjective in the sense of a feeling experienced by a subject and subjective in the sense of idiosyncratic—only this subject has this idea—are two different meanings of the word subjective. Medicine holds a third sense of subjective—your *statement* that you feel feverish is also considered subjective; that is, your words, in general, are considered by doctors to be subjective. That is strange, because "objective" generally refers to something that can be known in common like the empirical facts noted above, and observers can certainly hear and understand the words. "Yes," responds the physician, "but what the words *mean* is not something outside observers can hold in common, and that is why they are considered subjective." Philosophers do not share this meaning of subjective and they are often confused when they hear physicians speak about subjective versus objective, particularly since physicians tend to use "objective" to stand solely for that which can be measured, and that is certainly not the philosophical meaning. The reason the meanings are considered subjective may be that they are buried inside the subject, but in that case the core temperature of the body would be subjective because it, too, is buried inside the subject. (A scientist might answer that the core temperature is measurable and is not in the subject, it is in the body—at best a puzzling distinction.)

To the contrary, both the meaning of the patient's words and the temperature of the patient's body are *objective* and can be determined by others. While the patient's *feeling* of feverishness is irreducibly subjective, the patient's *report* of the symptom is objective; it is something that is part of shared reality and can be examined. The utility of a report of feverishness will depend on the use to which it is put. If used as the sole measure of body temperature, it will be deficient in both accuracy and precision—elevated body temperature may be present in the absence of a feeling of feverishness, and a feeling of feverishness may or may not be present in the absence of elevated body temperature and these relationships (between feverishness and elevated body temperature) can vary. It remains true, however, that when patients report that they feel feverish, then (even if they are believed to be lying) their reports of feverishness remain *objective facts* to be explained or used. The same truth holds for reports of all symptoms. What may be in doubt is their relationship to changes in the working of the body. If the patient reports being short of breath, the physician must elicit the precise meaning of that report before it is clinically useful. But when *attentive* clinicians elicit symptoms, their reliability as indicators of changes in body function can be assessed. In this regard symptoms are no different from most other clinical information that is considered objective by physicians.

Values

In discussing the kinds of information in the texts from Shakespeare, Melville, and Conan Doyle, I noted that in addition to empirical facts about the characters, there are facts in the moral dimension. Cassius is envious, Captain Graveling is tirelessly responsible, and Holmes is determined. These are moral characteristics in that they represent human behaviors that range from good to bad. What people believe to be the right or the wrong thing to do is a function of their moral values. But values is a more inclusive term than morals, because the word moral is usually reserved to describe behaviors of people toward other people or their concerns. Yet individuals also *value* a crunchy apple, a lovely child, and a sturdy chair, none of which judgments are in the moral realm (especially if we confine the world "lovely" to the child's appearance rather than behavior). In fact, it would be difficult to find anything of interest to humans about which they did not express some value—some measure of desirability or its opposite. Similarly, it would be virtually impossible to find some aspect of human existence that was not influenced by human values.

Modern medicine appears to be an exception. Medicine has established its scientific status in this century by aggressively expunging notions of value from its vocabulary. When medicine embraced science, it adopted the view that because science is value free, a medicine based on science also had to be value free. The philosophers who provided the underpinnings of twentieth-century science agreed that whereas a statement of empirical fact says something real, a statement of value is not a real statement at all because it has no cognitive meaning—by which they mean that it cannot be reduced to a factual basis. At best, they said, such a statement expresses the speaker's feelings. The idea of ridding medicine of feelings and personal opinions as sources of evidence was very appealing. Now the impersonal, value-free evidence of science would replace the opinions of authorities or prestigious doctors; the words of the neophyte would have equal weight with those of the expert when based on the demonstrable facts of science. This shift of emphasis toward scientific evidence and away from personal authority has been one of the important reasons for medicine's advances in this century.

For all its apparent attractiveness, however, a value-free medicine is a contradiction in terms. Evidence based on values enters medicine in at least five distinct ways: (1) The values of society are important determinants of medical care. The desire for health is itself a value, and the health of some groups (children, for example) is valued more than others (the aged). (2) Medical care plays a part in achieving the goals of both sick persons and the healthy. Goals are statements of value, and they must be weighed against each another to decide on the best course of medical action. (3) Physicians, personally and as professionals, hold values that have an impact on the care they provide. They believe some symptoms, diseases, or courses of action either more or less important. They have well-established ideas of what is normal and what is abnormal—and such terms are, in themselves, value laden. Physicians have distinct ideas about what is good medicine or doctoring and what is bad medicine or doctoring. (4) Persons, sick or well, do not exist apart from their values, and it is obvious that persons cannot be known or described by value-free facts. (5) Understanding wholes and wholeness is inextricably linked to values. Wholes are not mere things, they are systems that fulfill themselves or achieve their aims with varying degrees of completeness. The ideas necessary to understand such concepts are inevitably linked to value, as when we think of the athlete's body and compare it to our own. Sometimes the values in these various aspects lie along the axis of right and wrong and are in the domain of medical ethics. For all its importance, however, the moral is but one facet of the realm of values. Values, then, like scientific facts, are essential to the clinician's knowledge of sick persons. But where methods of reasoning about facts have a long history and a well-developed basis, thinking about values and morals seems more problematic, partially because scientific facts are usually referred to as *objective* whereas values are considered *subjective.*

Probabilistic

In recent years the probabilistic nature of medical facts has become clear. (A probabilistic fact is one that it is impossible to know with certainty.) When an electrocardiogram shows a certain abnormality, the squiggles on the electrocardiogram paper are indubitably on the paper, just as a report of shortness of breath is unquestionably a report of shortness of breath. However, the abnormal squiggles on the paper are no longer considered absolute evidence of heart damage; the relationship is now considered probabilistic. There may be heart damage but no change in the electrocardiogram, or the abnormal squiggles may be present in the absence of damage to the heart. The same probabilistic relationship exists between virtually all test results—even X rays—and the bodily events they purport to reflect. Whenever facts are known through the mediation of another agency—the state of the heart as mediated by the electrocardiogram—an element of probabilism enters knowledge.

In this view of medicine, information about a patient's values assumes greater importance. Just as patients' reports of their symptoms must no longer be incorrectly viewed as subjective (and therefore "useless"), knowledge of patients' values may be objectively considered to reflect the actual values of the patient *within certain probabilities*. There is a fundamental difference between value information and what it reflects about the sick person and the symptoms or signs of illness and what they reflect about the body. When physicians say that the abnormalities of an electrocardiogram or stress test reflect (with a certain degree of probability) abnormalities of the coronary arteries, they have no doubt as to what they mean by an abnormal coronary artery, or that what they mean will remain consistent—a rose is a rose is a rose is a rose. On the other hand, what is meant by the statements that Sherlock Holmes has sharp and piercing eyes, that Cassius scorns his spirit, and that Captain Graveling is prudent? Such statements are often called value judgments, a term that usually has a negative connotation. Sir Douglas Black, president of the Royal College of Physicians and later of the British Medical Association, wrote a monograph in praise of scientific medicine containing a brief section in response to the charge that scientists are cold people:

> The belief that scientists are cold detached people has the nature of a value judgment, and as such cannot be rigidly proved or disproved—there being, for example, no objective measure of 'coldness' or 'detachment' in terms of which we could categorize a group of scientists. The problem is in no way solved by discovering individual scientists who give an impression of aloofness in personal contacts, any more than it would be by discovering scientists of notably warm personality. My own view is that there are 'cold' and 'warm' people in every walk of life. . . .
>
> Neither as an undergraduate nor as a university teacher was I aware that students in the scientific faculties were notably less extroverted or idealistic than those in other faculties(5).

Sir Douglas goes on to quote others about the passion and intensity of scientists, this one's "lively originality" and that one's "sacred fury." While the first sentence of the quotation impugns value judgments, the remainder of the section is filled with judgments about value. Sir Douglas, like the rest of us, cannot do otherwise, because he, like the rest of us, must characterize things in order to make choices and act. Why did you pick this muffin rather than that, this article of clothing, that apple, read such and such a book, ask George rather than Bill to come to dinner? Because of properties each has and which you variously value.

Yet Sir Douglas' criticism of value judgments has validity despite the fact that the term is usually applied only to negative statements—we do not usually accuse someone of making a value judgment when that person tells us how wonderful we are. Is a "fast" car the same "fast" as a "fast" sailing ship? Is a "prudent" sea captain similar to a "prudent" restaurant captain? Clearly these words have meanings that depend on the situation. However, despite their relative nature, the words of value that Shakespeare uses have meanings that are constant enough for us to comprehend after three hundred years. In literature (and in ordinary discourse), then, words of value seem quite adequate to their task. How can that be?

Victor Borge, a comedian and pianist, has a funny routine in which he "composes" music by cutting and pasting bits of sheet music by the great masters. Spying a tiny piece of paper that has fallen to the floor, he picks it up as if it were the keystone of his composition. Then he raises his hand to play what he has found—plink—one note! Value terms, like musical notes, have little meaning and less use unless considered with their fellows in their natural environment. The first step in comprehending their effectiveness is to remind ourselves that, as with all language, we are trained from early childhood in the use of words that describe values as part of our education in successful communication. The basic rule of conversation is that speakers must be understood. Thus, from infancy on we learn how to communicate our attitudes and values so that they are understood first by our family and then by others. Communication is an amazingly redundant process. The words we use are underscored by the syntax, the nonword parts of speech including pause, tonal emphasis, pitch, and speech rate as well as the expressions on our faces and our body language.

The second reason that value terms provide useful information is that when a statement of value—of attitude, opinion, interest, concern, or judgment—appears in a conversation, it is never merely an isolated word or phrase. There is always other information that causes the listener to agree or to doubt. In this fragment of a conversation, the doctor, after listening to the patient, renders an opinion of value.

> *Patient:* Well, there has been—I try not to let anything worry me—but my husband died because he was a worry wart, and I said now I'll never die of a heart attack. But, uh, the thing is, now, see, my son, he has a place down in Breezy Point and he took the family and his wife—
>
> *Doctor: Breezy Point is which way? The Rockaways?*
>
> *Patient:* Yeah, And I'm all alone in the house—not that I'm afraid, but the thing is, you hear so many sudden deaths—you know what I mean? And I'm all alone. And I fell—gee, I could—and I have to watch my step, too.

I fall easily if I'm not—don't watch my step. So I don't, uh—seem to, uh . . . I'm a little upset and, uh, 'cause every once in a while I get a pain up in my . . . up here, you know. [She and the doctor have a short interchange about her blood pressure and whether it is rising. Then she returns to the complaint about her son.]

Patient: I have an idea he had shared it with the dau—my daughter-in-law has some sisters out on the island, out in Bay—Hampton Bays and that. But what harm would it have been? I thought he was going to call me before he left yesterday morning, and he didn't.

Doctor: *I wouldn't, uh—in your place, I wouldn't be that meticulous. Too grown up for this . . . right? Don't let those little things get on your nerves.* (6).

Meticulous? The doctor, (whose native language is not English) used the wrong word. The assessment of value he was expressing was inappropriate in the circumstances, and the reader immediately knows his word is wrong. Each of the following words—hurt, uncharitable, aggrieved, unaccepting, faultfinding, injured (and others)—would have rendered a judgment of value about her statements and each might have been correct, but each represents a somewhat different evaluation of her attitude. We know it is the wrong word, not by judging the isolated word "meticulous" out of context, but by its place in the conversation and the context of the world in which the conversation took place.

The third reason that words of value work in literature and conversation is that their meanings depend on their subjects. If we employ the adjective "velvety" in reference to fabric, the mucous membrane of the mouth, the surface of a tumor, the fur of some animal, or a quality of fine wine, we are obviously speaking about five different qualities, only one of which is an attribute of ". . . soft dense pile produced by weaving into a single cloth an extra warp which is looped over wires and later cut" (OED). The meaning of the adjective arises not only from the word itself but from the things it modifies. We have concepts and ideas about fabrics, mucous membranes, tumors, animal fur, and wine that include characteristics of the physical sensations they cause when touched. Velvety, as it refers to each of these things, is distinctly different. No one would mistake the velvety feeling of velvet for the velvety feeling that you get when you stroke the inside of your cheek. It is parsimonious—and practical—good luck that language uses the same word for these different objects—imagine if you had to know a different word for every single thing that feels velvety. So when Herman Melville writes that Captain Graveling is prudent, we know precisely what he means to the extent that we know about sea captaincy.

Melville does not merely tell us what Captain Graveling is, however, he also tells us what he is not. Captain Graveling is not foolhardy, careless, heedless, innattentive, or lackadaisical. The author has constructed our picture of Captain Graveling, and the word "prudent" is but one step in that process. It is a process because as we read *Billy Budd,* our concept of sea captains (and thus also of prudent) is continuously enlarged. The assessments of value by Shakespeare, Melville, and Conan Doyle are comprehensible to us because of what we know of human behavior and the dimensions their characters give to the value terms.

It follows from this that the more you know about something, the more precise will be your knowledge of the values associated with it and the greater your ability to evaluate an individual example of the thing. "Isn't this a wonderfully crunchy apple?" said the man about a Washington State Delicious. "I don't think they're so crunchy, they're a little mushy," said the listener. "Now, a Granny Smith, that's a crunchy apple." "I never ate a Granny Smith," said the man. We already knew that because if he had, his standard of crunchy apple would no longer include the Delicious. When the woman with asthma comes into the emergency room late in the course of her attack, requiring much more treatment than would have been the case had she arrived sooner, the inexperienced physician says, "How can anyone be so stupid?" The more experienced physician says that the patient is not dull-witted but, in common with many sick people, had managed to remain unaware of her breathing difficulty until it overwhelmed her—a typical reaction to illness rather than a sign of low intelligence.

We still must deal with the basic difficulty of values, as stated by Sir Douglas. The characteristics, properties, and attributes of patients—their personalities and their behavior—allow no objective standard by which they can be measured and compared with each other or across time. How are we to know which one of those valuations mentioned in the text following the dialogue of the doctor and the complaining mother best fit her? The same criticism can be applied to many of the attributes of person discussed in the previous chapter. Physicians would devalue the doctor's opinion—even if he had used an appropriate word—by branding it subjective; it is his personal opinion arising from his internal, private measures of value. However, when the same doctor tells his colleagues that the patient has a systolic heart murmur, they will not consider the information subjective. In fact, in a current article about heart murmurs and in the accompanying editorial, the word subjective is never mentioned(7)(8). The doctors would say that the heart murmur is objective, as is the size of a patient's liver as palpated and the shadow of the heart on a chest X ray. Two facts put in doubt, once again, the utility for medical practice of medicine's ideas about subjectivity versus objectivity. The first is that while it is true that heart murmurs and livers and heart shadows are there for all to observe (and thus objective, by any standard), the doctor's judgment of these things is personal. As Alvan Feinstein showed many years ago, doctors frequently disagree in their assessment of such objective information. The second fact is that the woman's behavior, described by the doctor as meticulous, is also there for all to observe. The information on which he based his value assessment is objective, just like the heart murmur.

It is fair to say that we trust doctors' assessments of heart murmurs much more than their value assessments about patients. They are trained to listen to the heart, and their training has provided them with standards against which to measure what they hear. These standards, formulated from their knowledge of heart murmurs, are internalized in memory, but they can also be found in textbooks and discussed with colleagues who share a language of description. Further, heart murmurs are never isolated pieces of information. They exist in patients whose hearts have other characteristics that can be heard, seen on X ray, and studied by electrocardiography or echocardiography. These patients have a history that is also consonant with or contradictory to what has been heard through the stethoscope.

Physicians' knowledge of values is not formalized in the same fashion, they have not been trained in assessing values, there is no textbook to which they may refer and there is no formalized shared language of values in medicine that will allow discussion with colleagues. It is not surprising that their assessments of value are not on a par with their assessments of heart murmurs. To improve the quality of physicians' knowledge and use of value information is a three-step process. (1) Recognizing that people do display their values in their presentation to the world, their language use, or in other behaviors. (2) Learning to assess this information in a manner that both accurately and precisely reflects the patients' values. (3) Learning to reason about values in a logical manner.

People Display Their Values

A person's values, both negative and positive, are apparent in the things that are important to them: their interests, concerns, what they respond to, and the relative weights they apply in making choices. Since people constantly make choices, live in a world shaped by their choices, act on their interests and concerns with varying degrees of intensity, and cannot, in fact, be totally neutral to their world for even a moment, it follows that people constantly display their values in every facet of their existence. But are these their "true" values? It could not be otherwise, since even a consciously fabricated set of values must bear some relation to the person's values—otherwise why the choice of one set of counterfeit values over another? Furthermore, since values are displayed in every moment of existence, it is inconceivable that they could all be under conscious control. It is the case, however, that persons' values may not always be consistent with each other, that values exist on many levels, that some are more enduring than others, and that they may change with circumstances.

These realities—that values can be so changeable and may be inconsistent—give rise to the belief that information about values is of limited utility. In clinical medicine this issue surfaces when patients express a desire not to be resuscitated in the event of a cardiac arrest. Should such patients later lose consciousness or be otherwise unable to express their wishes, doctors often believe they should be resuscitated despite their earlier wish, "in case they changed their mind." It is true that there are things about which we change our minds—tastes change. And it's also true that when illness is severe, people often discover what is really important to them—another way of saying that values change or change in priority. Because of this it would be foolhardy to believe that because one knows a person's values, the knowledge is eternal and unchanging. Since the body also changes, physicians understand the importance of keeping abreast of the changes with up-to-date test results and repeated examinations. Yet most people do not think of the changes in the body as transitory in the same way that values are believed to vary. There are surface phenomena, such as skin temperature, and physiologic parameters, such as blood pressure, which change from minute to minute or day to day, but there are other bodily features, such as bone structure, which change very slowly. The same with values: some superficial likes and dislikes are as changeable as the wind, while basic personality, expressed by values, is remarkably constant.

People, in their presentation to the world, do display their values for others to see and know. Furthermore, information about values should be considered in the same light as information about the body. Some of it is rock solid, some inconstant, but none of it is merely random variation unrelated to the person as a whole or the entire spectrum of the person's values. Here, as in all our other dimensions, we are of a piece. A recent billboard advertisement shows a bearded man contemplating a frosty glass of beer as he says, "Guinness Gold. If only my father had lived to see it." If his father's only relation to beer was to drink it (if he was not, for example, the owner of the Guinness Brewery), then we are led to believe that his father's values were such that beer played a very important part in his life.

Learning To Assess Values

The crucial fact is that information about their patients' values is there for doctors to discover. They must acknowledge the need and then train themselves to be attentive to the facts that reveal values—at least as attentive as they are to the sounds that come up the tubes of their stethoscopes. Since it is clear that to know about a person's values is to know so much of importance about the person, it must be assumed that the major reasons that physicians do not discover their patients' values are the same reasons why they do not know who their patients are. In relation to moral values specifically, the social prohibition against open criticism of persons often prevents physicians from forming a seemingly critical idea of their patient's values. At the same time, however, physicians have a number of categories of value judgments relating to patient behaviors that are seen to impede doctors' work or reflect on what doctors consider patients' inherent ignorance. Assessments of a patient's values must be sharply distinguished from such negative value judgments—which, I suppose, are as inevitable here as in every other walk of life. The task is not to listen to sick persons talking and come away with an assessment of their values (in the same way that one might assess their immune status) and then make pronouncements that one is "type A," another "brave," or a third "neurotic." To do that would, in the best of circumstances, create another set of generalizations of doubtful value like a diagnosis of arthritis for someone with back pain. Our interest in patients' values comes from the desire to individualize medical science and reinstate the concept of disease in this particular sick person in order to care for *this person.*

The existence of a world of facts underlying values makes it possible to teach the ability to appreciate the values of another person *apart from the observer's opinion of those values.* As part of a classroom exercise in the introductory lecture of a course in history taking for medical students, a tape recording was played of a patient giving the history of his illness to a physician. The students took a test with questions about the facts provided by the patient and a place where the student could record an opinion about the kind of a person he was. A large list of adjectives (which frequently serve as statements of value) was given to use in characterizing their opinions. At the beginning of the course, the students' ability to remember the factual information offered by the patient was poor, and they differed greatly in their value assessments of him. At the end of the course the test was repeated. Their accuracy in reporting what they had heard was greatly increased, and their assessments of the patient had become quite uniform. The students' experience supports the beliefs that attentive listening—skilled observation in general—is attainable through training, and that judgments of values based on trained observation are consistent and reproducible.

By being attentive to speech and carefully observing presentation and behavior, one can discover how a patient relates to his or her body, medical care, doctors, hospitals, family, medications; what is most important and what least, what is most frightening and what least—in other words, how these objects or events are valued. As these facts of value are learned (and thus the patient increasingly appreciated), the physician is more able to act in the patient's best behalf as seen by the patient. Judgments of value in this sense are the opposite of value judgments in the colloquial sense. Obtaining this information is a difficult job that demands skill and patience but, unlike mind-reading or guessing, the information is there to be obtained. Assessments of values—of opinions, attitudes, desires, fears, hopes, and concerns—is a process that takes place over time and allows checking and cross-checking when necessary. As with all information in medicine, the degree of certitude will vary but is open to amplification by questioning and probing. If you want to know whether you are correct in your assumption of what I believe is important, ask me—and, if the information is vital, ask me again tomorrow and the day after, and check with my family. Ask yourself whether what you hear is consistent with the rest of what you know of me. If my behavior ten years ago, last year, last month, and yesterday are all consistent with my expressed desire not to be resuscitated after cardiac arrest, accept my decision as authentic and enduring *even if, by your lights, I am being foolish.*

Values as the Subject of Reasoning

Values can also be the subject of reasoning in the same way as other facts(9). Reason has many meanings, but it is generally accepted as the intellectual faculty that helps us construct necessary connections, inferring from the past to the future, relating content provided by knowledge, memory, and the senses. The faculty to reason does not depend on what is reasoned about—which is why reason can be applied equally to facts about values and emprical facts. [Although certain reasoning processes—typically those that deal with religion, faith, or the mystical—are wrongly described as irrational or may seem obscure or flawed, the ability to reason about such things remains intact(10)]. Therefore, including information about values as part of the body of clinical information in no way detracts from the validity of the clinical reasoning process.

The aspect of reasoning involved in making inferences about the future requires further comment. Accepting my values as consistent (e.g., those that led to my refusal of cardiac resuscitation) justifies the prediction that when they are tested, my values will not have changed. "You cannot be claiming," the skeptic might reply, "that information about values allows firm predictions in the same way that scientific facts lead to predictions. That would be ridiculous." The skeptic is correct. In considering this, however, it should always be kept in mind that truly scientific predictions are *not* about the future in the sense of tomorrow or next week. They pertain to any circumstance, past, present, or future, in which the same conditions hold that the scientific statement describes. In a chapter entitled "The Character of Generalizations in Social Science and Their Lack of Predictive Power" in *After Virtue,* Alisdair MacIntyre details why human behavior can never be as predictable as the behavior of (say) molecules of a gas. Two of his four reasons particularly concern us here.

The first is that radical innovation is possible, leading to previously unforeseen possibilities. Suppose, for example, that a new device is invented that permits a patient who has been resuscitated to return to an active life with complete cardiac and pulmonary support provided by a device as small as a camera. Would the values he or she expressed a year ago about resuscitation still hold true? While that particular supposition may be unlikely, it is true that technological innovation has an unpredictable effect on patients' attitudes. A second reason is that things happen that cannot be foreseen. It is not so much that my values have changed as it is that the situation is so different from what I believed it would be that my previous attitudes, although well known to my physicians, are no longer the relevant information. For example, the patient had pushed forward the date of heart surgery in order to be able to participate in a conference he felt was vitally important to his professional future. On the way to the hospital, he was hit by a taxi and sustained serious injuries. His professional future seems less important to him now than the possibility that he will not walk again. This is the kind of contingency with which doctors are very familiar.

Do these obstacles along with those to knowing who a person is discussed in the previous chapter preclude predictive inferences based on values? Not at all, because if they did you would not be able to live your life in a social world—daily life requiring, as it does, so much prediction (in the sense of guessing about tomorrow) based on the values of other people. Reasoning about values, if it is to be an effective part of clinical medicine, requires the understanding that it is a process that takes place over time. Ultimately, however, facts about values will never permit predictions of scientific validity. But how is this different from other aspects of medicine, where the management of uncertainty remains a crucial clinical task? Discerning values and reasoning from them effectively require expertise. As learning about patients' values becomes a legitimate part of a doctor's job, medical schools will deal with the problem of teaching the process, a vocabulary will develop to support discussion among physicians, and doctors will become as expert as they are about feeling for an enlarged liver.

Aesthetics in Medicine

We also know about persons by aesthetic means. When we say that someone does not look right to us, comment on how gracefully a young person runs, or note that Shakespeare's characters "hang together," we are making aesthetic assessments. To speak about aesthetics in the context of medicine may seem strange, but I believe that it supplies a necessary dimension of knowledge.

The term aesthetics is itself a problem. In its usual sense, aesthetics has to do with beauty and the continuum between the beautiful and the ugly. This will not bring us closer to its use in medicine, so I propose to substitute the term harmony for beauty and harmonious for beautiful. The word order suggests itself as a companion to harmony, as stated in the *Oxford English Dictionary's* definition of beautiful as "attractive or impressive through expressing or suggesting fitness, order, regularity, rhythm, cogency, or perfection of structure." A similar example of the use of aesthetics can be found in Rudolf Arnheim's book, *Entropy and Art:* "Order is a necessary condition for anything the human mind is to understand. . . . Order makes it possible to focus on what is alike and what is different, what belongs together and what is segregated. When nothing superfluous is included and nothing indispensable left out, one can understand the interrelation of the whole and its parts, as well as the heirarchic scale of importance and power by which some structural features are dominant, others subordinate(11)." It should be remembered, in this context, that what is concerned with harmony and order is also logically related to disharmony, disorder, and chaos. Aesthetic information may seem far from science but that is not the case. In recent times mathematicians have gone beyond their tradiational concern with arithmatic, algebra, geometry, and calculus, and have been increasingly concerned with seeking patterns, order, and chaos with both the mind and the eye(12).

We know whether something is harmonious not primarily because of thinking about it, although that is possible, but because of the pattern to our eyes, the sound in our ears, the feel in our hands, and even the smell. The information in the aesthetic dimension is primarily sensory, but our response to the information is a "feeling about." Aesthetic feeling is, therefore, ineluctably subjective—but this does not mean that it is idiosyncratic or random.

Bernard Bosanquet identifies three characteristics of aesthetic feeling that remove it from the ephemeral. First, it is a stable feeling. When we have an aesthetic experience, whether in the contemplation of a beautiful object or the experience of the completeness of something, the aesthetic feeling does not disappear. It is not like an appetite that becomes sated. It is also stable in the sense that tomorrow in the same circumstances the aesthetic feeling will reappear. Second, aesthetic feeling is relevant to the object or event that evokes it—it is irrevocably attached to that object or event. The special quality of particular aesthetic feeling is "evoked by the special quality of the something of which it is the feeling, and in fact is one with it(13)." Third, it is a feeling that can be, and usually is, held in common. It can be shared, discussed, illustrated, and educated. These three properties of aesthetic feeling—*stability, relevance, and community*—are necessary for artists to do their work. Poets need us to respond not merely to the meaning of their words but also to their rhythm; graphic artists require that their shapes and colors evoke consistent responses; composers depend on the common (within their culture) human reaction to certain combinations of sounds. The opening notes of Beethoven's Fifth Symphony have a universal effect on the listener who has been exposed to the Western tradition of music, one that has been constant over two centuries. The symphony would have a different effect if the interval between the opening third and fourth notes were either greater or smaller, or if the fourth chord of the opening bar was higher in pitch than the preceding three(14). The uniformity of response to such a specific aspect of what S. Alexander calls the aesthetic impulse suggests that it is objective as well as subjective.

The belief that matters of aesthetics are subjective comes from supposing them to be mere states of mind. The feelings or thoughts evoked by an object or event are certainly private, but the object of reference is not. The color red may be sensed slightly differently by each of us, but all of us who are not color-blind are able to act in a consistent fashion when asked to distinguish red from green(15).

The fact that aesthetic knowledge can be shared is particularly important in the context of medicine, because it means that even the nonmeasurable can provide a stable basis for clinical opinion and action. That aesthetic feeling provides different information than that provided by scientific measurement and that aesthetic information is dependable in its own right can be shown by reference to optical illusions. No matter how often you have been told that the logs in Figure 1 are the same size, and even if you measure them as you look at the picture, they continue to appear different. The illusion, although subjec-

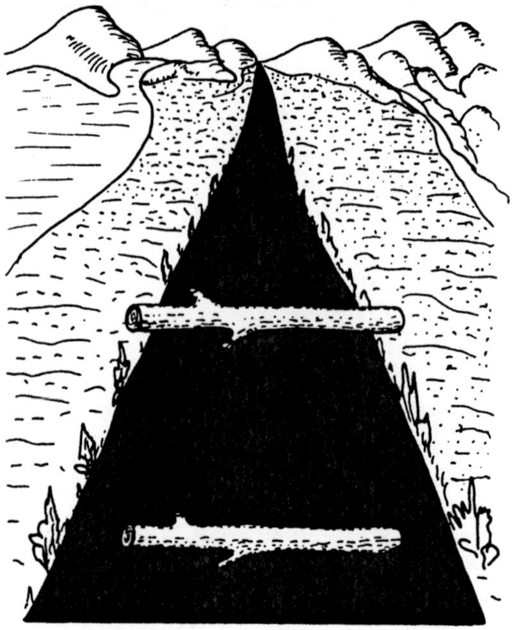

Fig. 1. No matter how often you have been told that the logs are the same size, they continue to appear different. Optical illusions, although subjective, are shared and stable (from Lloyd Kaufman, *Perception: The World Transformed,* New York: Oxford University Press, 1979. Reprinted with permission.).

tive, is shared and is stable. These lines by William Wordsworth make the same point.

> My heart leaps up when I behold
> A rainbow in the sky:
> So was it when my life began,
> So is it now I am a man;
> So be it when I shall grow old,
> or let me die!
> The child is father to the Man;
> And I could wish my days to be
> Bound each to each by natural piety.

No matter how consistent aesthetic feeling may be, it has been considered individual and subjective and thus necessarily excluded by medical science in its search for general knowledge about human biology. For medical science to progress, every trace of the personal had to be removed, as illustrated by the contrast between the seventeenth-century illustration of biomechanics—the body as a machine—and the contemporary illustration from a textbook on biomechanics (Figures 2 and 3). The same point is made by contrasting an old anatomical illustration with one from a modern anatomy book (Figures 4 and 5). In the contemporary illustration, art is used to tell us a truth about the body for which the written presentation of facts is insufficient. The facts represented—spatial relationships and structural order—are aesthetic, but the information resides primarily in the picture. Another example of the

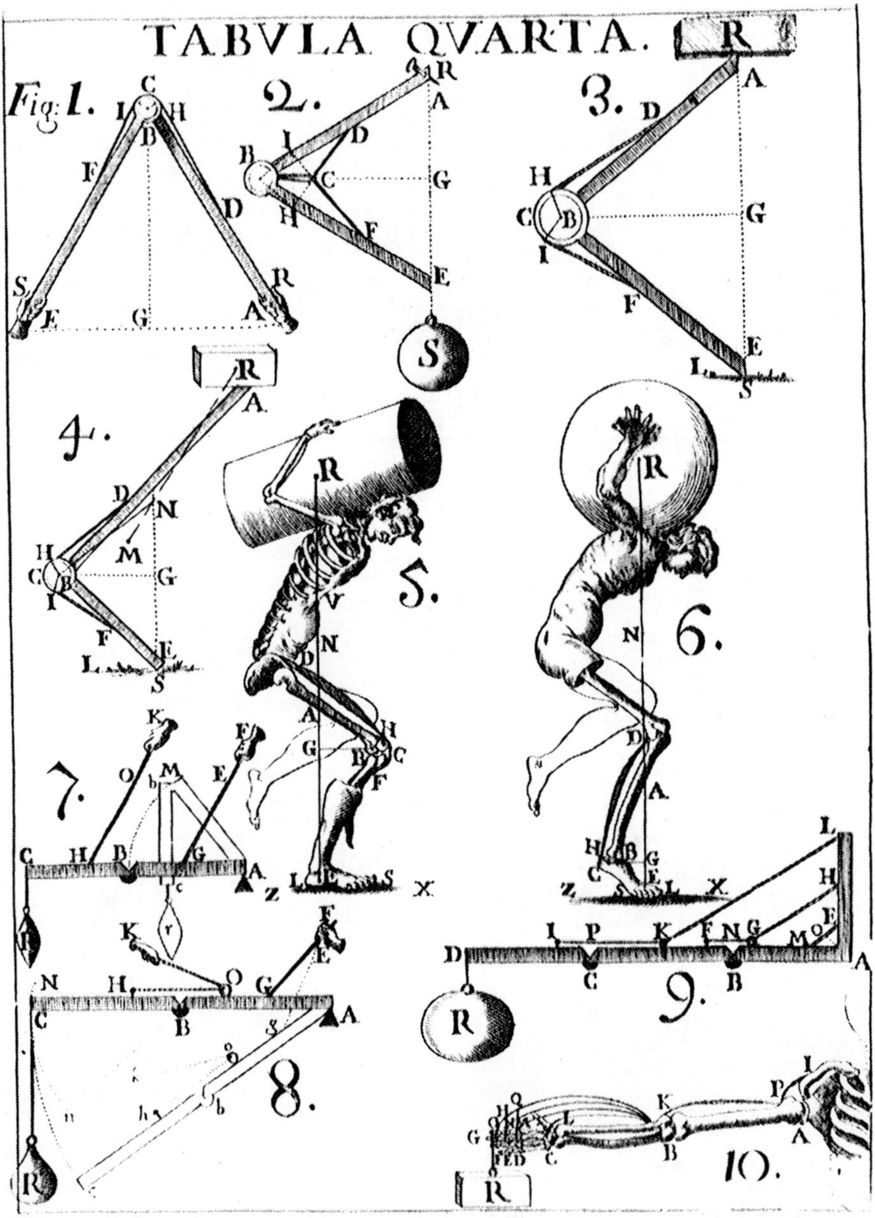

Fig. 2. The body as a machine, but still personalized, in the seventeenth century (from Giovanni Borelli, *De Motu Muscullorum,* Rome 1680).

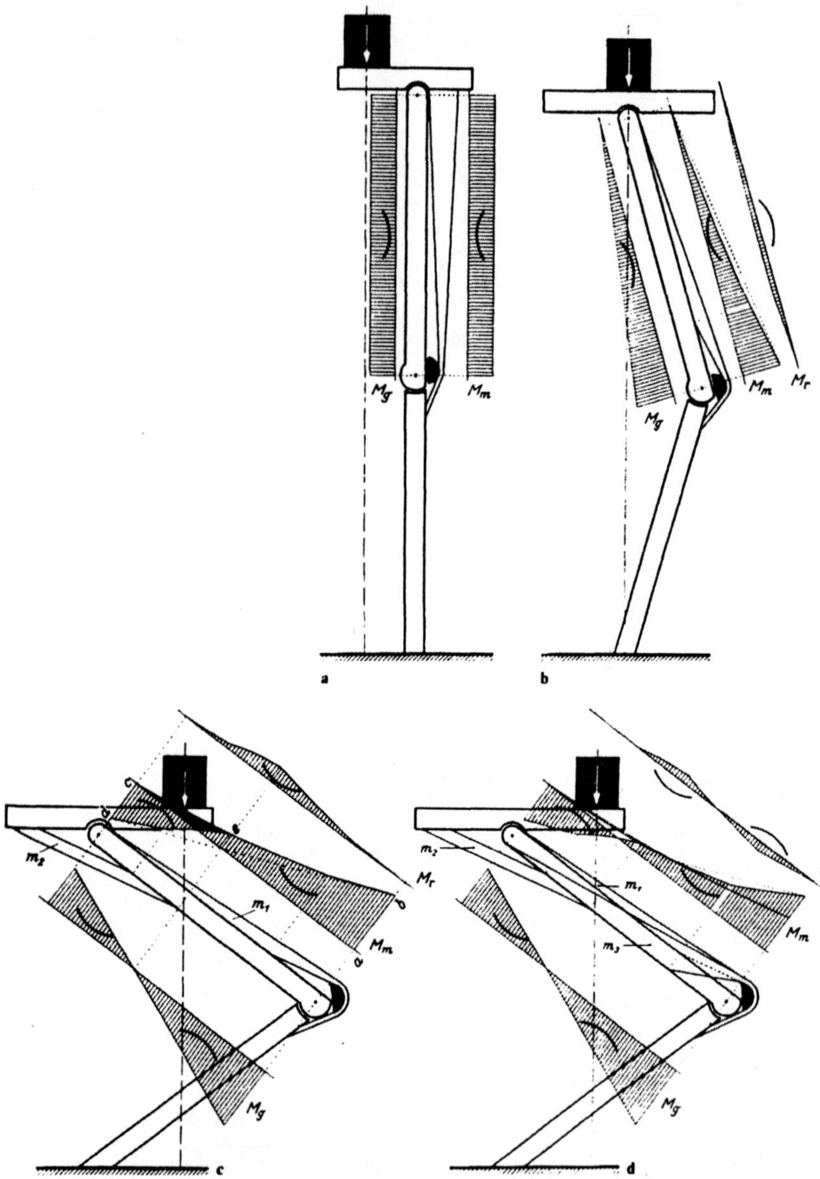

Fig. 3. The body as a machine, depersonalized, in the twentieth century (from F. Pauwels, *Biomechanics of the Locomotor Apparatus,* Berlin, Heidelberg, New York: Springer-Verlag, 1980. Reprinted with permission.)

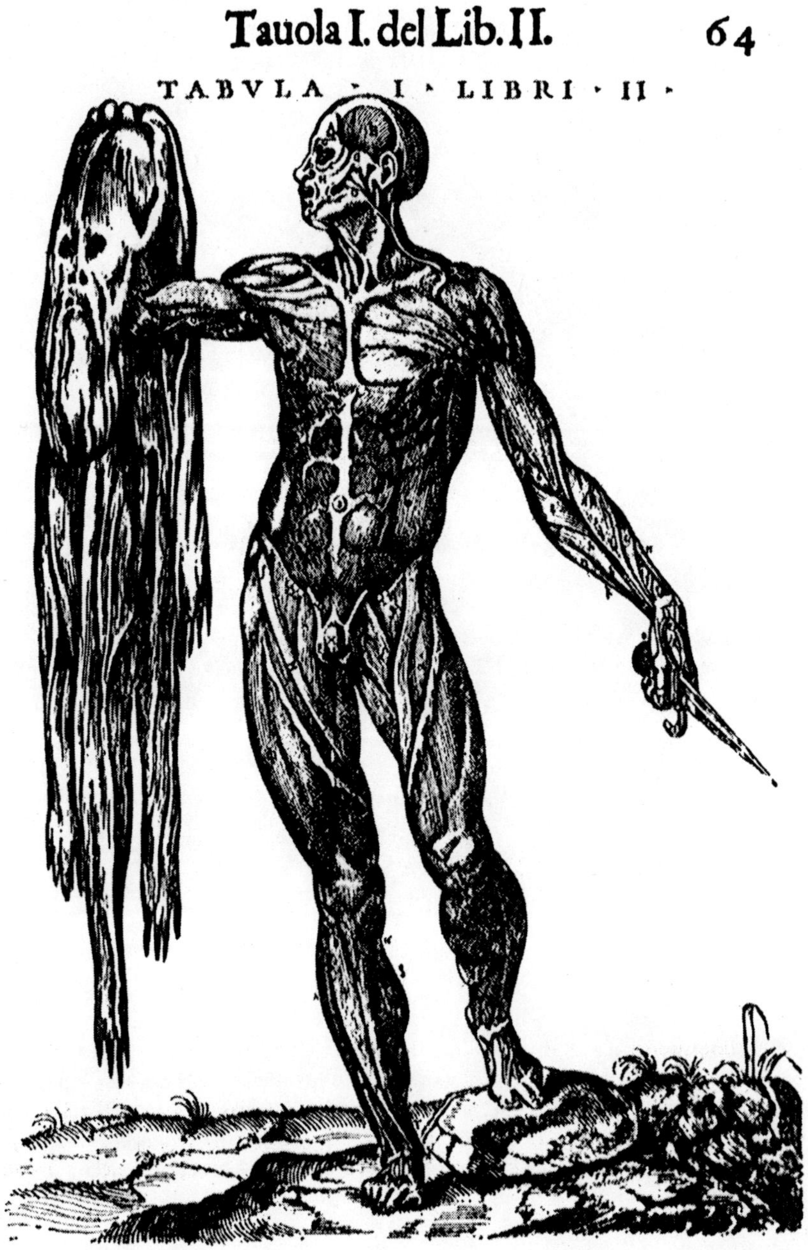

Fig. 4. The muscle man. A seventeenth century woodcut of the anatomy of the muscles that is rich in personal details (from Juan Valverde di Hammusco, *Anatomia del Corpo Humano,* Rome: Antonia Salamanca and Antonio Laferj, 1559).

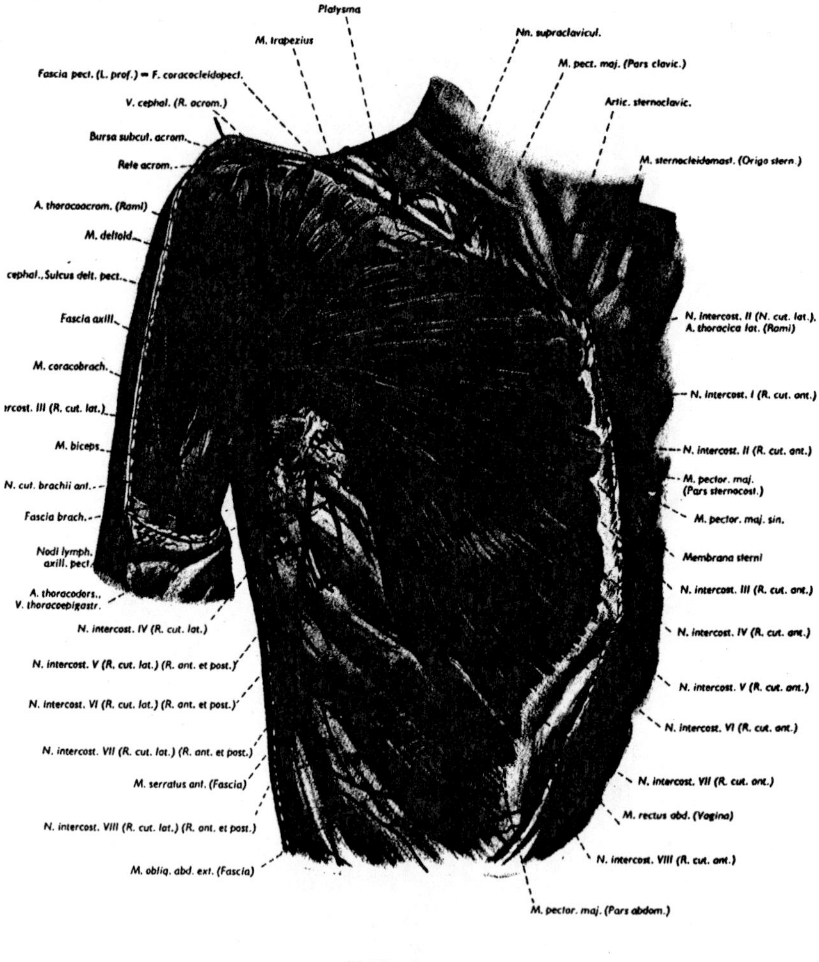

Fig. 5. A contemporary anatomical illustration is used to tell truths about the body for which the written presentation of facts would be insufficient. The facts—spatial relationships and structural order—are aesthetic but the picture is depersonalized. (Reproduced with permission from E. Pernkopf, *Anatomy: Atlas of Topographic and Applied Human Anatomy, Third Edition,* Copyright 1989, Baltimore, Munich; Urban & Schwarzenberg.

aesthetic difference between old and new anatomical illustrations is seen in Figure 6. In this old woodcut of the anatomy of the urinary bladder, the picture of water flowing under the bridge in the background is used to tell us a truth about the body that is metaphorical rather than literal. The picture may appear rather heavy-handed to us, but we must remember that it was done in

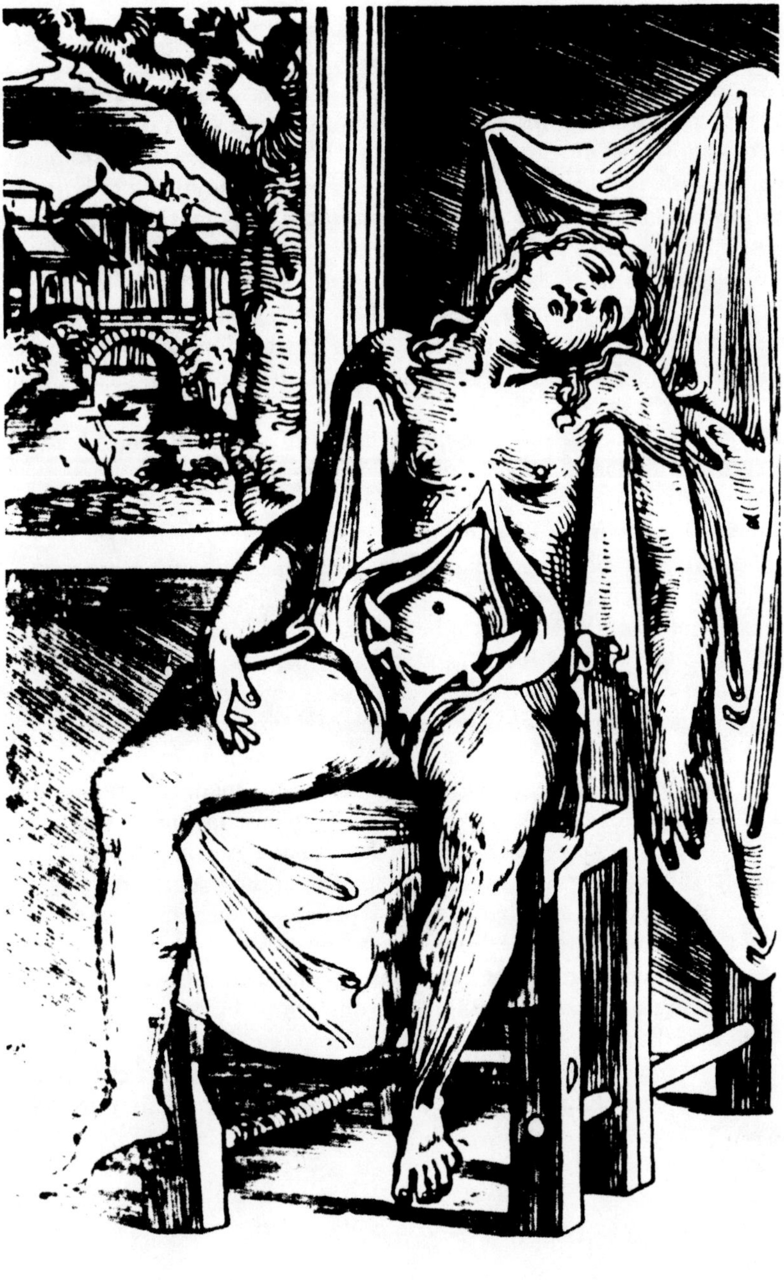

Fig. 6. An old illustration of the anatomy of the urinary bladder. The picture of water flowing under the bridge tells a truth about the body that is metaphorical rather than literal (from Jacopo Berengario, *Isagogae Breves,* Bologna, 1523).

an era when people had very little anatomical knowledge. No similar illustrations are found in modern texts.

Charles Hartshorne has described life as a work of art. We must remember that just as a work of art can be beautiful, it can also be garish, flat, uninspired, chaotic, a "chromo," or even ugly. Within an aesthetic frame of reference, individual values or behaviors and even autonomy are important not in themselves but rather for their function in the self-creation of a person, of a lived life. From the same perspective the passage of time can be portrayed in more human terms. Remember, when considered frozen in time or even as though there were no time, individual facts about a person or a body make sense. But a frozen moment of time is an abstraction; instead, the events of our lives unfold over time. What we care about—our fears, desires, concerns, likes, and dislikes—are displayed in our actions and reactions to this or that situation. In this "real-time" concatenation of moments, the idea of person achieves the human dimension of self-legislation.

One is always in a process of becoming; every second, every minute, hour, and day. The person one is becoming is constituted from: (1) what one was; (2) the circumstances of the moment—the presence of other people, the setting, the presence of disease—almost everything going on in one's internal and external world; (3) one's inherent aim, interest, or purpose at the moment, since the process is not random. It is here, in the moment-by-moment choices that determine the person, that human authenticity and independence have true meaning. Choice is the essence of the process.

We must look at life's choices in a minute-by-minute, hour-by-hour, and day-by-day time scale to understand how sickness, medical care, and hospitals fit in, and how an aesthetic viewpoint can help us. Obviously, most people do not believe that sickness, disability, or death have any place in their purposes. However, illness, infirmity, suffering, and impending death are facts of fate—they are among the things that happen to people—and because of this, they are part of the circumstances of the moment from which persons constitute themselves. Effort is required, when one is ill, to make choices that are in harmony with the being one was before illness. Much must be denied, and fragments, precious and little, must be seized upon to help remain within the rhythm of the earlier lived life. In these circumstances, choices that reflect one's true self—aesthetically consonant over time, independent and autonomous—are most difficult.

The Aesthetic "Correctness" of the Person's Story

There is a knowledge of person that can only be considered in aesthetic terms, the "correctness" of the story of the person's life. The storyteller's art is, in part, the ability to create a well-rounded picture of character as the tale unfolds. As in the excerpts by Shakespeare, Melville, and Conan Doyle the author may give us a brief of the character, but the true measure of the writer's skill lies in the manner in which the character is progressively revealed as the story proceeds. As characters are fleshed out, we must (if the author is successful) accept each new detail—even if it surprises us—as both fitting together with what we already know and as teaching us more about the person and about life itself. If what we learn from the next page does not fit what we have read in previous pages, we impeach both the character and the author. The judgments we make are aesthetic.

Medicine abounds in stories, as Katherine Hunter has so well documented. Physicians tell stories about patients to other doctors and, as Charles Bosk has shown, use stories about colleagues to serve the purposes of moral regulation. However, the essence of all that is believed to be antithetical to modern scientific medicine is captured in the phrase anecdotal medicine. The limitation of medical scientists has been to associate the individual storyteller with irreducible subjectivity and, consequently, with knowledge that cannot be shared. Both associations are incorrect. If the storyteller's knowledge did not have a public dimension, we could not participate in it. *The Death of Ivan Illytch* by Tolstoi remains one of the best "textbooks" on the dying person that has ever been written because it plumbs the universal aspects of sickness, death, and dying of interest to us all.

The problem, it seems to me, is not that medicine is currently too ancedotal, but that perhaps doctors do not know how to tell a good story. A single case history properly described is an invaluable teaching aid. It does not teach about the pathophysiology of pneumonia and it should not be used to choose the best therapy, but it can tell about the interaction of the person and the pneumonia. Stories are also an excellent experimental tool. In teaching ethics to medical students, actual case examples are in themselves indispensable, but it is when the case is changed in one detail or another that the students can really see the effects of various elements on decision-making(16). Storytelling is a skill that can be taught and learned. When medical students develop the skill of telling the story of particular patients' illnesses, they will both see the place that patients and their particulars play in illness and be able to convey the information to their colleagues.

Aesthetics and the Ugly

The most immediate role of aesthetics in medicine is to show us the ugly and disordered. Figure 7 shows a wound that is considered ugly by all observers. The same wound a few days later may also seem ugly to you (Figure 8). Doctors may agree that the first abdominal wound is ugly, but they would likely disagree about Figure 8. Most surgeons, I think, would agree that Figure 8 shows a pleasing wound. Why is it aesthetically pleasing to them while it is ugly to laypersons? It is not merely that they have grown accustomed to ugliness, because, as Bosanquet points out, aesthetic feeling is stable. One may become acclimated to living amid ugliness and disorder, but the ugly will not thereby become beautiful and harmonious. Surgeons see beauty in an apparently ugly wound because their knowledge alters their perception

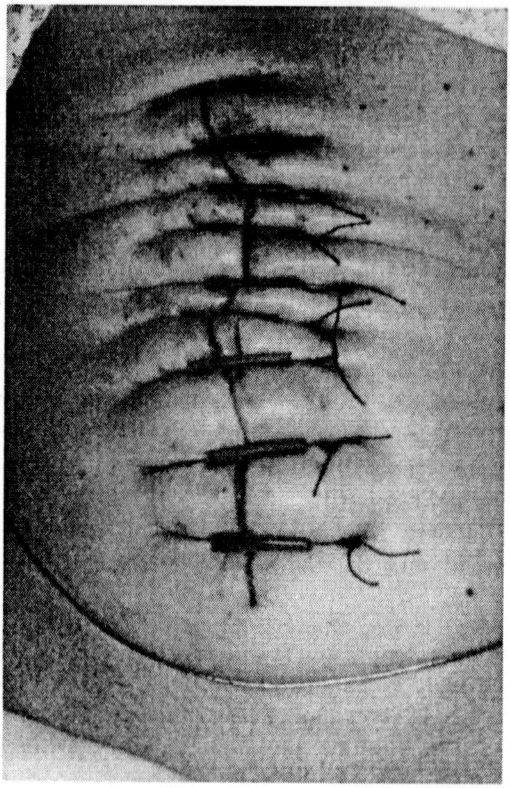

Fig. 7. An abdominal wound that all observers find ugly (photograph by the author).

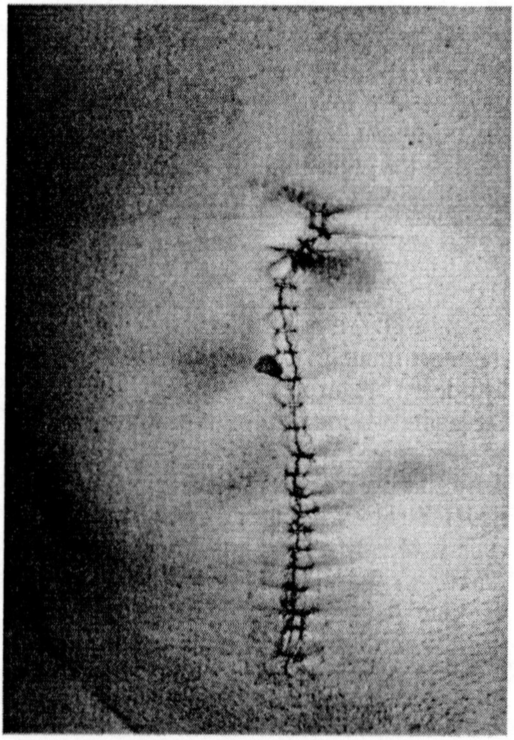

Fig. 8. Knowledge alters aesthetic appreciation. Most surgeons would agree that this is a pleasing wound because it is healing properly (photograph by the author).

of it. The expert eye observes the wound to be healing properly. Rather than disorder and disharmony, the wound in Figure 8 reveals the orderly process of healing. Frequently, beauty is seen by the experienced because they are able to discern the harmony that evades the novice.

My interest in the place of aesthetics in medicine was sparked by what I learned from Charles Stegeman, professor of fine arts at Haverford College. He volunteered to teach drawing to medical students at The Medical College of Pennsylvania and demonstrated that students who do poorly in anatomy do not draw as well as those who are successful in their anatomy classes. Unsuccessful anatomy students, he found, are often unable to pictorially represent the world around them—specifically, the human figure. He believed that this was due to their inability to appreciate spatial relations, and he showed both that drawing skill could be taught by teaching an appreciation of these relationships and that gaining that appreciation improved the students' performance in anatomy. (His experience is quite convincing to skeptics who believe that drawing cannot be taught to the inartistic. As he points out, however, because he can teach someone to draw an accurate representation of the human figure does not mean that he can teach them to draw so that their work brings tears to the eyes of the beholder.)

Among the medical faculty Professor Stegeman worked with was a pathologist who showed him microscopic slides of diseased and normal tissues. To the amazement of the pathologist, Stegeman was consistently able to distinguish diseased from normal tissues. He showed how the relationships of the structures of normal tissue were orderly while in diseased tissue they were disorderly or even chaotic. Professor Stegeman obviously brought highly developed capacities to his microscope viewing. First, of course, like all good artists he could notice completeness of detail in what he looked at (artists simply see more than untrained amateurs). In addition, he had a developed interest in the problem of spatial relations. Finally, he had a belief in the orderliness of nature.

There are physicians who would challenge Charles Stegeman's with slides on which he could not recognize the presence of disease. But we do not require that he be a pathologist—that skill is not what we as physicians lack. What Professor Stegemans's perceptions illustrate is the vital importance to clinical medicine of understanding the aesthetics of relationships. Clinicians, as I have pointed out, treat whole sick persons based primarily on knowledge, about parts—molecules, organelles, cells, and organs. Unfortunately, there is no systematic method for describing how to look at parts and understand wholes. If that were not enough, the difficulty does not stop there—even understanding whole persons is insufficient. People have relationships, and these relationships affect them both when they are well and sick. Persons live in families, and the nature of the family has an impact on the sick person. Families (and people) live in communities that also have an effect on the sick and their care. Understanding the impact of these dimensions on the lives of the sick and the well and how they interact is clearly important in caring for sick persons. George Engel, an internist, brought to the attention of the medical community the idea that illness is a biopsychosocial phenomenon and cannot be completely described in any lesser terms. It is not that patients with diseases also have psychological or social problems, the sick are sick in all dimensions simultaneously.

We are faced with the knotty problem of the relationship of a whole to its parts. We want the physician to know the sick person—the whole sick person—who has come for help. Yet, in the best of circumstances and with the best clinicians, the person is presented part by part. It is in this area that aesthetics has a part to play because I believe that the unity of the individual can best be seen as an aesthetic unity. Bernard Bosanquet writes, "it is not uncommon to take a work of art as an example of the compulsion by which the nature of a whole controls its parts, simply because this control, *which is the essence of individuality,* lends itself to analysis in a work that is pervaded by an especially harmonious unity" (emphasis added)(17). This point can be most simply illustrated by the pictures of the willow seen in Figure 9. First look at the vein pattern in the closeup of a willow leaf, and notice the resemblance to the whole leaf. Then see how the same pattern is repeated in the arrangement of willow leaves on a small branch. Finally, observe the pattern continued in the whole tree. You will see this same relationship of part to whole in many trees and plants. The relationship is present also between naturally growing objects and their environment. As you walk in the woods and fields, see how shrubs and plants "fit" where they grow. To further make the point, walk into a different environment, deep in the woods, for example, and in your mind's eye place there some of the shrubs from the meadow. They will probably seem out of place. Figure 10 shows a tree covered with tent caterpillars. Notice how its disorder stands out among the harmonious. As you do these mental experiments in aesthetics, avoid explanatory statements because they will interfere with your ability to see. You may be tempted to explain the phenomena by saying that our eyes are accustomed to these settings and their occupants or by pointing out that the plants or shrubs have adapted to their environments, and so on. These interpretations are irrelevant to the importance of aesthetics in relating part to whole.

The same applies to humans. Look at your hands and those of others. See how they "fit" their arms and how they would appear wrong on another's arm. This is also true of the feet to their legs. As foot to leg so leg to body, and so on. In Figure 11 notice how clothing can affect appearance. The clothed backs are strikingly different from the naked ones. When we put on clothing, we belong not only to ourselves but come into unity with the group.

Persons are always in some relationship to other persons, as can be seen from the couple walking in Figure 12. Look at other pictures of couples and observe how they pose in relationship to each other so that two people form one unit. (When that is not the case, the disharmony can be quite striking.) When a group of persons consider themselves in conflict with the larger community, they will often proclaim their dissent in values by dressing in a way that clashes with that of the dominant society. The currently popular punk rock style, the long hair and beards of the male hippies of the 1960s, and

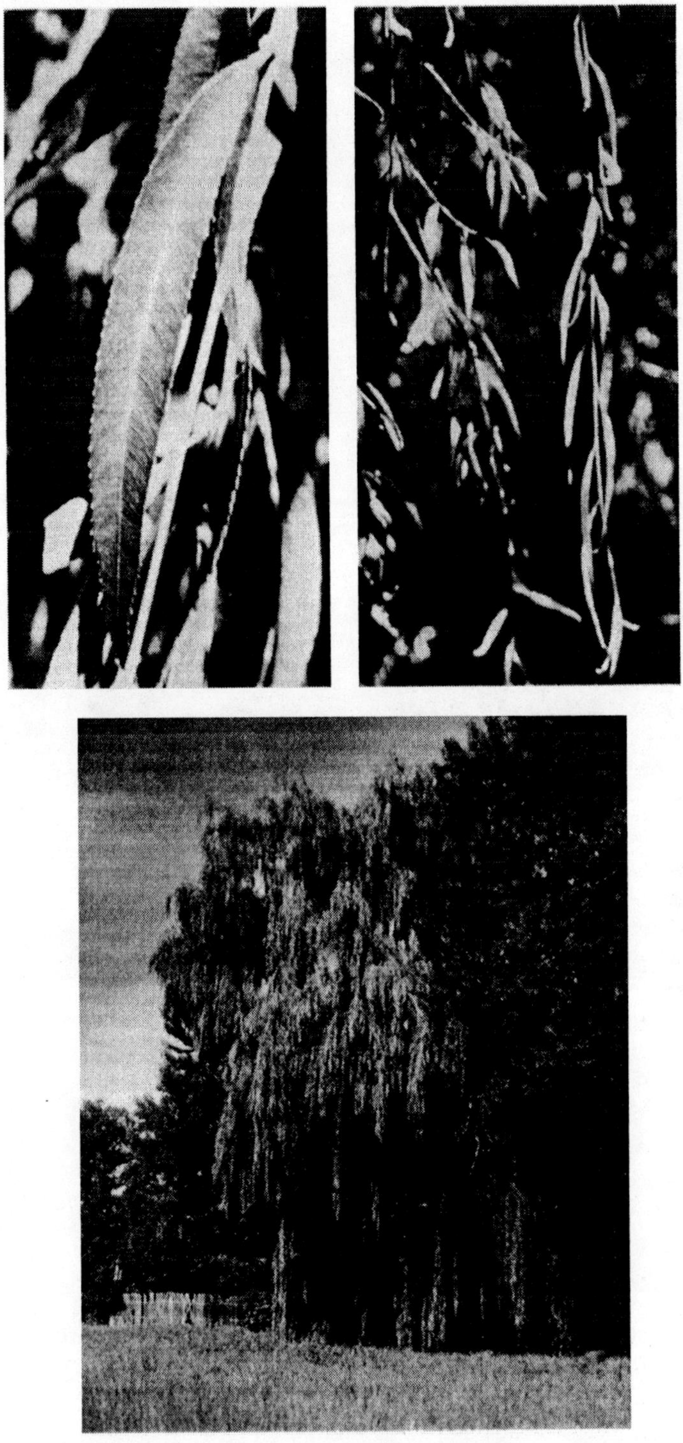

Fig. 9. The relationship of part to whole can be shown aesthetically. The pattern of the leaf and its veins is duplicated in the pattern of the leaves on the branch and in the pattern of the whole willow tree (photograph by the author).

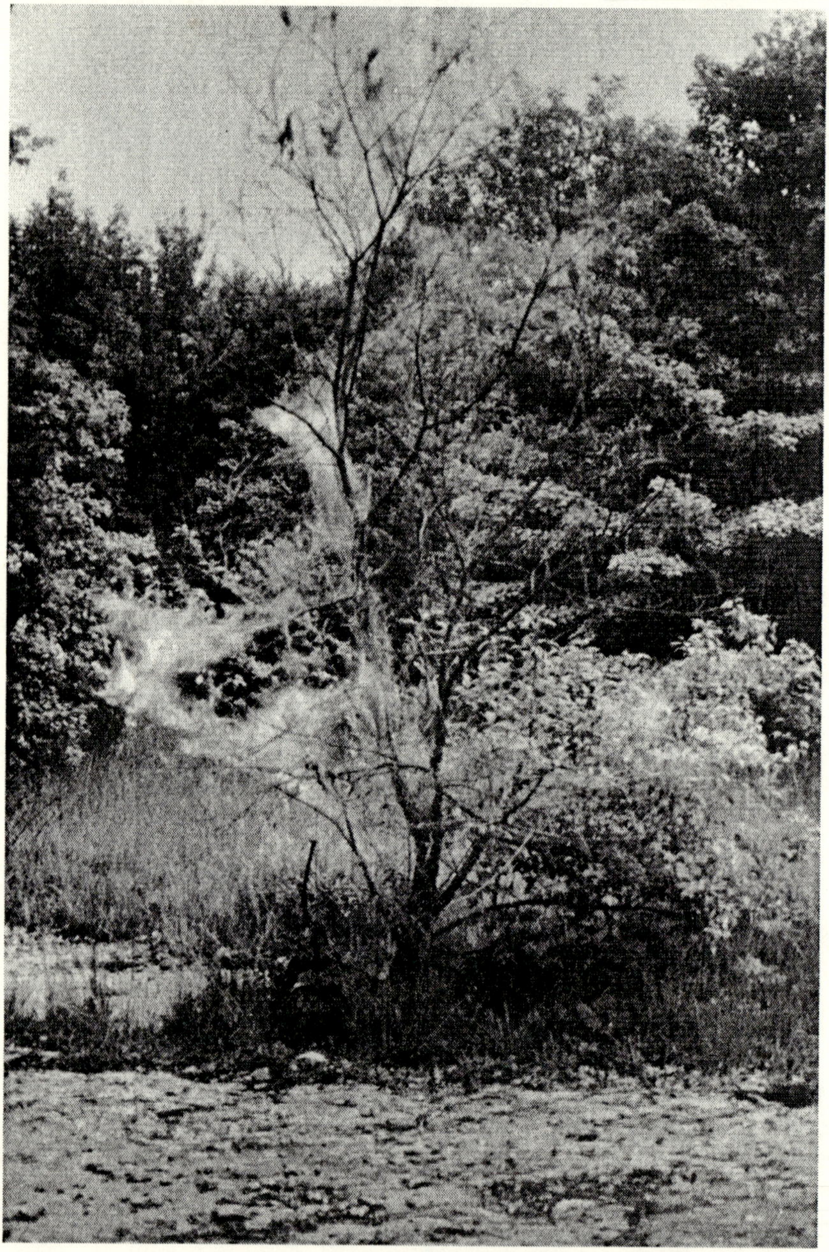

Fig. 10. A tree covered with tent caterpillars. Notice how its disorder stands out against the harmony of its environment (photograph by the author).

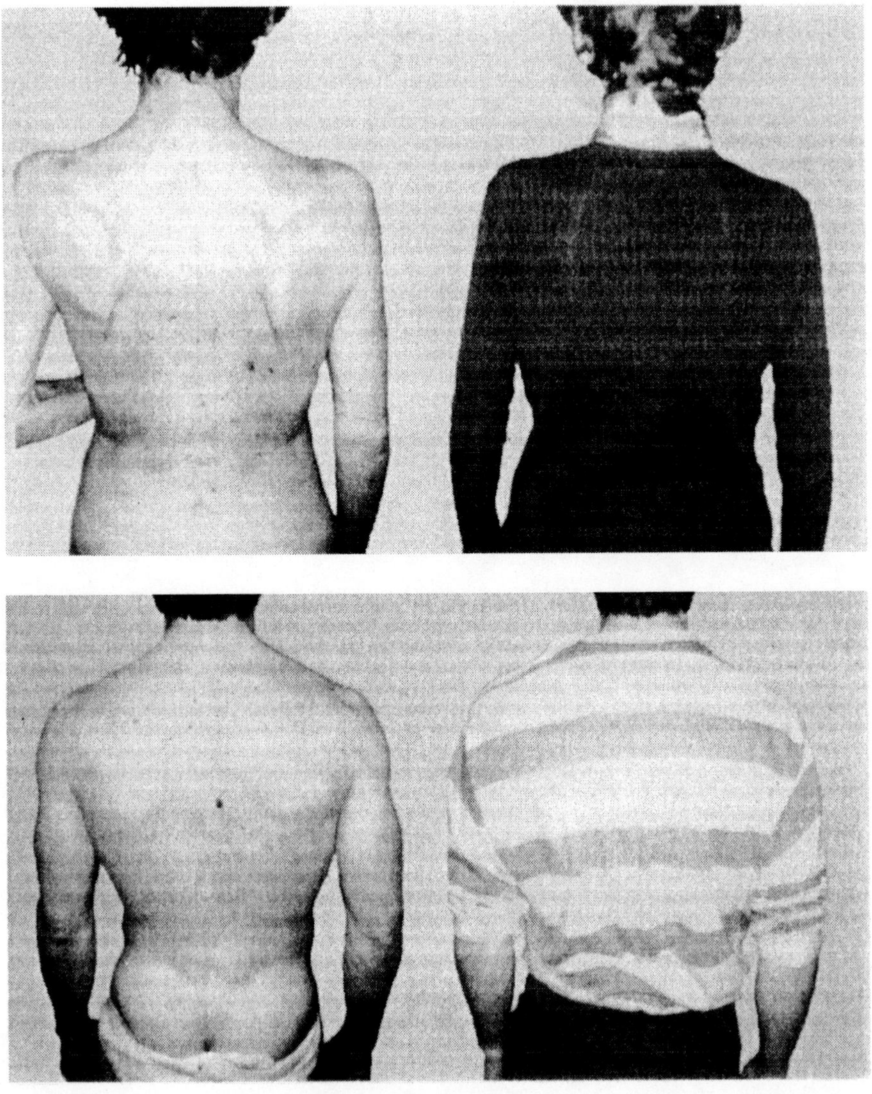

Fig. 11. See how clothing can affect appearance. The clothed backs are strikingly different than the naked backs of the same persons. When clothed we belong not only to ourselves but come into unity with the group (photograph by the author).

the T shirts and jeans of the women's liberation movement of the late 1960s and 1970s are examples. But even in these instances a positive aesthetic relationship is maintained between the protesting and the dominant styles. As the dissenters' values are assumed by the dominant culture, their clothing and demeanor are also adopted(18).

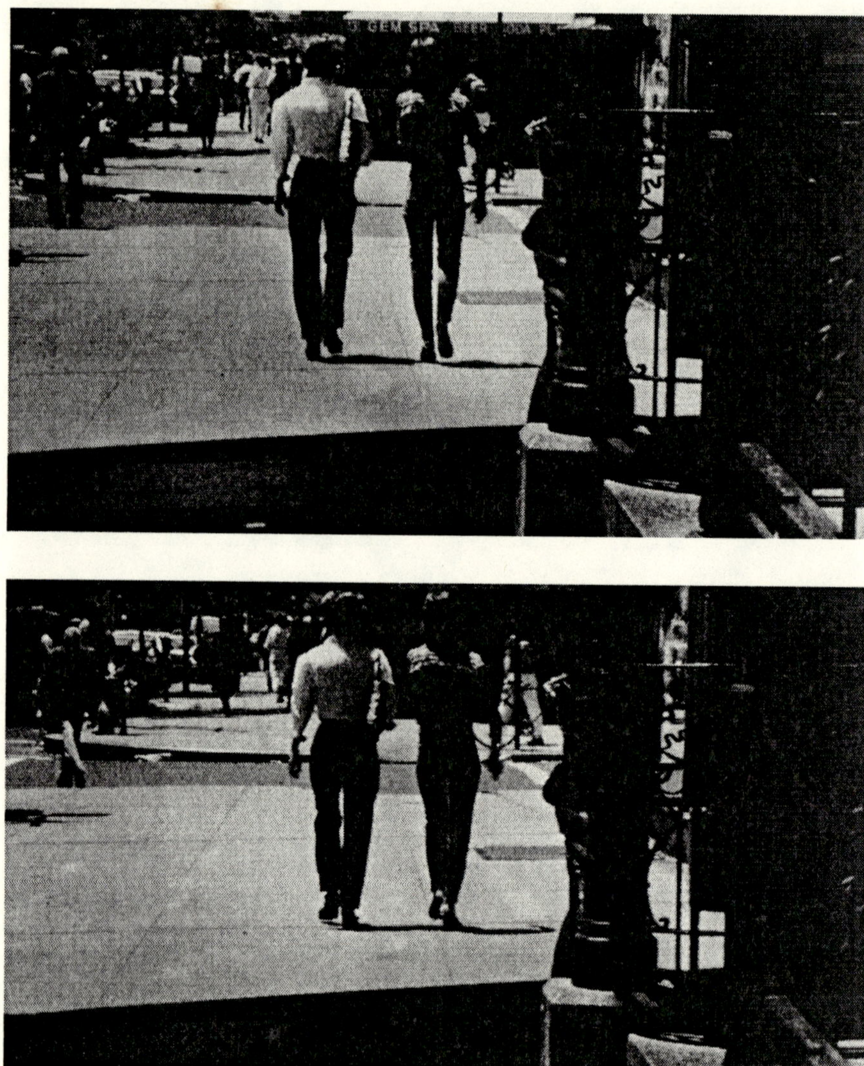

Fig. 12. Persons are always in some relationship to other persons. These pictures of a couple walking together show how they form one unit (photograph by the author).

The aesthetics of style and demeanor is a complex subject, because dress and demeanor are so often employed as group and status markers that require recognition and compliance in order to serve their function. On the other hand, when true social pathology is present, disorder reigns. The point is illustrated by the dress of "bag ladies." Indeed, one's attention is frequently drawn to people on the street who display obvious mental pathology by their dress and presentation of self that clash aesthetically with the observer's expectations, not merely as a result of their shabbiness.

Even in large groups we always maintain ourselves in relation to others. Crowds are usually thought of as disorderly groups, but this perception is generally untrue. As people stream across a busy street when the light changes, the truly striking thing is not the disorder, but the order. We accept the orderliness of a flock of birds flying south in the winter or the synchronized swimming of a school of fish without realizing that humans in large groups are also orderly. As we are in relationship to each other, we are to our environments. Look around the areas of your town or city where the comfortable live and notice the concord. In contrast, the slums are usually not only dirty, but disorderly. The walls of this or that building are splashed with graffiti, garbage abounds, there sits an old car on flattened tires or with broken windows. Oases of prettiness or neatness are in contrast with the general untidiness. Consider the disorders of the human condition: war, communal strife, group conflicts, family breakdown, the diseases that follow from social instability, and individual sickness. These disorders are frequently found together—with disorders in higher levels of organizations accompanied by disorder in lower levels. It should not be surprising, therefore, that just as the poor carry a greater burden of disease and greater family and group strife than the comfortable, so their environment reflects their difficulties. We humans are of a piece; what afflicts a part, afflicts the whole, what disorders the whole disorders the parts.

Knowing Suffering

In earlier chapters I showed how suffering is the distress of whole persons whose intactness is threatened or disintegrating. Pain or shortness of breath, for example, are bodily symptoms that lead to suffering when they threaten to overwhelm the whole organism. A whole organism is not whole in merely the biological sense. The individual sick person, the subject of medicine, is not only this particular boundaried object that at this moment you see before you. The wholeness or individuality of suffering extends beyond the confines of the body. We know the person by *all* of the information we collect about that person. A sense of time is necessary for suffering; more than a future, there must also be an enduring past. I must have some sense of how I am constituted and what I can do to fear the loss of a piece of myself—and for that I must have a past. The person's idea of self must include others in order for the person to know what he or she can do or be. We are what we are in part because of what we are not and what we cannot be or do; we gain this knowledge because there are others with whom we can compare ourselves. Self-knowledge is also constituted of the reactions to oneself of others. Our sense of self (and, thus, the whole) must include the world around us; knowledge of abilities and projected future actions would otherwise be meaningless.

There are important impediments to full awareness of the suffering of others. To know in what way others are suffering demands an exhaustive understanding of what makes them the individuals they are —when they feel themselves whole, threatened, or disintegrated as well as their view of the future, the past, others, the environment, and their aims and purposes. Given its almost infinite complexity, this may appear impossible; after all, we usually do not even know these things about ourselves. Perhaps, then, most beliefs, about the suffering of others are really ideas about the seriousness of the threat—pain, shortness of breath, or isolation. The person contemplating the sufferer knows that he or she would suffer in similar circumstances. But the threat or distress that causes one person to suffer may not be a source of suffering in others. Because of this, errors are made. Some people, on the other hand, deny themselves the freedom to express their pain or suffering for fear of distressing friends or family. There are others whose heroism and sense of transcendent purpose free them from suffering, even in the presence of terrible pain. On occasion the suffering of others is denied when it should be obvious. For all these reasons, even knowing that others are suffering may be difficult or even impossible. And, yet, compassion is a fact. It appears possible to truly know whether another suffers based on the correct interpretation of words, vocalizations, and gestures. However, this is most often true of acute suffering; chronic suffering also exists and elicits the compassion of others. There is the possibility that a direct transfer of feeling exists where one senses the distress of another even in the absence of other cues. But even if true, this would still be a perception requiring interpretation like any other perception, and for interpretation it would look to other information and evidence in support.

We must understand that compassion exists in degrees. It can vary from the generally compassionate feeling for the person who appears to be suffering, to the full expression of compassion for *this* suffering person. To know others to the degree required for the depths of human compassion requires a knowledge not only of the empirical facts of their existence through time, but also of their values as displayed in their presentation of self, their speech and their behavior. Their purposes and their aims become known in the retelling of the past and their moment-by-moment choices and behaviors. Finally, to know others as the whole persons they are demands an aesthetic sense of wholes and parts—in the moment and over time. Since, in suffering, disruption of the whole person is the dominant theme, we know the losses and their meaning by what we know of the person who confronts us. This is what one person knows of others out of compassion for their suffering.

References

1. Shakespeare, William. *The Tragedy of Julius Caesar.* I. ii, ll. 191–211.

2. Melville, Herman. *Billy Budd, Foretopman.* in *The Works of Herman Melville.* 1924. London, Bombay, Sidney, Constable and Co., Ltd. Vol. 13.

3. Doyle, A. Conan. A Study in Scarlet. 1893. London, Ward, Lock and Bowden, Ltd., pp. 17–18.

4. Harris, Errol E. *An Interpretation of the Logic of Hegel.* 1983. New York, University Press of America, p. 33.

5. Black, Sir Douglas. *An Anthology of False Antitheses.* 1984. The Neuffield Provincial Hospitals Trust, p. 25.

6. Cassell, Eric J. *Talking with Patients. Vol. 1: The Theory of Doctor Patient Communication.* 1985. Cambridge, Mass., MIT Press, p. 84.

7. Lembo, Nicholas J., Dell'Itallia, Louis J., Crawford, Michael H., and O'Rourke, Robert A. Bedside Diagnosis of Systolic Murmurs. *NEJM.* 1988. 318:1572–78.

8. Craige, Ernest. Should Auscultation Be Rehabilitated. *NEJM.* 1988. 318:1611–12.

9. Stuart, Henry W. Valuation as a Logical Process. In *Studies in Logical Theory.* Edited by John Dewey. 1903. Chicago, University of Chicago Press.

10. Blandshard, Brand. *Reason and Analysis.* 1964. La Salle, Ill., Open Court Pub. Co., p. 25.

11. Arnheim, Rudolf. *Entropy and Art.* 1971. Berkeley, University of California Press, p. 1.

12. Steen, L.A., Editor. *On the Shoulders of Giants.* 1990, Washington, D.C., National Academy Press, p.2.

13. Bosanquet, Bernard. *Three Lectures on Aesthetic.* 1915. London, Macmillan. 1968. New York, Kraus Reprint Co., p. 4.

14. Zuckerkandl, Victor. *The Sense of Music.* 1959. Princeton, N.J., Princeton University Press, p. 11.

15. Alexander, S. *Beauty and Other Forms of Value.* 1968. New York, Thomas Crowell, Chap. X.

16. Cassell, Eric J. *The Place of the Humanities in Medicine.* 1984. New York, The Hastings Center, p. 21.

17. Bosanquet, Bernard. *Logic: Or the Morphology of Knowledge.* 1911. Oxford, The Clarendon Press, Vol. II, p. 235.

18. Cassell, Joan. *A Group Called Women.* 1977. New York, David McKay, pp. 88–92.

12

The Clinician's Experience: Power Versus Magic in Medicine

Science and Art

TRADITIONALLY, THE PRACTICE of medicine has been divided into its science, concerned with disease, and its art, associated with the actual care of patients. As in many a tense marriage, arguments have been advanced about the differences, similarities, and mutual need of each of these aspects for the other. In these discussions, when the concern is that the needs of the sick are being overlooked in modern scientific medicine, the importance of empathy, compassion, communication, and other humane qualities of physicians are stressed. When its protagonists fear that science is getting short shrift, they point out the impossibility of understanding the processes of disease in the absence of science, and they demonstrate the superior precision of thought brought to clinical medicine by the basic biological and physical sciences. In a recent essay, Marsden Blois acknowledged both concerns as he discussed the need for a kind of vertical reasoning that would integrate the mathematically exact molecular insights of the hard sciences with the more complex but far less precise knowledge of the social sciences(1). This is analogous to the story of the rabbi who was asked to judge which of two disputants was correct. The rabbi listened at length to the first one and said, "You're right." Then he sat down with the second and after hearing him said, "You're right." After both had left, the rabbi's wife said, "You told both of them they were right. They can't both be right." "You know," the rabbi said, "You're right."

In the case of the art of medicine versus the science of medicine, however, both seemingly opposed points of view *can* be correct, since they are concerned with two different things, although they seem in opposition because both perspectives are incomplete in themselves. There is no question that if you want to treat sick persons based on the mechanisms of disease—and any other way would be inadequate—then science is essential to medicine. On the other hand, if you want to treat sick persons as the persons they are—and any other way would be inadequate—then art is essential to medicine.

Sick persons, unlike livers or enzymes, do not meet the criteria as objects of science. They cannot ever be completely known or known apart from the knower, and they cannot be measured solely in the objective terms of science. They never exist isolated in space. Their behavior is influenced by where they are. They are ultimately individual and therefore inevitably different one from another. They are never and cannot ever be isolated in time—all persons sick and well are influenced by the times in which they live and all have a history and a future both of which are essential to understanding them. Persons are ultimately moral—the words "good" and "bad," "right" and "wrong" derive their meaning from their applications to persons and their concerns.

Medical science is focused on the here and now, this moment in which the object of science exists. (Although as persons, medical scientists, like the rest of us, may have their eyes focused on the practical outcome of their work or even fame and fortune.) The art of medicine, on the other hand, is always focused on the future—what will happen to the patient, what he or she wants to make happen or prevent—because it is only the future that counts for the patient. (The future, it should be remembered in this context, starts a moment from now.) Part of the future is how the disease will behave. To know that, it must be known how the disease has behaved in the past—its tempo and its character and (the term fits) its "personality." Another aspect of the future is how the patient will behave, act, think, speak, care, and respond, which can be predicted by learning what the patient did in the past.

One other characteristic distinguishes the clinician from the medical scientist. Scientists are primarily discoverers of the secrets of nature seeking knowledge, whereas clinicians are expected to act on their patients' behalf. People go to doctors because they want something done for them. If the doctor makes an important discovery, that is fine, but the patient expects action.

I believe that to resolve the problem of art versus science in medicine, we must understand that the truly successful clinician must respect both aspects. Knowledge, whether of science or compassion, does not do things to patients—clinicians do. This is the corollary of the truism that doctors do not treat diseases, they treat patients. The disputation between art and science in medicine merely reflects a world that has been chopped up into artificial pieces. There are no diseases that exist outside of sick persons, there are no patients without doctors, and there are no clinicians without patients. The situation is like the story of King Solomon and the two women who claimed the same child(2). If the child had been divided in two, each woman would have had a piece—but there would have been no child. Dividing up clinical medicine by reducing it to one or another of its aspects may satisfy the disputants, but then the thing that most people mean when they speak about medicine disappears. When I speak of medicine I mean that complex whole made up of patient, doctor, disease, and the knowledge of medicine that cannot be understood apart from the real physical and social world in which it is imbedded. What is necessary for us to understand, however, is how these two kinds of knowledge—abstract knowledge of medical science and the knowledge of the art of medicine—can be combined and brought to bear on the patient's illness.

The Importance of the Clinician's Experience

The doctor-patient relationship creates bonds that set clinicians apart from medical scientists. The distinction between them is heightened by the directions in which clinicians must organize their thinking and the ways in which they develop a view of sick persons. Although in his book, *The Double Helix,* James Watson seems anything but the dispassionate scientist in search of the truth—he and Francis Crick hotly pursued not only the secret of DNA but a Nobel Prize as well—it is an undeniable fact that whatever passions came to the surface during their research, their scientific revelations can be known by the reader to the same extent that they are known by Watson and Crick themselves. However, this is not true for clinicians; first of all, they must control their passions if they are to do a good job and, second, what they discover about their patients can be only partially shared with others, partly because, as I will show, some of the knowledge is inseparable from the clinicians themselves.

We expect the ethical physician to act in the best interests of the patient, as the patient defines these interests, and within the constraints of the illness, the limits of medicine, and the exigencies of the setting. To fulfill these obligations the physician must know the nature of the illness—both the disease and how it is manifested in the particular patient—as well as how the patient defines his or her best interests. The physician must also possess medicine's knowledge and know to what extent and how it is to be applied in this particular circumstance. Each aspect of the knowledge expected of the physician has both a didactic and experiential basis. The knowledge the clinician employs in the care of patients is integrally bound up with the actual experience of caring for patients. I do not only mean that clinicians must have knowledge born of experience in addition to theoretical knowledge, although that is true; in addition, the knowledge employed in caring for a particular patient will be appropriate for *this* patient to the degree that the actual experience of the patient becomes part of the clinician's knowledge. This implies that the clinician cannot know the patient, the illness, or the circumstances without true awareness of the patient's experience. This is one of the meanings of the word "empathy"—the infusion of the patient's physical, transcendent, affective, and cognitive state into the doctor's knowledge of the patient's experience of illness. Direct experience with the sick plays such an important part in the training of physicians that it is amazing what little part experience plays in the theory of medicine.*

*In the teaching hospitals of the United States, the intern—the least trained physician—is most often given primary responsibility for the patient. At this writing, when private patients are

Why Experience Has a Bad Name

From Classical Greece to the present, the most respected road to true knowledge has been reason. Immediate experience as a source of knowledge is still suspect (with the exception made by some for events such as divine revelations). Real knowledge was considered possible only about essences and forms, with knowledge from sensation thought to be of lesser value because of its changeable nature(3)(4). Experience was despised as makeshift and uncertain. Critics of experiential knowledge also believed that sensation, from which we know what we have experienced, was unreliable, as manifested by such phenomena as optical illusions. In our era, the objective knowledge of science is considered most useful while experiential knowledge is tainted by subjectivity. However, the real problem, according to this point of view, is not experience, but humans—the subjects of experience. *Persons* are not to be trusted because they are considered vulnerable to emotions and passions, which distort reason. Growing alongside the rise of science and positivism in this century, however, has been the movement to return the person to the center of the intellectual stage. This trend is prominent in medicine, but it is apparent in the arts and politics as well. Remember, as we look to the experience of the clinician, particularly empathic experience, as a source of knowledge for the care of sick persons (in its ethical as well as conventionally medical dimensions), that we carry the traditional suspicion of experience as a threat to reason.

The Relation of Knowledge to Experience

Experience is one of those concepts everybody knows about but rarely examines. It is so central to clinicians, however, that we must look at it closely. To start with, we must be rid of two common notions. The first is that children and what are usually called primitive peoples are more open to their experience than modern adults. This idea is linked to the belief that to be closer to nature is to be closer to experience—as though standing near the cascading waters of Niagara Falls provides more experience than standing at 42nd Street and Broadway. Nothing intervenes between modern humanity and its experience that does not come between the innocent and their experience—not recorded music, kitchen machines, communication devices, or motorized transit. For one and all, ideas stand between experience and its appreciation.

A second common belief is that direct unmediated awareness of experience is both normal and desirable and more often found among children and

---

cared for in most university medical centers, the attending physician (the patient's private doctor) is not permitted to write orders on the patient's chart. This is to allow the intern to gain experience. This incoherent oddity of modern medicine (which patients cannot believe when they find out about it) extolls the value of experience while denying its benefits.

primitive peoples—and, the notion continues, modern adults have lost this awareness. Nothing could be further from the truth. As both Whitehead and Collingwood have made abundantly clear, true awareness of the sea of sensation, if possible at all, is an act requiring extreme self-discipline. Whatever we experience, we experience as something—a this, not a that—therefore experiencing, like perception, is a cognitive act. As pointed out previously, Bosanquet would say, I see something, and my idea about it reaches out to form it while it comes back to further form my idea. If, as I believe, Bosanquet is correct, then the larger and more fully formed is the idea or concept that reaches out to give form to the perception (as long as it remains true to the perception), the more complete the perception will be—the more information it will contain. I look at a sick person and I see vastly more than a medical student sees. I see the expression on the face and in and around the eyes, the skin color, the turgor of the skin, whether care has been given to general appearance, the dry and cracked lips, whether the mouth is held open, the hygiene of the teeth. The smell of the person registers in my nose, the patient's affect is apparent to me, details of the bed, the bedside table, and the room crowd into me. The neophyte student may perceive little more than his or her own repugnance. I hear a violin while you, a violinist, hear a Stradivarius. The more acutely trained our senses are, the more completely we encounter experience. The more information we encompass within the perception before interpretation completes the act, the richer is the experience. Infancy and primitive innocence offer none of these advantages. To the contrary, the more that I have experienced something, the more will I experience it. Behind the beauty of the child's wide-eyed innocence lies the wonder of learning, not of experience.

A confusion seems to exist with the word experience when used as a quantitative expression. Sometimes the phrase "more experience" is employed to imply diverse experience, and sometimes it means merely the greater amount of experience someone older has compared to someone younger. Sometimes we contrast experience and innocence, as though we can have one only at the expense of the other. On other occasions, as when my wife was awestruck at her first experience of the Washington cherry trees in bloom but blasé in succeeding years, we speak of the excitement of first experience as though the experience has changed. The cherry trees in bloom represent the same experience, but her experience of them is different because *she* is different for having experienced them the first time. The lack of clarity in these expressions derives from a poor understanding of the relationship of the individual to his or her experience. Sometimes experience means that which is experienced, sometimes the individual's response to that which is experienced, and sometimes the knowledge gained from experience.

While the words experience and perception are sometimes used interchangeably, experience usually refers to something more fully formed, an integrated collection in space and time. Yet the word experience refers to things even larger, as in "The experience of sickness" or "The experience of a lifetime has taught me that . . ." What is it that experience broadens if not knowledge? Experience extends our knowledge by giving us more of it, by creating within us new categories of knowledge. "Before I visited Japan I never realized that you could make a beautiful flower arrangement with just a few flowers." "Before I took the course in medical ethics I never realized what the word 'autonomy' meant or how important it was." Experience also gives greater breadth to existing concepts. One man's vast experience of food has given him sophisticated tastes: "Once you try a really good French Bordeaux, a California red will never seem as complex again." These examples imply that experience can train the senses, that the new knowledge that comes from experience may alter the body. Experience unquestionably changes bodily functions as diverse as bladder function and javelin throwing—physical training is a form of experience.

One aspect of our experience of others deserves special comment. We do not formally acknowledge (because we cannot explain) the transmission of information from person to person that seems not to have been perceived in the usual manner. Yet such information plays an important part in our knowledge of others. It is one element of compassion and essential to empathy and is obviously present among members of a family, those who are emotionally close to the sick and those who care for them. It plays a part in the doctor-patient relationship(5).

The complexity of personal experience arises from its richness, the kinds of information that are apprehended, and the kinds of knowledge to which this information leads. In any but the simplest experiences—and in probably none of the kind that interests us here and leads to clinical action—empirical facts do not exist alone. There will also be elements of value, emotion, and aesthetics stimulated by the circumstances that become part of their perception by the subject and influence the knowledge that results. The word *meaning* captures the element in the subject's apprehension of experience that is larger than perception. The meaning that is assigned determines under which category(s) of knowledge the experience will be subsumed (e.g., is the problem "medical" or "personal"). Meaning and the concepts and beliefs of which it is formed inevitably contain terms that are used in assigning importance, and importance is a statement of value. Simple experiences are more or less important than other simple experiences. Complex experiences have parts that are more or less important than other parts. This hierarchy of values pervades all meanings, although it is incorrect to assume that there is only one hierarchy or that all the values are coherent.

Experience provokes emotion (feeling), mild or strong, and this enters into the meaning and the assignment of value. There is no participation in experience without feelings being produced. We use this common observation as a test of whether someone has truly been a participant or merely an observer; the implication is that happenings can be experienced in differing degrees and participation is an emotionally active state. If the knowlege derived from the experience is free of feeling, it is less truly representative of the experience. If the patient speaks with considerable feeling about a headache, but the doctor listening fails to register that feeling, then the doctor has not understood the meaning of the headache to the patient. As we all know, however, we are often unaware of the emotion produced by situations, but lack of awareness does not necessarily diminish the effect on us or our actions. Emotions are frequently translated into values, and the intensity of the descriptive language employed or the importance assigned to incidents may result from their emotional effect. As discussed in the last chapter, aesthetic knowledge is also a vital part of experience. The meaning of even ordinary words involves physical sensation, emotion, and spiritual feelings as well as the cognitive. There is no reason to believe that experience is less richly endowed with meanings or that the knowledge of the person who has experiences has a narrower compass.

Theory, of course, or the knowledge found in textbooks of medicine, is *not* filled with values, aesthetics, or emotion even though, being scientific or medical, it has its origin in experience. Theory is theory and textbook knowledge is what it is, in part, because it is abstract, generalized, and free of the "contaminations" of individual persons. The universal knowledge of medical science is useful, however, because it can be applied *appropriately* to individual patients. When it is applied, theoretical or abstract knowledge must somehow reacquire these elements of value, aesthetics, and emotion if it is to be true to the experience of the individual patient and doctor. The solution to the problem of applying the abstract to the particular must lie with the individual physician, because it is not disembodied science or scientific knowledge that is applied to patients, but the knowledge of a particular physician. When a doctor knows something in relationship to a particular patient, elements of value, aesthetics, and emotions have once again become a part of abstract knowledge because, as Bosanquet pointed out, knowledge and experience are in a *reciprocal* relationship. Unfortunately, knowledge of medical science and technology are often applied *inappropriately* to particular patients by individual doctors. Even when poorly used by individual physicians, values, aesthetics, and emotions become mixed with the knowledge; it cannot be otherwise. In view of this, and assuming that the doctor has a good grasp of medical science, what determines when knowledge is appropriately or inappropriately employed, or, in the language of the previous chapter, what determines whether abstract disease knowledge is properly reparticularized? The simple answer is that abstract knowledge will be properly applied—reparticularized—to the degree that the physician comes to know the person and the sickness through his or her experience of the patient.

The key—which is not simple—is in the relationship of knowledge to experience. To go back a step, we know what we are experiencing because of concrete ideas that are applied to experience. For example, the physician says the patient's legs are edematous or, listening through a stethoscope, that there is a loud heart murmur. But abstract concepts also are employed to interpret experience, as when doctors talk about heart failure, coronary heart disease, or kidney failure, to describe what they believe is wrong with a patient. These more theoretical formulations are put forward because they are believed to best interpret the experiential information that comes from the patient, the doctor, or the tests. It is tempting to explain the process of interpreting experience as occurring within a hierarchy of ideas, each level more abstract than the one before. But discussions of medicine based on formal disease notions provide little evidence for such a process in everyday medicine. Experts discussing a case in a conference may start at the particular facts of the case and then, ascending step by ever more abstract step, present the evidence for the cogency of their favored theories, but rarely do physicians reason in that fashion about their own patients. On the contrary, the theory more often seems to provide the basis for deciding which facts (what aspects of the experience of the doctor and patient) are pertinent to the conclusion. George Santayana offers a clue to this puzzle:

> The whole machinery of our intelligence, our general ideas and laws, fixed and external objects, principles, persons, and gods, are so many symbolic, algebraic expressions. They stand for experience; experience which we are incapable of retaining and surveying in its multitudinous immediacy. We should flounder hopelessly, like animals, did we not keep ourselves afloat and direct our course by these intellectual devices. Theory helps us to bear our ignorance of fact(6).

Santayana invites us to conclude that it is not the relationship of knowledge to experience but *the relationship of the subject to experience* that is crucial in determining how knowledge is applied to experience. My earlier discussion of the immediacy of experience made it appear that all of us are constantly aware of all our surrounding experiences. Such active involvement is the exception. Let this excerpt from a poem by Rupert Brooke make the point:

> Then, the cool kindliness of sheets, that soon
> Smooth away trouble; and the rough male kiss
> Of blankets; grainy wood; live hair that is
> Shining and free; blue-massing clouds; the keen
> Unpassioned beauty of a great machine;
> The benison of hot water; furs to touch;
> The good smell of old clothes.
> (from "The Great Lover")

We would not require poetry to celebrate immediate sensory experience if it were something to which we always paid heed. It is not. We need poetry, the frequent (but incorrect) references to children and primitives, and the formidable path of mystic experience to remind us of the difficulties of becoming contiguous with the experience at hand. Instead (again), concepts and ideas stand between the world and our experience of it. Rupert Brooke's descriptions helps illuminate the relationship of the subject's knowledge to his or her experience.

One way of thinking about the blanket of Rupert Brooke's poem is that it is at once a warm bed covering, a household linen, a domestic article, an artifact of Great Britain's manufacturing capacity, a commodity in international commerce, and a contribution to the nation's economy. In no step in the ranking of these ideas in which blankets play a part and that are each further removed from the "kiss of blankets" is knowledge complete that does not have an experience of some particular blanket, but in each the importance of the blanket is different. Of course we can think about blankets in other ways. Rupert Brooke's blanket is *also* not as snuggly as a down comforter, coarser than a silk coverlet, painful against a sick person's fevered skin, too small to shield the car, poor protection against the rain, and too hot for summer. Each of these ideas also requires both experience and knowledge of blankets as part of some personal pursuit. Different purposes require different knowledge because out of the mass of raw experience to which we are exposed we tend to be aware of (and thus require knowledge of) only what interests us. So it is with doctors and patients. Anything a patient says or that is found by examination can be interpreted in more than one way depending on the doctor's knowledge and interests.

Let me conclude this section on the relationship of knowledge to experience by reiterating certain points. Raw unmediated experience is an exceptional state. Our knowledge usually tells us what we have experienced. What knowledge we apply, whether grand theory or simple idea, depends on what purpose we are pursuing. In all cases, there is a reciprocity between experience and knowledge—knowledge interprets our experiences while experience enriches our knowledge. As experience is converted into abstract knowledge it loses the values, emotions, and aesthetics always present in human experience. When knowledge is applied, it reacquires values, aesthetic factors, and emotions, but this does not guarantee its proper application because, ultimately, we are guided in our experience by our pursuits and the skills and knowledge that serves their purposes—thus purposes also reciprocate with experience and knowledge. This complexity suggest that physicians be explicitly trained *how* best to experience and learn from their experience.

A Case in Point

When Frances Heath came to her physician because she was short of breath and had swollen ankles (again), it did not take more than a few moments to confirm that she had heart failure (again). Frances Heath hates to take diuretics (water pills) because they make her urinate so much that it is difficult for her to leave her apartment. So when she has been feeling well for a long time, she begins to forget them or puts off taking them from day to day. Gradually she reaccumulates edema fluid (swelling of her ankles) and then, to her surprise (because it always seems to creep up on her), she is sick again. You may wonder why she does not simply restart her medication. But what happens is that she gets frightened about her breathing and reminded of how alone she is, and that, as much as her shortness of breath, drives her into the physician's office.

It is generally accepted that the physician's task on first seeing such a patient is to make a diagnosis—to find the name of the thing that afflicts her. The diagnostic task is much more complex than that(7). At this point, however, we are interested in the relationship of knowledge about medicine to the experience of the clinician who sees Frances Heath and the patient herself. Frances Heath has developed heart failure on the basis of long-standing coronary heart disease. The genesis of coronary heart disease, its variants, its anatomy, biochemistry and physiology, the determinants of the onset, course and outcome of the disease, and medical and surgical treatment have been the subject of intense study for many decades and have totally transformed the treatment of the disease and the expectations of those who have it (see Chapter 6). The doctor treating this patient—any doctor trained in Western medicine—possesses this knowledge to a greater or lesser degree. The experienced practitioner has, in addition, knowledge amassed from years of experience treating similar patients.

Hospital residents completing their speciality training, and to a lesser extent senior medical students, have the same body of knowledge without the benefit of as much experience. When medical students learn about diseases they assimilate not only facts about the origins, pathology, and pathophysiology of diseases, but also the characteristic signs and symptoms. In their discussions of disease states, textbooks list the symptoms and signs and the frequency with which they appear, and it is on these that students will begin to depend for learning how to make a diagnosis. The text, *Signs and Symptoms in Cardiology* edited by Lawrence D. Horwitz and Bertron M. Groves, provides an excellent example(8). The chapter on congestive heart failure starts with a definition: "Heart failure is a condition in which the ability of the heart to pump blood is inadequate to meet the metabolic needs of the body." This is followed by a short discussion of the theories of heart failure and a longer discussion of its pathophysiology, followed by a section entitled "Clinical Presentation" in which first the symptoms and then the physical findings characteristic of congestive heart failure are considered. In a modern text such as this, the authors relate the symptoms and signs to the cardiac abnormalities.

However, patients with congestive heart failure like Frances Heath not only display symptoms and signs of their failing hearts; like the rest of us, they present to the observer an almost infinite number of physical features that can be seen, felt, heard, smelled, or even tasted in addition to all the characteristics of their person discussed in previous chapters. Furthermore, people may be short of breath for many reasons. They may have no disease at all, congestive heart failure, emphysema, asthma, a collapsed lung, fluid in the chest, fluid in the abdomen, pregnancy, clots in the lung, or anxiety attacks, and all of these may present singly or in combination. Swelling of the ankles occurs when no disease is present, in liver disease, kidney disease, tumors of the abdomen, malnutrition, protein abnormalities, trauma, pregnancy, or varicose veins, singly or in combination. Since diseases are processes, they always have a beginning in which it would be difficult to distinguish their presence from normality. They also almost invariably have several components, some more abnormal than others.

The findings on physical examination, such as the sounds heard through the stethoscope when examining a patient with congestive heart failure, may also be present in other diseases or even in the absence of disease. A vast number of symptoms or abnormalities are discovered on examination that are virtually never found in the absence of disease but a few are so specific that they earn the title *pathognomonic*—diagnostically specific. Diseases usually manifest themselves by more than one symptom or sign. It would be surprising for congestive heart failure to produce only shortness of breath without any other manifestations. Consequently, in making the diagnosis of disease, physicians characteristically expect a cluster of symptoms and physical findings. But even here, the same cluster may be shared by more than one disease. The results of laboratory, X-ray, and other technical diagnostic methods, although they may add an important measure of certainity, often share these ambiguities.

The Advantage of Experience

With this as a background, the great advantage of teaching medicine at the bedside is clear. Learning from sick patients in hospitals supplements the theoretical and abstract knowledge of textbooks. Medical students and house officers on the wards of teaching hospitals the world over learn several distinct things: how to collect information from patients (from observation, the history, physical examination, and tests), how to make diagnostic and therapeutic judgments based on that information, how to deal with the inevitable uncertainities and ambiguities of clinical medicine, and how to cope with the difficulties that arise because diseases occur in sick persons. The kind of experience the students and house officers have is related to their purposes and their concepts. Although, as we know, they look to their experience with the patient to provide the information on which to make diagnoses, they cannot be open to the actual immediate experience of their patients or their own experience in relation to the patients *because they do not yet have the theory or knowledge that would lead them in that direction.* Following their textbooks and their teachers, they organize their experience conceptually so as to divide the patient into a collection of manifestations of disease on one hand and patient behaviors on the other. This is the equivalent of the distinction between the science and the art of medicine. As we have seen repeatedly, these are artificial divisions that are put to lie by the everyday experience of sickness and medical care. Consequently, the evidence of everyday experience that points up the error in this view of medicine must itself be denied or set aside as nonmedical—which is what students, house officers, and their teachers do. As George Santayana says, "Theory helps us bear our ignorance of facts." This does not impugn ignorance to these individuals as individuals, but to the barrenness of the theory that guides them.

The rather dramatic picture of the doctor faced with making a diagnosis and deciding on treatment for a sick patient is only a small part of medicine inside or outside the hospital. Brief encounters on the telephone or face to face and even looking at X rays or test results bring into play the process of diagnostic and therapeutic thinking. Remember that the doctor is expected to act and is always trying to decide what should be done (including nothing)(9). If the patient's symptoms change or something new happens, what does it mean? Is new action necessary? Should the drugs be changed? Is an operation appropriate? What about another test? Should the original tests be repeated? Is it all right if the recently ill person flies to Los Angeles? Should the couple see a fertility expert? Would the doctor write a letter excusing the patient from jury duty? Should the patient be called about not keeping the appointment? Is a consultant necessary? What should be told to the patient, the spouse, or other doctors? New questions arise over time, even when things are going well. What is happening? Is something threatening the patient? If so, what is it? Must some additional action be taken? This aspect of medical care is not discussed as much as the more formal process of simply naming the disease; moreover, fitting it into the artificial divisions of the science and the art of medicine would require mental acrobatics. Although textbook concepts, theory, or abstract medical knowledge are useful, physicians must call upon other types of knowledge to supply the answers.

In light of what I have said about the narrowness of present training, why are physicians eventually able to act appropriately in these circumstances? The answer is simple. Doctors learn these things from experience. After their training and in the early weeks and months of practice, they are continually required to make judgments. These experiences are inseparable from their experience of their patients. Soon the problem of making diagnoses, deciding (with their patients) on appropriate actions, learning how to write the endless letters of excuses, permissions, and requests for information, making referrals, and answering the seemingly endless telephone calls about virtually anything and everything become their professional life. This is the experience of the clinician. These medical experiences and their required responses may be exciting, dangerous, worrisome, life-threatening, boring (very rarely), funny, mind-boggling, frequently challenging, sad, unhappy, and almost invariably interesting. As the years go on, clinicians become experienced—they have acquired the knowledge born of experience—and competent to deal with an increasing range of problems related to sickness. They know what drugs, treatments, and surgeons (and other specialists) can and will do what and with what outcome. They learn the dangers of falling behind the latest knowledge and determine how best to keep up. They become both generous and wary. They know when their efforts will pay off and who will or will not benefit from what they do and say. They know what patients they can get along with and those they had better avoid. They learn the politics of medical care in and out of their hospitals. Doctors learn the dangers and rewards of the sometimes intense intimacies of medical care. They learn how to be efficient and practical, run an office, get along with staff and colleagues, live the family and social life of a physician. They become experienced clinicians.

From experience clinicians learn about the body, the behavior of disease, and human behavior—particularly in relationship to illness. They require this knowledge in order to treat sick persons. The experience they learn from is largely the experience of others. Ideally, they must experience the experience of their patients. When the doctor first sees a patient, much of the illness has already occurred. Yet the facts of the past are as crucial to the clinician's tasks as the facts of the moment. The past must be known in order to recreate the interactions of persons and biology that are the process of the illness. The early symptoms, what happened in the body, the tempo of events, environmental circumstances, and what the person did or did not do now exist almost solely in the memory of the patient. To understand how the patient will behave, act, think, speak, care, and respond, the clinician must know the patient in the past. These facts of the past—"the history"—are obtained by careful questioning until what happened and the responses of the patient to those events have been re-created within the clinician—until the clinician has experienced the patient's experience. Remember that knowledge and experience are always in a reciprocal relationship—clinicians find the erudition that allows them to make sense of patient's experiences in their general knowledge of the world, their medical knowledge, and in their knowledge of themselves. As we saw in the previous chapters, the information on which the process of re-creating the past is based is value laden and cannot be separated from the aesthetics of parts to wholes—the whole patient, the whole of patient and doctor, and the whole of patient, doctor, and setting.*

The Physician as the Instrument

The facts of the heart can be seen separately from the physician, but the instruments that learn from the experience of others are physicians themselves—it is impossible in the nature of things for them to separate themselves from the process. Information about the patient that is being acquired, evaluated, and utilized and which enters into value and aesthetic assessments may also include feelings, body sensations, and even the spiritual (transcendent). This kind of information is so much an intimate part of the clinician that its origin in the patient is difficult to distinguish from the normal, jumbled onrush

*Doctors are not alone in this method of inquiry. The academic discipline closest, in this respect, to being a clinician is not a science, however, it is history. Clinicians and historians are always going into the past in order to dig out recordable, archival facts. Yet both must attempt to get inside the people whose history they seek in order to understand the world in terms of that person.

of internally generated feelings. This again raises the difficult problem for physicians of the subjective nature of knowledge born of experience. Let me make the point with what is generally regarded as the most problematic of experiential information: knowledge of feelings and emotions.

A perception even of one's inner feelings is, as previously detailed, a cognitive act. It is an interpretation and, as such, requires thought, but not necessarily conscious thought. For example, one might be sitting with a very angry patient and begin to act angry toward the patient. The inner perception of feelings of anger will have taken place below awareness; like most such feelings, they intensify to become a state of anger which, looking outside for justifications, becomes angry behavior. On the other hand, in the same situation one might perceive one's angry state and respond by inwardly saying, "Why am I angry?" The response might be to shortcut the process and avoid the angry behavior. Or, alternatively, at an earlier stage one might perceive the feeling of anger, ask, "Why do I feel anger?" and, in response to the self-query, neither become nor act angry. In fact, thinking about the feeling of anger, one might realize that no true outer cause of anger existed and correctly posit that the source of the feeling of anger might be the angry feelings of this person sitting opposite, in which case the behavior that followed would be not to act angry, but to discover why the other person is angry and determine what should be done about it.

The warnings go back to Plato: The experience of the clinician produces knowledge tainted by emotion and passion. Science was meant to rescue medicine from this problem yet science cannot solve this problem. *There is no alternative to using this kind of experiential knowledge in medical care—understanding and accepting that fact is the beginning of the solution to the problem.* The pall has not hung over experiential knowledge only; distrust has also focused on the subject who has the experience. Centuries of trying to disengage the subject from knowledge born of experience have not led to success. The next step in solving the problem lies in remembering that only another person can empathically experience the experience of a person. In medicine the subjects of experience are the patient and the doctor. Only the physician as a person can empathically experience the experience of a sick person. *It must finally be accepted, therefore, that there can be no substitute for the physician as a person.*

To meet the challenge posed by the need to relieve suffering, medicine requires the introduction of a systematic and disciplined approach to learning from experience and the knowledge that comes from it, not artificial divisions of medical knowledge into art and science or strained and unreal analyses of objectivity versus subjectivity. Physicians who use knowledge born of their experience have not necessarily become hopelessly subjective, nor have they lost their objectivity. The difficulty is not experiential knowledge, which can be objective; the problem lies in how physicians manage such information.

R. G. Collingwood writes about thinking about knowledge from experience:

> The act of thinking, then, is not only subjective but objective as well. It is not only a thinking, but it is something that can be thought about. But, because (as I have already tried to show) it is never merely objective, it requires to be thought about in a peculiar way, a way only appropriate to itself. It cannot be set before the thinking mind as a ready-made object, discovered as something independent of that mind and studied as it is in itself, in that independence. It can never be studied 'objectively,' in the sense in which 'objectively' excludes 'subjectively.' It has to be studied as it actually exists, that is to say, as an act. And because this act is subjectivity (though not mere subjectivity) or experience, it can be studied only in its own subjective being, that is, by the thinker whose activity or experience it is. This study is not mere experience or consciousness, not even mere self-consciousness: it is self-knowledge. Thus the act of thought in becoming subjective does not cease to be objective; it is the object of a self-knowledge which differs from mere consciousness in being self-consciousness or awareness, and differs from being mere self-consciousness in being self-knowledge the critical study of one's own thought, not the mere awareness of that thought as one's own(10).

The information on which judgment and action are to be based ranges from the numerical readout on a cardiac monitor or the consideration of an X-ray film to an inner feeling properly interpreted as arising within the patient and empathetically picked up by the doctor. At one extreme the facts are grandly objective and public and at the other extreme private, achieving their objectivity only through the difficult effort of self-knowledge. Some facts meet any criterion for scientific knowledge while others are values themselves, or aesthetic feelings. Some knowledge on which judgment is based exists for all to share while other knowledge is inseparable from the clinician even if it can be shared. The task of giving each kind of evidence equal weight in the process of judgment is forbidding. For example, during a routine examination a physician felt a mass in the patient's abdomen that he thought was a large spleen. A radioactive liver and spleen scan was ordered, yielding normal results. Some months later the patient returned with abdominal pain and again the physician felt what he believed was the large spleen. This time a CT scan was ordered, which again showed a normal spleen. However, the left kidney was greatly enlarged, accounting for what the physician had felt. The original information from the physician's hands was correct; interpreting it as an enlarged spleen was an error. The objective test that seemed to contradict what the hands felt was unfortunately given greater weight, and an alternate interpretation was not considered. It is extremely common, but unwise, to put aside the information from our senses because it is contradicted by what we believe or by other sources of fact that appear more reliable. The skill in medical judgment is not only accepting as evidence facts from within but by rigorous self-examination and self-knowledge, giving such information as much objectivity and weight as externally objective evidence.

Experience Mediates Between Science and Art

Now I can answer the question posed earlied in this chapter: Assuming that a doctor has a good grasp of medical science, what determines when such knowledge is appropriately or inappropriately employed or when abstract disease knowledge is properly reparticularized? The best circumstances for correct application of knowledge or theory are present when the clinical picture is as fully known as possible in all its details. In discussing attentive listening I described this as separating the observation from the interpretation—hearing what a person *says* prior to interpreting what the person *means.* In clinical medicine this involves knowing not only what the heart sounds like or the electrocardiogram looks like, but all the relevant details of the patient and the patient's illness. The troublesome word is *relevant.* Clearly, one cannot know *all* the details. The reciprocity of experience and knowledge permits step-by-step sounding out of the details and fitting them and the knowledge to each other in a process that extends over time. This is part of the dialectical reintegration of knowledge to produce a new and higher level whole discussed in the previous chapter. The enemy is allowing theory to obscure the facts through premature closure of the experience. In order to learn from experience and use their knowledge of medicine appropriately, clinicians must be open to and even immerse themselves in the immediacy of their experiences and the experiences of others. Of some clinicians we say that they have had twenty years' experience, others have had one year of experience twenty times. The former were engrossed in their experiences, which they allowed to teach them, while the latter placed their knowledge as a shield against experience.

Thinking of experience as a teacher is not a new attitude, but one that is difficult to attain and maintain. I believe, however, that it can be taught, that students of medicine can learn how to be subject to their own immediate experience. They can be taught how empathic experiencing is achieved. They can learn the the self-discipline and self-reflection necessary to clinical self-knowledge.

The Experience of Uncertainty

The more clinicians are open to experience, the more they are beset by uncertainty—the hallmark of clinicians is their ability to tolerate uncertainty. Thirty years ago the sociologist Renee Fox wrote a chapter called "Training for Uncertainty" that appeared in *The Student Physician,* a volume about the training of medical students(11). All these years later, and despite the fact that uncertainty and risk are central concepts in the new fields of medical decision making and clinical epidemiology, the issue has still not been specifically addressed in medical education, although it underlies many of the problems of current medicine from high cost to depersonalization(12).

Even when there is little doubt about the disease, as with Frances Heath who has advanced congestive heart failure, doubt will attend other facets of the illness that have a bearing on treatment. When deciding on actions to take, choices among alternatives are always present. *It cannot be otherwise.* In addition, of course, are the uncertainities that arise because the individual clinician's knowledge may be lacking and because medical knowledge in general is necessarily incomplete. Finally, medical judgments always deal with actions that will have consequences in the future. Because the future is involved, another element of uncertainty is introduced. The key to understanding medical judgment is knowing that it is fundamentally the management of uncertainty.

In practice, uncertainty can be put out of mind in several ways. The first de-individualizes the patients to make them more like the textbook case, Mr. or Mrs. Everycongestiveheartfailure. When the patient says that she is short of breath, the idea of congestive heart failure comes immediately to the physician's mind and begins to guide observation. But rather than carefully observing, the inexpert see only what they expect to see on the basis of their theory. Evidence to the contrary is dismissed, and the case for their chosen diagnosis, in this instance congestive heart failure, is flimsily constructed. Facts that deviate from the usual instance are either suppressed or dismissed.

Pretending to a certainty that does not exist is another solution that marks the inexpert. A heart murmur is heard and pronounced to be of such-and-such a type—all doubt is erased by fiat. Similar transformations into certainty are forced on virtually all the information, no matter how shaky it may actually be or how removed from the actual experience of doctor or patient. The case that is finally constructed may bear little relation to the facts of the particular patient.

Redefining the problem to eliminate uncertainty is also common. For example, instead of acknowledging the difficulties presented by Frances Heath *and* her congestive heart failure, the problem can be defined so that her negligence about her medications is seen as the sole problem. By terming it negligence, the physician can believe that his or her responsibility is diminished. After all, what does it matter what is wrong with her? If only she had taken her medications she would still be fine.

Shrinking the problem to even smaller dimensions is a fourth method of dealing with clinical uncertainty. Whatever doubt we have about Frances Heath and her congestive heart failure we resolve by getting an echocardiogram (a "sound" picture of the heart that can show, among other things, how effectively it is pumping blood) or some other test—as though the case and its problems can be reduced to questions solely about the pumping effectiveness of her heart. In the case of Amos Unger and his chest pain discussed in Chapter 9, first the treadmill exercise test and then the coronary arteriogram were made the crucial issues in deciding what to do for him, as though what was the matter with him was the equivalent of what was the matter with his tests. This is an extremely common modern strategy for solving the uncertainty problem—reduce the problem to one for which there is a test and then make the test results decisive. It may be difficult to see why such a strategy is faulty. The tests may reveal disease of the coronary arteries either through physiological demonstration (the treadmill exercise test) or indirectly by X rays (the arteriogram). However, the clinician's question is not only whether disease as measured in this manner exists, but what should be done for the patient.

The fifth and perhaps most common method for reducing uncertainty is to accept the uncertainty of today with the idea that as time passes, it will resolve itself. Temporizing actions are commonly part of such a strategy. But serious illness or its threat may make it extremely difficult for the patient or the doctor to sit on their hands while times passes. I remember reading once that the best action in the face of a certain kind of convulsion in children was to walk around the block slowly smoking a cigar. Inexperienced physicians have the most difficulty doing this because they tend, like sick persons, to see every threat as looming in the moment and requiring immediate action.

Ed Basalt represents such an example. While playing baseball he was struck in the lower back by a hardball. It hurt for a few days and then the pain went away. About a week later the pain returned and Mr. Basalt saw his physician. Examination revealed some tenderness over one of the bones of the spine which the doctor believed was a bruise. Mr. Basalt was not convinced by the explanation that his recent increase in activity had brought the pain back. What else could conceivably be the matter, he wanted to know. He continued to press his physician and discovered that tumor or infection of the bone were very unlikely but possible. He wanted to have an X ray, but when he discovered that early infection of the bone would not show up on an ordinary X ray, he continued asking questions until he discovered that the (then) new technique of nuclear magnetic resonance scanning was the best diagnostic technique. He did not want to follow the doctor's suggestion that he wait two weeks to see what happened to the pain (which was not severe); he wanted a nuclear magnetic resonance scan (despite its $900 cost). The scan was negative and the pain disappeared spontaneously.

Unfortunately, as the degree of certainty achieved in the first four methods becomes greater, the physician becomes more remote from the actual sick person and the sick person's problem. The doctor's increased certainty has not lessened the uncertainty that surrounds the patient. After the tests it is certain that Frances Heath's heart does not pump adequately. But she did not come to the doctor only because her heart is a failing blood pump. She was forced to the doctor by forgetting her medication and the fear created by her shortness of breath. Keeping her well requires solutions to the latter problems as well as the former.

Uncertainty and Power

As we have seen, no certainty is possible about what actions are in the best interests of sick persons. Correct action requires an informed doctor who knows as much as possible about the sick person and the illness through immersion in the clinical experience. Until this is done, the four central tasks of clinical medicine—discovering what is the matter, finding the cause, determining the treatment, and predicting the future—will fall short of their mark. Knowledge of the empirical facts of the body—of human biology—makes it possible for the clinician to know what is the matter with the heart; knowledge about persons in general and this person in particular make individualizing disease feasible.

Herein lies the danger to the doctor. Turning back toward the patient in order to gain the knowledge necessary to act on behalf of *this* sick person exposes the physician to the uncertainties that beset the patient. Let the doctor ask more questions, observe more closely, listen more acutely, and more information will be forthcoming. Let knowledge from feelings enter the process and let the clinician carefully intuit—still more evidence will be forthcoming. But although many uncertainties are resolved, more will be exposed. This is because past or present facts of any particular illness—sick person *and* disease—will always be richer in detail and more complex in their interrelationships than the concepts of disease or understandings of person the doctor employs to perceive and understand these facts. This is one meaning of the saying, "The individual is unknowable." A basic tension exists. Withdrawal from the patient is rewarded with certainty and punished by sterile inadequate knowledge; movement toward the patient is rewarded with knowledge and punished with uncertainties. The fact remains, however, that to disengage from the patient is to lose the ultimate source of knowledge in medicine.

Why should the physician fear uncertainties connected with the patient's illness? Because, as discussed earlier, the relationship between physician and patient is such that what endangers the patient threatens the physician(13). The greater the doctor's participation in the patient's experience and the closer the doctor comes to the patient to acquire the information about disease and person, the more the doctor is connected to the patient. The closer the doctor, the greater the trust of the patient and the stronger the bond. The solution to the problem of unresolvable uncertainty is to use the time that inevitably passes in each illness to acquire ever more information about patient and disease; during that time the bond between doctor and patient is also growing. Relationships, like illnesses, are not events but processes. The stronger the bond, the greater the threat to the physician from what endangers the patient.

We know the dangers to the patient: deepening sickness, disability, suffering, and death. What are the dangers to the physician? On the surface, the worst that can happen is that he or she is wrong—fails to do the right thing or makes a mistake. If the blunder is large enough, the error is exposed for all to see. The withdrawal of colleagues' respect and the censure of laypersons is not a small matter; fear of this dogs the actions of young physicians, who are also haunted by the current specter of malpractice litigation. However, the danger to physicians was present long before malpractice suits. Experienced doctors are aware of how rare such public errors are; they know that most of their mistakes will never be known, even to themselves. More important, doctors are endangered by the rupture of their relationship with the patient, injuries to their pride, the constant deep-seated fear of inadequacy, evidence that they are losing their skill or nerve, damage to their medical knowledge, and, finally, loss of their ability to know and understand. One might cynically cast all these aside except the last as merely injuries to vanity. Ultimately, what is really important is the central knowledge one knows with one's whole being. Facts and fragments—even large portions—of this knowledge can be exhibited, taught, shared with others, and objectified. But the structure of the knowledge and its interrelationships throughout cognition, feeling, and being are a part of the person of the doctor—of every knower(14). This is why to teach well is to show the way to knowledge and help the student change rather than to merely transfer facts, concepts, or skills.

What is endangered in the physician by the threat to the patient can be summed up in one word: *power.* Physicians are powerful people. They are able to walk in the world of sickness, suffering, and death with seeming impunity. They have power over life and death. Because of this power they are accorded special status in every culture, whether they are called physicians or shamans. Presidents obey their suggestions and commanders of armies heed military surgeons. As doctors gain experience, they gradually come to inhabit the power that goes with their work. The most personally unprepossessing physicians command authority. Otherwise brave people are fearful on entering a physician's office and joyful at good news once there, as though the physician's words (rather than the fact of sickness or its absence) had power over them. And they are correct—the doctor's words *do* have power over them.

It is strange how hard people work to avoid using the word power in regard to themselves. I told an audience of senior medical students that they were about to become among the most powerful people in their culture. You would have thought I was foretelling leprosy. They squirmed with discomfort at the idea and offered synonyms they found more tolerable—for example, "knowledgeable," "skillful," "influential," and "authoritative." They were equally uncomfortable at the suggestion that most of these words stood for reasons for their power but were not synonyms for the power itself. I wanted them to begin to understand that with power go responsibilities—one of which is actively training themselves in the proper use of their power.

The students' unhappiness at the word power is mirrored in modern medicine, which has ceded to science the power of the clinician. Personal power in medicine implies hand-holding, charm, bedside manners, and subjectivism. The idea that a physician can lay aside his or her personal power and still care for the sick is an illusion. The power goes with the profession; it is an ineradicable aspect of clinical medicine. The miracles of modern medicine—drugs and therapeutic or diagnostic technologies—have no power; doctors who use these things have power. Science has no power, only scientists do. I believe that scientifically trained doctors who do not develop their personal powers will remain half-doctors. Or worse, even scientific doctors without trained and disciplined personal power may develop "magical" feeling—they may believe that their hands have acquired magical powers, that they can produce effects through the intervention of forces or powers about which they have no systematic or learned knowledge, whose effects they cannot predict and which do not follow the usual causal rules. In a doctor (although not in a patient), magic is the enemy of therapeutic power, because the healing powers of a physician, which are born of the doctor-patient relationship, operate apart from the technology and come from within the physician.

In *The Healer's Art,* I discussed at length the characteristics of sickness apart from the disease that causes them(15). I showed that the sick become disconnected from their ordinary world, find that their everyday reasoning fails them, suffer a breakdown in normal feelings of indestructibility, and lose control over themselves and their world. Earlier we saw how these same features of illness carried further produce suffering in acute or chronic illness. In *The Healer's Art* I made a distinction between the healing and curing function of physicians to show how a sick person could undergo the technology of cure or even be cured but not become well again because the work of healing had not been done. In their role as healers, physicians help reconnect sick persons to the world of the well, restore the competency of reason by providing explanations of events, provide alternative means and sources of control, and start patients on their way back to a sense of omnipotence. In all these acts, the doctor as healer helps provide a route by which the sick patient may regain the autonomy lost to sickness(16). The therapeutic instrument in healing is indisputably the doctor.

The conditions for healing are met when there is a sick person, a healer, and a relationship between them. Consequently it is possible for healing to take place without the physician knowingly acting as a healer. (It follows that in the same circumstances, the antithesis of healing can also take place.) As a result, when physicians do not acknowledge the phenomenon of healing, learn about it, and use it consciously and systematically, then things will happen to patients that will seem inexplicable. When baffling things take place with patients—especially, but not only, when they are good happenings—doctors may get those magical feelings mentioned above—they may believe they have willed these events into being.

Magic (as here defined) is inextricably and inversely related to personal power. As one begins to know systematically how to produce an effect (one need not know how it works), the ability shifts from being magical to exerting personal power. I want to make two categorical statements about the personal therapeutic power of physicians. First, healing powers consist only in and no more than allowing, causing, or bringing to bear those things or forces for getting better (whatever they may be) that already exist in the patient. Second, virtually all a doctor's healing power flows not from control over the patient, but from the doctor's self-mastery—which is why to surrender, lose, or fail to maintain mastery over one's self is to reduce or give up one's healing powers (though not one's power to harm). This is why magic, which seems to call on forces external to the doctor, defeats the doctor's power. Modern clinicians are not required to depend solely on their personal powers of healing because their mastery of it gives them the power of modern scientific medicine. But, the power resides not in the science and technology but in doctors. As with their healing powers, their power to cure requires the same systematic discipline and self-mastery. To the extent to which they fail to maintain their knowledge, their mastery over it, and their responsibility for it, they lose their therapeutic power. The art and the science of medicine exist in peaceful partnership within the clinician to the degree to which they are controlled by the clinician.

Diagnostic and therapeutic power in clinicians is directly proportionate to their ability to tolerate uncertainty. Uncertainty is intrinsic to the nature of diagnosis and therapy. To help reduce uncertainty one must know more. To know more means to have obtained information from differing sources and of disparate sorts. It means to be submerged in the experience of patients and patients' experiences—in the experience and knowledge of medicine. Knowing more is not sufficient. The physician must reason about scientific concepts and knowledge from experience—facts, values, and aesthetic constructs changing over time—in the service of a fundamentally unknowable individual patient. It requires reconstructing the past and positing a future. From all this evidence, inference must lead to an action that seems more correct than all other alternatives. To seek certainty itself is ultimately to abandon the patient; to pretend to oneself a nonexistent certainty is to retreat into magic.

In the experience of uncertainty in which they are forced to live their lives, physicians must become their own instrument and acquit their power and its responsibility by staying on the long road to self-knowledge.

References

1. Blois, Marsden S. Medicine and the Nature of Veridical Reasoning. *NEJM* 1988; 318:847–51.

2. 1 Kings 3:16.

3. Collingwood, R. G. *The Idea of History.* 1956. New York, Oxford University Press, p. 20ff.

4. Collingwood, R. G. *The Idea of Nature.* 1960. New York, Oxford University Press, p. 11.

5. Pellegrino, Edmund, and Thomasma, David. *A Philosophical Basis of Medical Practice.* 1981. New York, Oxford University Press, p. 115.

6. Santayana, George. *The Sense of Beauty.* 1955. New York, Dover Publications, p. 78.

7. Pellegrino, and Thomasma, *op. cit.,* Chap. 6.

8. Horwitz, Lawrence D., and Groves, Bertron M. *Signs and Symptoms in Cardiology.* 1985. New York, Lippincott, Chap. 11.

9. Pellegrino and Thomasma, *op. cit.,* p. 124.

10. Collingwood, *The Idea of History, op. cit.,* p. 292.

11. Fox, Renee C. Training for Uncertainty. In *The Student Physician.* Edited by Merton, Robert K., Reader, George and Kendall, Patricia L. 1957. Cambridge, Mass., Harvard University Press.

12. Gordon, Deborah. Clinical Science and Clinical Expertise. In *Biomedicine Examined.* Edited by Margaret Lock and Deborah Gordon. 1988. Dordrecht, Kluwer Academic Publishers, p. 261.

13. Cassell, Eric J., The Conflict Between the Desire to Know and the Need to Care for the Patient. In *Organism, Medicine and Metaphysics: Essays in Honor of Hans Jonas on his 75th Birthday.* 1978. Boston, D. Reidel Publishers.

14. Heidegger, Martin. *What Is Called Thinking.* Trans. by Gray, J. Glenn. 1968. New York, Harper & Row.

15. Cassell, Eric J. *The Healer's Art.* 1976. Philadelphia, Lippincott. 1985. Cambridge, Mass., MIT Press, Chap. 1.

16. Cassell, Eric J. The Function of Medicine. *The Hastings Center Report* 1977; Vol.7, No. 6 (December).

EPILOGUE

The Care of the Suffering Patient

IN THE SPRING of 1980, Lily Sterns, then sixty-one, called about vaginal bleeding. She was reluctant to see her gynecologist because of her fear of cancer, but she went anyway. An endometrial biopsy disclosed a cancer of the uterus and the gynecologist advised her to have a hysterectomy. It was probably only minutes after they left the gynecologist's office that her husband called to ask who, "anywhere in the world," was the best doctor for her condition; they wanted a second opinion. The gynecologist I suggested agreed with the recommendation. She, her husband, and two grown daughters came to my office to discuss the matter. They ended by deciding that there was no choice but to be operated on. The prospect of surgery was particularly repugnant to her. She was the kind of woman generally characterized as delicate and sensitive; she was more than usually modest and avoided direct reference to body parts or bodily functions. When I first saw her years earlier she had talked at length about her bad experience with gall bladder surgery when she was younger. She returned to that event repeatedly in her questions about the hysterectomy.

Lily Sterns did not like physicians and visited me infrequently—then only when she was ill. In common with many of her friends and acquaintances, she thought doctors used drugs and chemicals too frequently and that they were not sympathetic with the body's self-healing tendencies. She was careful about her family's nutrition and believed strongly in the importance of natural foodstuffs and the avoidance of food additives and similar chemicals. Because of these beliefs, even before the surgery, she and her husband began exploring alternative cancer therapies. Jack Sterns brought in a book on "metabolic" treatments for cancer(1), which I read, because his friends had told him of a clinic in Germany where they could go for such treatments. After much discussion, and despite her dread, they agreed again that she should be operated on. I did not object to their consulting a physician who offered nutritional therapies for cancer.

On the basis of the diagnosis of endometrial cancer and what we know of Lily Sterns it can be anticipated that her surgery and subsequent illness might be accompanied by suffering. Her dread of surgery could not be allayed and did not seem fully explained by her beliefs about medicine and doctors. Anticipated hospital procedures, surgery, post-operative care, and diagnostic and therapeutic activities for the malignancy could be expected to repeatedly violate her way of dealing with her body and its functions and her strongly held beliefs about nutrition, "chemicals," and natural defenses against disease.

The relief of Lily Sterns' suffering starts with anticipating its occurrence and beginning measures for its prevention. The first presupposition of treatment in such patients should be that no matter how optimistic the diagnosis nor how minimal the disease seems, they may ultimately suffer. In fact, that possibility should underlie even the initial conversation about the symptom (here, vaginal bleeding) that starts the cycle of medical care. The second presupposition is that what happens to Lily Sterns throughout the illness, no matter how many days or years it may last, can be influenced by the physician's actions from the first minutes of treatment. Doctors already act on these two presuppositions in relation to disease with every person who comes to them for no matter how minor a symptom. They are always alert to the possibility of serious disease and aware of the importance of their every action. If they enlarged the scope of their thought about these presuppositions to include the person and the possibility of suffering, they might prevent or treat suffering as well as disease. Moreover, this would keep the treatment or prevention of disease from being an inadvertent cause of suffering.

Unmitigated dread of sickness or surgery is not rare and it should not be taken lightly. It is one of the reasons why patients delay seeing physicians for symptoms which they *know* are serious or life threatening. Dread, other phobias, or behaviors that patients feel make them different or "strange" should be acknowledged and accepted. Because suffering inevitably involves isolation from others, the risk of suffering is increased whenever something that is of great importance to the patient is dismissed, trivialized, or considered a psychiatric symptom or "crazy." Patients cannot usually articulate convincing reasons for their dread and it rarely responds to simple reassurance or even full explanations. It is helpful, however, for the patient to know what is going to happen in whatever detail they wish. I asked Lily to come and see me before surgery and listened at length to her fears. I explained in detail what would be involved in her admission to the hospital, pre-operative tests, and examinations by the house staff. I answered all her questions as well as I could, making it clear that I was trying to reduce her uncertainty, not promising that matters would be as I predicted. I *promised* that I would not abandon her. In modern group practices, such assurances may not be practical, but it is possible to introduce the patient to the other physicians who will be participating and, in the presence of the patient, review the specific fears or uncertainties of special concern. In that fashion, the other doctor(s) becomes a party to the acceptance of the patient's idiosyncrasies.

The operation revealed that she had (endometrial) cancer and that it had spread into the muscle of the uterus. Despite the frightening diagnosis she was surprised and pleased by how little difficulty she had with the surgery. Mrs. Sterns and her family were dismayed when radiation therapy was advised. They sought several opinions, but the doctors' advice was confirmed. Three weeks after surgery she started radiation therapy, which continued for five weeks. Because of her slight build she was only mildly ill during the radiation. As she had been forewarned, diarrhea started during the third week. Although she found it particularly repugnant (she soiled herself on a number of occasions), she had plenty of medication to control the symptom. She tried a number of nonphysician remedies but I urged her to use the tincture of opium because it was her ability to continue her everyday life that seemed to me more important than avoiding medications. Homeopathic and similar treatments, I pointed out, had not been designed with the severity of radiation enteritis in mind. She worked out a set of therapies—a kind of compromise between my recommendations and her other beliefs—depending on the severity of the diarrhea.

Patients should be prepared for the difficulties to come by knowing what is likely, why it happens, and what will be done should the event occur. Doctors, naturally enough, do not like to think of themselves as making their patients sick or causing great distress. Thus, they may minimize the unpleasant effects of their treatments or imply that they rarely see such things happen. The result is to shift the blame onto the patient as though it is some weakness within patients that make them sick from the radiation. It is not helpful to either downplay nontherapeutic effects of treatments to ensure patients' consent or to provide a list of possible nontherapeutic effects so complete it would frighten anyone. Both put lie to what should be the physician's essential message—we are in this together. Lily Sterns' diarrhea largely subsided after a few months.

Eight months later she was admitted to the hospital because of intestinal obstruction. At operation recurrent cancer was found within her abdomen. Chemotherapy with cis-platinum, a drug new at the time, and hexamethylmelamine was advised. She rebelled at the thought, but despite her resolve not to take "chemicals" which she believed would "undermine the body's immune system," she agreed. At the same time she started a "macrobiotic" diet and a regimen of coffee enemas. She had a terrible time with the cis-platinum. She vomited awfully when she got the cis-platinum and then it was almost two weeks before all vomiting and nausea disappeared. During that period she ate little and was extremely weak. In the ensuing two weeks she fearfully anticipated the next treatment, sleeping little and eating poorly. Thus, although she was only in the hospital for two days out of each month, she was sick almost the entire month. Her suffering had started and the situation was intolerable. Using hypnosis, an attempt was made to solve the problem. Hypnosis can be a wonderful adjunct in patients with serious disease. It cannot stop vomiting in situations like Lily Sterns', but it can markedly reduce the part played by painful memory and frightened expectation. In hypnosis, her chemotherapy was likened to watching telephone poles from the window of a train. They (the treatments) are not there until they suddenly "arrive" and then they quickly disappear. In addition it was possible to deal with her fear that it was her own emotional weakness that would ultimately cause her death. Although weakness, some nausea, and poor appetite lasted for a brief period postchemotherapy, the problem had greatly lessened as had the anticipation of the next treatment. Her invalidism ceased and she resumed her everyday activities.

After twelve cycles of chemotherapy Lily Sterns had a "second-look" abdominal exploration to determine if she had residual malignancy that would require continued chemotherapy. She did, but her subsequent difficulties were not primarily related to cancer. Post-operatively she developed a severe infection with high fevers requiring intravenous antibiotics. Her intestines did not return to function and she could not eat. Fecal fistulae (holes in the large intestine traversing through the skin) developed and intestinal contents drained continuously through the openings. She continued to receive antibiotics and then total parenteral nutrition (a system for providing adequate calories and nutrients intravenously) was begun. She gained weight and her strength slowly returned.

As new problems occurred and she overcame them, she began to believe that she was not the weak and fearful woman that had always been her self-image. Instead, she found reserves of strength and bravery within herself and was proud of her achievements. It was sad, she thought, that it took serious illness to reveal her depth and strength. She told me that she wanted to live and was fighting for that, but she believed that she would probably die. Even though the thought saddened her, she said, in a way it was worth it because her children and her husband were so proud of her, and she had set a good example, for her daughters. When she developed pain in her lower abdomen that required increasing amounts of narcotics, she asked whether hypnosis might be useful for its relief. She had "conquered" the problem with the chemotherapy and thought she could control her pain. I taught her how to put on "pain-free panty hose," made a cassette tape of the pain control exercise that she could listen to when alone, and showed her daughter how to help her. Controlling the pain by herself increased her sense of achievement. She remained in the hospital for five weeks until the fistulae healed completely and she was maintaining her own nutrition.

Soon after leaving the hospital, although she tired very easily, she was "in command" again of her family and her home. When the fistulae opened up again, and fecal drainage started, she did not want to return to the hospital. She knew that she was going to die, she explained to me, but she had things to do with her family that could not be accomplished in the hospital. Home hospice services were not yet available in New York, but her daughters took over, learning to care for her and for her draining wounds. She returned to her bed only a few days before she died, eight weeks after discharge from the hospital, in June 1982.

Such illnesses are marked by the number and severity of their symptoms, the toll on the patient, family, and friends, and the quantity, complexity, and cost of their medical care. Our modern era is conspicuous for the great numbers of such cases. I have illustrated the problem with a patient with cancer, but the same potential for long-lasting illness and suffering is present with heart failure, chronic pulmonary diseases, patients requiring kidney dialysis, and many other diseases. The essential point about these patients is not the chronicity of their illnesses—chronic illness has always been present—but the long duration of severe and demanding sickness such as was previously found only with acute diseases. The survivors of such illnesses—primarily the family (the patients rarely live)—seldom have good memories of their medical and hospital care. Instead, they remember inadequate pain relief, deficient information from "truth dumping" to half truths and lies, long waits for simple services, an endless parade of (to them) unnecessary tests and procedures, impersonality, changing hospital house staff, and tangled chains of command ("who is my doctor?"). This is unfortunate because these patients usually require *and get* enormous dedication and skill—they receive the best that modern hospital care has to offer.

It is a sad fact that serious illness is attended by sorrow and pain. Worse when medical care fails to relieve them, it is *even worse* when medical care adds to the suffering. There are three goals that, if met by the actions of physicians and other caregivers, would, I believe, promise better care and result in greatly reduced suffering of patients and their families. They are simple—almost self-evident. As with many simple things, they are difficult and often burdensome, particularly for physicians. The first aim is that all diagnostic or therapeutic plans be made in terms of the sick person, not the disease. The second is to maximize the patient's function, not length of life. The third goal is to minimize the suffering of the patient and the family. These aims are interlocking because they arise from the more basic idea that physicians and other caregivers should focus primarily on the best interests of the sick person rather than treatment of the disease. Since sick persons generally know best what is in their interests, what aspects of function matter most to them, and when they are suffering, these goals require working closely with patients and their families.

Therapeutic courses of action in the care of the terminally ill that at first may seem strange are made coherent by these objectives. Some examples may be useful. In a patient with (even widespread) metastatic cancer in the bones, it would be wise to use radiation therapy to treat an area of disease in the spine to avert paraplegia, even though the treatment would have no effect on the progression of the disease. Palliative treatment such as this permits death from a more tolerable effect of the disease. A dying patient who is uncomfortably short of breath because of anemia severe enough to reduce oxygen transport is given blood transfusions even though she has decided not to be treated with antibiotics for her life-threatening infection. In a permanently bed-bound patient with diabetic gangrene, the foot is allowed to mummify (an old-fashioned treatment) rather than subjecting the patient to amputation above the knee. Patients with brain tumors are commonly treated with cortisone-type drugs to aid in the control of their neurological symptoms. When their tumors recur and they become irreversibly comatose, the cortisone-type drugs can be abruptly stopped with the knowledge that the disease rebound that occurs when steroids are rapidly withdrawn will hasten the comatose patient's death. In other words, choosing a more comfortable mode, time, or place of death is a suitable therapeutic goal when death is near.

It must be absolutely understood that decisions regarding such courses of action are to be made by the patient. The patient, using the knowledge and advice of the doctor, must decide what goals (not what treatment) meet his or her best interests or purposes—*no one else can know that.* Patients bring to the decision-making process what their aims are (within the constraints of fate) and physicians bring their knowledge of what can be done and how. On the other hand, it is not only unnecessary, but may be cruel, to discuss the medical details by which the patient's purposes are realized. The primary issue is not whether the patient agrees to this or that specific drug, treatment, or operation, but for the doctor to understand the implications and expected outcomes of each treatment for the patient's aims. For example, an eighty-two-year-old woman was advised to have radiation therapy after a mastectomy. She was unhappy at the thought—especially after she heard about the nontherapeutic effects. She was able to come to a decision, however, after she heard that without radiation there was an increased chance (but not a sure thing) that she would get a local recurrence. And that treatment was not usually as satisfactory after recurrence. She was also told that without the radiation, in the worst case, she would probably live between two to four years before cancer would cause her death. Doctors are frequently reluctant to present options in this light because they are too well aware of the possibility of error in their estimates. On the other hand, this is the way they come to their own decisions, and it seems reasonable that patients should have the chance to make judgments in a similar manner. Discussions with patients, if at all possible, should be made at a time when they are able to express themselves clearly about *the things that matter to them.* Some patients may have to be forced into these conversations "kicking and screaming." Nonetheless, physicians have an absolute and unremitting responsibility to understand their patients' aims—and come to terms with them—no matter how much time and how many attempts are required. (Doctors would do no less to stop bleeding.)* Legalisms, bureaucratic requirements, and formal consent forms are not an adequate substitute for such discussions.

"What if the patient has a change of mind?" Doctors sometimes ask me about the weight that should be given decisions that have been arrived at

*I do not mean that patients should be told the facts of their disease if they do not want to hear them. On the other hand, if decisions about treatment must be based on both the facts of the disease and the purposes of the patient, then patients need sufficient information so that the decision does, in fact, represent their best interests as they see them. On rare occasion such discussions may have to be indirect, metaphorical, or almost completely nonverbal. By whatever method of communication, however, patients must, in their own terms, know the problem, the alternatives, and be able to express their preferences.

earlier in the illness. It is up to the physician to decide (with the sick person) what voice best represents the patient, the earlier or later. If the patient seems to have had a change of heart, it is reasonable to consider whether the later desire is consonant with what has gone before—in the illness and the patient's life. As an illness is a process, the care of sick persons must include an ongoing dialogue about their goals. When the focus of medical care is the sick patient, therefore, such problems seldom arise because at every twist and turn of the illness, doctor and patient will understand the importance of keeping their common purpose attuned to the new circumstances.

Patients' with illnesses such as Lily Sterns' usually die. Rarely, they will get better, but even then it is most unusual for them to return to normal work or recreation. With skillful treatment, they may go home again to their place in the family. Physicians and other caregivers are so accustomed to the importance of their work that they tend to forget that medical care is irrelevant and distracting in normal life. To return someone to function is to approximate as closely as possible the behavior of the healthy. For this to occur it is essential to reduce the intrusiveness of medical care. Hospital stays must be cut to a minimum and visits to the doctor's office made as infrequent as possible. To accomplish this telephone calls are greatly increased, house calls are necessary, home-care services are employed, and the family taught how to provide care.

More is involved than merely changing the type and place of medical services. Healthy and fully functional people do not keep their eyes on the clock to know when their next medication is due, worry about each spoonful entering their mouths, or watch their every action lest harm come. It seems evident that the sick person's function and freedom to take part in everyday life are constrained by the body. In fact, everyone is held back by the limitations of the body. Watch young children, where inabilities arising from the limits of their bodies are omnipresent; they do not act angry at their bodies, fearful of them, or as though their bodies get in their way. As they grow up we know the dangers of overprotection and instilling fear. Instead we applaud their early attempts to achieve physical mastery and in so doing we empower them in relation to their bodies. In contrast, recall the care of sick persons where bodily constraints and fears are constantly emphasized. Danger from or harm to the body is frequently stressed to the point where the person is obliterated by the body. Gradually, the patient also utilizes the body to limit the freedom of others until the body becomes the arena of interactions. It is not the *the lived body,* however, that overwhelms the person and takes center stage, but fear of the body and fear of damage. What *could* happen instead of what is. Sick persons must be empowered in relation to the body—freed from fear and from bondage to the body to the degree possible. To accomplish this they must be provided with knowledge, medications, and other tools to control the manifestations of disease and the support needed to behave normally despite them. It is necessary to bolster the strivings of the sick to be the most fully functional persons they can be—even those who will soon die.

Doctors worry that this kind of care increases risks to the patient. Wound infections occur, patients fall, there are medication errors, diabetic control may suffer, congestive heart failure may occur because of dietary lapses. It has been my experience over many years that when working closely with patient and family, these risks can be minimized so that they do not occur with greater frequency at home than in the hospital. In these circumstances, patients are usually *much more* comfortable and happier. Most important, suffering is usually greatly reduced. Modern physicians frequently believe that serious disease can *only* be treated in the hospital. That is not the case. Experience with hospice care has shown that even serious problems such as intestinal obstruction can be cared for at home. (Home care should not be approached with ideological zeal. There are some patients and families where it is inappropriate and they should not be forced into situations where they will fail.)

The subject of risk is important to this kind of medical practice. If patients are placed at increased risk, legal precedent has made physicians responsible for those risks. In this era of frequent malpractice suits, the idea of accepting increased risk makes doctors understandably nervous. To physicians I say that if they are truly afraid of a lawsuit from a particular patient, the kind of care I am describing will not work for that patient. Concern about legal action from all such patients is simply not realistic. When doctors are afraid of certain risks, they sometimes "cover themselves" by warning the patient of the danger. "Dumping" the burden of the risk on the patient can be destructive. Fear is as disabling as disease. For example, telling patients with metastatic cancer in the bones that they must be careful lest they fracture their hips serves no purpose at all except to frighten the patients into immobility. On the other hand, there are risks that must be heeded. The need for that will be better met when probabilities determine the behavior of patient and doctor rather than merely possibilities. It is the patient who wants protecting, not the doctor or hospital.

Medical care, tuned to the specific needs of a particular patient with a particular disease in particular circumstances, requires that physicians acquire a high degree of knowledge about all three. Foretelling what is going to happen—prognostication—always essential, must become a finely tuned skill. Patients and families are constantly worried that they will not know what to do if some emergency occurs so they must be kept prepared for what is about to happen next. When one challenge after another is successfully met (no matter how unimportant they may seem to the doctor or nurse), the confidence of all is built up. Fear of weakness gradually becomes pride of strength. Surprises, bad enough in a hospital, can be a disaster at home. Good prognostication requires continued information and attention to detail, and is one of the reasons for frequent telephone calls. In addition, good telephone communication gives the necessary sense that the doctor will be there when needed. This continuing strong supporting presence by the doctor is central to the relief of suffering. It is a key element in the physician's trustworthiness. *Actively* minimizing or relieving suffering must be a primary part of treatment. As the previous chapters have made clear, suffering is an individual matter and *only the patient can be the final judge of whether he or she is suffering*. Because of their own distress the family may not be an adequate guide to whether the patient is suffering, but they may know the patient's physical symptoms, whether the patient has withdrawn, changed behaviors, or complained in a different fashion. Ultimately, to know whether a patient is suffering, you must ask the patient. The word suffering is employed by some patients to denote any pain or distress, while others will not reveal that they are suffering except to a careful, patient questioner. One begins to know with experience what questions to ask. Using your own reactions is a good beginning. If you believe, for example, that if you smelled like that you would suffer, then perhaps the patient's foul smell is a source of suffering.

Pain remains the most common source of suffering. Its relief—the relief of all symptoms—is the hallmark of care aimed at the relief of suffering. This is not the place to explore the reasons, but it remains true that adequate relief for severe and continuing pain is unusual in the modern hospital. There is no longer any excuse, however, for a doctor not to relieve pain because much has been written on the subject and there are good guiding texts (2)(3)(4)(5). If a physician will take the relief of a particular patient's pain as a challenge—vowing at all costs to make that patient comfortable—the pursuit of that goal will lead to every other concept and action necessary for the relief of suffering.

To alter the experience of pain, one can attempt to intervene at *any* point in the pain process—it is narrow-sighted to believe that pain can only be relieved by giving pain-relieving drugs. The source of pain may be removed or reduced. The sensation can be diminished with analgesics. Associated physical problems that exacerbate the pain, such as muscle spasm, can be relieved. Perception may be altered by any means from drugs to distraction. The meaning attributed to the perception can be changed by teaching the patient about the pain, providing new information, or demonstrating (if it is true) that the patient's ideas are incorrect. Patients who have been rolling in agony, believing their pain beyond relief, will often tolerate the same severe pain without complaint after they have been shown that it can be controlled. Behaviors in response to the pain can be altered. Finally, the person can be helped to change in ways that alter the threat and restore intactness. The great utility of hypnosis is the ability to use it to effect change at virtually any point in the pain process. The time scale of the interventions and their specifics depend on whether acute or chronic pain is involved. With pain of any severity, source, or duration, the central principle is that intervention can take place at any stage in the process of pain or suffering. Guided by that postulate, the possibility of relieving pain and suffering is vastly increased.

Other symptoms can be similarly controlled. To manage the physical symptoms that lead to suffering, doctors must not only "think pathophysiology" and "think body," they must "think person" as well. This will allow them to track the symptom from its origin in the disease to its association with the characteristics of the sick person that provoke suffering. When they do this, they will find that modern medicine has provided them with effective tools to intervene in almost any symptom at virtually any stage in its development.

There are patients whose pain cannot be relieved, illnesses in which symptom control is impossible, diseases in the face of which the best physicians are impotent. In such situations, *suffering must be relieved even if pain or other symptoms cannot be controlled.* The basic principle is that the intactness or integrity of the person must be restored. I must make clear that while one can know *that* another person is suffering, what *in the person* is the origin of the suffering cannot be fully known. Because of the privacy of suffering, the suffering person is always, to some degree, isolated from the rest of us. Suffering is a profoundly lonely state. The first step in restoring intactness is, therefore, to reach out to the suffering person to bring him or her back with the rest of us. You must communicate to the person that no matter what happens or how difficult it is, you are going to be there and help.

Suffering always involves self-conflict even when the source appears external. Because of this, making objective and conceptually separating the thing that seems to be the source of the suffering can help lift its burden from the patient. This is important because to objectify is to provide for joint ownership and sharing of the situation. For example, a man with recurrent cancer of the stomach was having trouble maintaining his nutrition. The intravenous parenteral nutrition catheter had become infected and he was trying to drink enough of the feeding solution to keep up his caloric intake. The liquid sickened him and try as he might he could not meet the nutritional requirement. His wife, seeing him, in her words, melt away in front of her, kept urging him to drink more. He communicated his desperation at failing his wife, his doctors, and himself—and dying (in his eyes) in the process. We cannot know all the wellsprings from which the personal meanings of this failure arise, and thus the fundamental origins of the conflict underlying his suffering are beyond our reach. But we *do* know about calories. Thus it is possible to demonstrate that while he seems to be taking in insufficient calories, he is getting more than (in his desperation) seems to be the case. Further, we understand and share his problem, we are sympathetic with it, we remove blame from him, and have some ideas he might try tomorrow (with which he agrees) that will improve things. We are also able to reassure his wife that he will not starve to death.

Any aspect of the person can be the locus of suffering—physical, emotional, social, familial, or private. But the intervention does not have to be directed specifically at those features of the person; it can take place as well in the world of shared reality. Merely putting the problem in words is part of the objectifying process. For the patient just described what was articulated was not that he feels himself to be failing his wife and himself—dying because of his own failures. How can we know that with certainty unless he says it? What can be stated are the difficulties with the feeding solution, its taste, the volume that must be swallowed, and the abdominal discomfort—the features external to the patient. Remember, that although suffering always involves self-conflict, its source is seen to be outside the sufferer. While the swimmer may be drowning because of failure of will, what is wanted at the moment is a life-preserver, not a psychological insight about willpower.

With more time and experience with the patient, we may begin to understand the wellsprings of suffering within the patient and be able to provide longer-term relief based on that knowledge. In searching for a psychological mechanism involved in the patient's inner conflict, we must be careful not to imply that the patient is at fault. Patients do not need us to point a finger in any manner—they blame themselves more than enough. Knowing that suffering may involve many aspects of the person allows us to direct our own efforts at support. Social contacts must be facilitated. Relationships within the family should be bolstered. Barriers to familial closeness erected during serious illness by, for example, untruths, false optimism, repugnance, and fear can usually be removed with little effort by teaching members of the family how to interact with a sick person. Physicians and other caregivers forget that many people are uncomfortable in the presence of sickness and its physical effects, even when the sick person is a loved one. Others are afraid to be with the very sick and dying because they are afraid of their own emotions (including the fear that they will not feel what they think they are supposed to). With a little bracing they can learn that sadness, tears, and pain are better now than later (when it is too late to interact with the sick person).

Patients, particularly very sick persons, need to talk about their illness and its effects on them. They need time entirely alone with their doctor's private ear listening only to them. Physicians are frequently uncomfortable with these conversations. They are afraid to encourage such talk because of the time involved and concern that topics will be raised that are emotionally discomforting or in which they have no expertise. Such fears are warranted, but what is the alternative? Assigning the task of listening to the patient to a psychiatrist or social worker may serve other functions, but it does not replace the patient's need to speak to the doctor caring for the disease. Sick persons usually do not make distinctions between the psychological and physical sources of their suffering. If the patient has cancer and the abdomen is bloated, its deviation from normal seems directly threatening. The fact that the *suffering* started because friends no longer visit or all outside social contact has ceased may not be apparent to the patient, family, or doctor because the social problem does not seem to have the destructive force of the cancer. To the patient the cancer and the social isolation have become conflated. The anger over helplessness and loss of control are transferred to the sick body. Where previously there was only weakness and perhaps some pain, now the body has become the source of the patient's suffering. The physical symptoms become unremitting.

If the physician should discover the grief over the social loss and be sympathetic, even compassionate (and both are important), the suffering will not give way. Because, in addition to attempting to resolve the social isolation, the physical problems must also be addressed; to the patient, the body has now become the all-powerful enemy. How can control over the body be demonstrated and the patient re-empowered when the presupposition of this discussion is that the physician can no longer control the disease or its symptoms? Because there is *never* a time when *nothing* can be done. A helpless patient whose physician is also helpless is a hopeless patient—a devastating state. A medication is changed, a new kind of bandage is employed, the timing of a treatment is altered—the patient *knows* the doctor is going to find some solution. The patient and physician are fused into an effective force, the very fact of which reconnects the patient to the surrounding group. When pain is absolutely intractable, the doctor will call a consultant; in another city or another country, if necessary. It is not essential to find one useless treatment after another, however, or to maintain the pretense that the patient will be cured when that is impossible. Patients who know they are going to die can still be helped to feel themselves in control. They are themselves, they have choices (their doctors have made that clear), they remain personally empowered until their death. While such self-containment without suffering is possible in the face of impending death, it is difficult when, for example, pain is overwhelming and unrelieved. In such circumstances, doctors must acknowledge to themselves the extent of the patient's suffering and then exhaust all possible remedies within their knowledge and the knowledge of others. Nothing less will do.

Fear is also a source of suffering. Actively preventing suffering requires understanding fear. Although fear may be inchoate in origin, it is almost always particular in its expression, a fear of this rather than that. Once identified, it usually responds to information addressed specifically to the fear. Here again, accurate prognosis supports the insistence on the real as opposed to the possible. Since fear, like suffering itself, requires the future, rooting someone in the present, as difficult as it is to achieve, may be meliorative. When fear does not respond to attempts at reassurance (typically, the same conversation is held again and again), it is because the underlying source of the fear has not been addressed. General reassurances of the "don't worry" type are worse than useless. Some people (e.g., Holocaust survivors or those abused in childhood) have lived with fear all of their lives. It is a *thing* that now attaches to this and now to that but it is independent of all the faces it takes. When such persons become ill, their fear may become overwhelming and in itself is the source of their suffering. We may not be able to understand such fear, but by its discovery alone we can become one with the sufferer in the battle against fear.

In this as in other aspects of the control of suffering, talking with patients, in conjunction with care of the body, is the treatment. While the dogged intention on any physician's part to relieve suffering will undoubtedly be effective, this is a special kind of communication. It is directed, for example, now at the patient, now at the body, and now at the relationship with the physician. It is purposeful communication that depends for its effectiveness on the way the spoken language works in medicine and on the special nature of cognition in sickness. As our knowledge of persons unfolds in coming decades, we will undoubtedly learn more about these healing functions of language.

The doctor-patient relationship is the vehicle through which the relief of suffering is achieved. One cannot avoid involvement with the patient and at the same time effectively deal with suffering. In fact, with patients who are suffering it is virtually impossible to be in their presence and remain indifferent. (Denial of their state, however, is possible). To be concerned is to be involved, at issue is the degree of the physician's active participation in the relationship. Every physician has the same fear—becoming closer to suffering patients, many of whom will die, surely promises pain, sorrow, and loss. Why would we not want to hold back, cover our feelings with a white coat, and hide behind incomprehensible technical language? Because, as understandable as self-protection may be, it renders useless the tools necessary for the care of the very sick and suffering. It is through the connection with the patient that information flows telling us what the patient is feeling and even what body sensations they are experiencing. Through the same bond we can provide the bridge over which the suffering person can return from the isolation of suffering. This endangered, fragile sick person knows that we can be trusted. He or she starts to become whole again and reconnect with the world through the relationship(6). It is also because of the relationship that the patient can accept a new reality that includes the illness and the physician who has objectified it.

This tells us the therapeutic advantage that physicians gain from the jeopardy of closeness to the patient, but not what is to protect them from legitimately feared emotional distress. Seasoned doctors and others who care for the dying can only say what experience will teach; the more completely open and unconcerned with self-protection the physician is, the less the emotional price of caring for the suffering and the greater the reward. It takes time, however, to learn this. To some this discussion may seem arcane. This is a consequence, I believe, of our present ignorance about the person. Current knowledge about the body would have sounded equally strange in a previous epoch. There is another reason that keeps us from appreciating the nature and importance of the close relationship with the suffering person. You may call it the "law of soft facts," if you wish. "Harder" facts drive "softer" facts into hiding. Numerical data puts in doubt evidence from the eyes and ears, which puts in doubt evidence from the other senses, which puts in doubt evidence from the feelings, which puts in doubt other transcendent information. It requires discipline and practice (and courage) to allow "soft" information, including that which flows across the bond with the patient, to have its due.

I have shown how making decisions based primarily on the sick person rather than the disease, maximizing function rather than merely length of life, and *actively* minimizing suffering lead to the prevention and relief of suffering. The certainty of knowledge we have come to expect from medical science is not here when we speak about the relief of suffering. Throughout its history, medicine is always solving new enigmas arising from sickness and death. As one problem is resolved, others appear. It is inevitable, therefore, that in the face of emergent dilemmas current medical technologies will be inadequate and the skills and concepts of physicians will fall short. Medicine cannot stay its hand, however, because sickness forever calls. It is the responsibility of physicians to care for the sick even with imperfect means in a sea of uncertainty. This is the source of their grace. Thus it has always been and thus it is now—the relief of suffering is the fundamental goal of medicine.

References

1. Bradford, Robert W. and Culbert, Michael L. *The Metabolic Management of Cancer.* 1980. Los Altos, Calif. The Robert W. Bradford Foundation.

2. Twycross, Robert G. and Lack, Sylvia A. *Symptom Control in Far Advanced Cancer: Pain Relief.* 1983. London, Pitman.

3. Foley, Kathleen M., Bonica, John J. and Ventafridda, Vittorio, Editors. *Advances in Pain Research and Therapy.* Vol. 16. 1988. New York, Raven Press.

4. Payne, Richard and Foley, Kathleen M. Editors. Cancer Pain. *The Medical Clinics of North America* Vol. 71 No. 2, March 1987.

5. Foley, K.M., The Treatment of Cancer Pain. *NEJM* 1985; 313:84–95.

6. Cassell, Eric J. *The Healer's Art.* 1985. Cambridge, Mass., MIT Press, Chap. 5.

Index

Printed in the United States
1643

9 780195 089127